Overlap of Respiratory Problems with Sleep Disordered Breathing

Editor

KRISHNA M. SUNDAR

SLEEP MEDICINE CLINICS

www.sleep.theclinics.com

June 2024 • Volume 19 • Number 2

ELSEVIER

1600 John F. Kennedy Boulevard • Suite 1800 • Philadelphia, Pennsylvania, 19103-2899

http://www.theclinics.com

SLEEP MEDICINE CLINICS Volume 19, Number 2
June 2024, ISSN 1556-407X, ISBN-13: 978-0-443-29372-6

Editor: Joanna Gascoine
Developmental Editor: Akshay Samson

Sleep Medicine Clinics (ISSN 1556-407X) is published quarterly by Elsevier Inc., 360 Park Avenue South, New York, NY 10010-1710. Months of issue are March, June, September and December. Business and Editorial Offices: 1600 John F. Kennedy Blvd., Ste. 1800, Philadelphia, PA 19103-2899. Customer Service Office: 3251 Riverport Lane, Maryland Heights, MO 63043. Periodicals postage paid at New York, NY and additional mailing offices. Subscription prices are $246.00 per year (US individuals), $100.00 (US and Canadian students), $283.00 (Canadian individuals), $292.00 (international individuals) $135.00 (International students). For institutional access pricing please contact Customer Service via the contact information below. Foreign air speed delivery is included in all *Clinics* subscription prices. All prices are subject to change without notice. **POSTMASTER:** Send change of address to *Sleep Medicine Clinics*, Elsevier Health Sciences Division, Subscription Customer Service, 3251 Riverport Lane, Maryland Heights, MO 63043. Customer Service: **Tel: 1-800-654-2452 (U.S. and Canada); 314-447-8871 (outside U.S. and Canada). Fax: 314-447-8029. E-mail: journalscustomerservice-usa@elsevier.com (for print support); journalsonlinesupport-usa@elsevier.com (for online support).**

Reprints. For copies of 100 or more of articles in this publication, please contact the Commercial Reprints Department, Elsevier Inc., 360 Park Avenue South, New York, NY 10010-1710. Tel.: 212-633-3874; Fax: 212-633-3820; E-mail: reprints@elsevier.com.

Sleep Medicine Clinics is covered in *MEDLINE/PubMed (Index Medicus)*.

SLEEP MEDICINE CLINICS

FORTHCOMING ISSUES

September 2024
**Multi-perspective Management of
Sleep Disorders**
Brendon Yee, Amanda Piper and
Stephen McNamara, *Editors*

December 2024
The Future of Sleep Disorders
Meir Kryger and Robert Thomas, *Editors*

March 2025
Pediatric Sleep-related Movement Disorders
Suresh Kotagal, *Editor*

RECENT ISSUES

March 2024
The Parasomnias
Alon Y. Avidan, *Editor*

December 2023
Sleep in Women
Monica Andersen, *Editor*

September 2023
Advances in Technology for the Sleep Field
Steven Holfinger, *Editor*

SERIES OF RELATED INTEREST

Neurologic Clinics
https://www.neurologic.theclinics.com/

Contributors

CONSULTING EDITORS

TEOFILO LEE-CHIONG Jr, MD
Professor of Medicine, National Jewish Health,
Professor of Medicine, University of Colorado,
Denver, Colorado, USA; Chief Medical Liaison,
Philips Respironics, Murrysville, Pennsylvania,
USA

DIEGO GARCIA-BORREGUERO, MD, PhD
International Medical Director Instituto del
Sueño, Calle Padre Damián, Madrid, Spain

ANA C. KRIEGER, MD, MPH, FCCP, FAASM
Chief, Division of Sleep Neurology, Medical
Director, Weill Cornell Center for Sleep
Medicine, Professor of Clinical Medicine,
Professor of Medicine in Neurology and
Genetic Medicine, Weill Cornell Medical
College, Cornell University, New York, New
York, USA

EDITOR

**KRISHNA M. SUNDAR, MD, ATSF, FCCP,
FAASM**
Clinical Professor, Division of Pulmonary and
Critical Care Medicine, Medical Director,

Sleep-Wake Center, University of Utah, Salt
Lake City, USA

AUTHORS

KORI ASCHER, DO
Assistant Professor of Clinical Medicine,
Division of Pulmonary, Critical Care, and Sleep
Medicine, University of Miami, Miller School of
Medicine

AMY ATTAWAY, MD
Respiratory Institute, Staff Physician,
Cleveland Clinic, Cleveland, Ohio,
USA

ELENA BARGAGLI, MD
Full Professor, Respiratory Diseases Unit,
Department of Medicine, Surgery and
Neurosciences, University of Siena, Siena,
Italy

SARAH BJORK, MD
Pulmonary and Critical Care Fellow, Division of
Pulmonary, Critical Care and Sleep Medicine,
Rush University Medical Center, Chicago,
Illinois, USA

JEANETTE P. BROWN, MD, PhD
Associate Professor (Clinical), Division of
Respiratory, Critical Care, and Occupational
Pulmonary Medicine, Department of
Internal Medicine, University of Utah
School of Medicine, Salt Lake City, Utah,
USA

LEE K. BROWN, MD
Division of Pulmonary, Critical Care, and Sleep
Medicine, Emeritus Professor, Department of
Internal Medicine, University of New Mexico
School of Medicine, Albuquerque, New
Mexico, USA

SARA CROCE, MD
Respiratory Diseases Unit, Department of
Medicine, Surgery and Neurosciences,
University of Siena, Siena, Italy

JANE C. DENG, MD
Professor, Pulmonary Medicine, VA Ann Arbor
Healthcare System, Division of Pulmonary and

Critical Care Medicine, University of Michigan Medical School, Ann Arbor, Michigan, USA

PETER DICPINIGAITIS, MD, FCCP
Professor, Department of Medicine, Albert Einstein College of Medicine and Montefiore Medical Center, Bronx, New York, USA

SAMUEL EPSTEIN, MD
Physician, Division of Pulmonary, Critical Care and Sleep Medicine, David Geffen School of Medicine, University of California, Los Angeles, Division of Pulmonary, Critical Care and Sleep Medicine, Greater Los Angeles VA Healthcare System, Los Angeles, California, USA

MANUEL HACHE MARLIERE, MD
Pulmonary and Critical Care Fellow, Division of Pulmonary, Critical Care and Sleep Medicine, Rush University Medical Center, Illinois, USA

OCTAVIAN C. IOACHIMESCU, MD, PhD, MBA
Associate Director, Clinical and Translational Science Institute of Southeast Wisconsin, Professor, Vice-Chair, Department of Medicine, Division of Pulmonary, Critical Care and Sleep Medicine, Medical College of Wisconsin, Milwaukee, Wisconsin, USA

DEEPANJALI JAIN, MD
Pulmonary and Critical Care Fellow, Division of Pulmonary, Critical Care and Sleep Medicine, Rush University Medical Center, Chicago, Illinois, USA

DALE JUN, MD
Pulmonologist, Division of Pulmonary, Critical Care and Sleep Medicine, David Geffen School of Medicine, University of California, Los Angeles, Division of Pulmonary, Critical Care and Sleep Medicine, Greater Los Angeles VA Healthcare System, Los Angeles, California, USA

CHITRA LAL, MD
Professor of Medicine, Pulmonary, Critical Care and Sleep Medicine, Medical University of South Carolina, Charleston, South Carolina, USA

BRIAN W. LOCKE, MD, MSCI
Visiting Clinical Instructor, Division of Respiratory, Critical Care, and Occupational

Pulmonary Medicine, Department of Internal Medicine, University of Utah School of Medicine, Salt Lake City, Utah, USA

ATUL MALHOTRA, MD
Professor, Department of Medicine, Division of Pulmonary, Critical Care and Sleep Medicine, University of California San Diego, San Diego, California, USA

JOSE M. MARIN, MD
Professor, Department of Medicine, University of Zaragoza School of Medicine, Zaragoza, Spain

MARTA MARIN-OTO, MD
Respiratory Department, Assistant Professor of Medicine, University of Zaragoza School of Medicine, Hospital Clínico Universitario, Zaragoza, Spain

WALTER T. McNICHOLAS, MD
Professor, Department of Respiratory and Sleep Medicine, St. Vincent's Hospital Group, School of Medicine and the Conway Research Institute, University College, Dublin, Ireland

REENA MEHRA, MD, MS
Respiratory Institute, Heart, Vascular and Thoracic Institute, Professor, Neurological Institute, Cleveland Clinic, Cleveland, Ohio, USA

ANDREA S. MELANI, MD
Medical Doctor, Respiratory Diseases Unit, Department of Medicine, Surgery and Neurosciences, University of Siena, Siena, Italy

OMAR A. MESARWI, MD
Associate Professor, Division of Pulmonary, Critical Care, and Sleep Medicine and Physiology, University of California, San Diego, La Jolla, California, USA

MADDALENA MESSINA, MD
Respiratory Diseases Unit, Department of Medicine, Surgery and Neurosciences, University of Siena, Siena, Italy

BABAK MOKHLESI, MD, MSc
The J. Bailey Carter, MD Endowed Professor, Chief, Division of Pulmonary, Critical Care and Sleep Medicine, Co-Director, Rush Lung Center, Department of Internal Medicine, Rush University Medical Center, Chicago, Illinois, USA

AVANTIKA NATHANI, MD
Fellow, Respiratory Institute, Cleveland Clinic, Cleveland, Ohio, USA

SANDA A. PREDESCU, PhD
Professor of Medicine, Division of Pulmonary,
Critical Care and Sleep Medicine, Rush
University Medical Center, Chicago, Illinois, USA

ALYSSA A. SELF, MD
Postdoctoral Fellow, Division of Pulmonary,
Critical Care, and Sleep Medicine and
Physiology, University of California, San Diego,
La Jolla, California, USA

SHIRIN SHAFAZAND, MD, MS, FAASM, ATSF
Professor of Clinical Medicine, Division of
Pulmonary, Critical Care, and Sleep Medicine,
University of Miami, Miller School of Medicine

AMANDA CAROLE STARK, PhD
Clinical Speech-Language Pathologist, Voice
Disorders Center, University of Utah, Salt Lake
City, Utah, USA

KRISHNA M. SUNDAR, MD, ATSF, FCCP, FAASM
Clinical Professor, Division of Pulmonary and
Critical Care Medicine, Medical Director,
Sleep-Wake Center, University of Utah, Salt
Lake City, USA

BERNIE Y. SUNWOO, MBBS
Associate Professor, Department of Medicine,
Division of Pulmonary, Critical Care and Sleep
Medicine, University of California San Diego,
San Diego, California, USA

MICHELLE ZEIDLER, MD, MS
Program Director, Division of Pulmonary,
Critical Care and Sleep Medicine, David Geffen
School of Medicine, University of California,
Los Angeles, Division of Pulmonary, Critical
Care and Sleep Medicine, Greater Los Angeles
VA Healthcare System, Los Angeles, California,
USA

Contents

Mechanical Interactions Between the Upper Airway and the Lungs that Affect the Propensity to Obstructive Sleep Apnea in Health and Chronic Lung Disease   211

Bernie Y. Sunwoo and Atul Malhotra

> Obstructive sleep apnea (OSA) is a common disorder characterized by repetitive narrowing and collapse of the upper airways during sleep. It is caused by multiple anatomic and nonanatomic factors but end-expiratory lung volume (EELV) is an important factor as increased EELV can stabilize the upper airway via caudal traction forces. EELV is impacted by changes in sleep stages, body position, weight, and chronic lung diseases, and this article reviews the mechanical interactions between the lungs and upper airway that affect the propensity to OSA. In doing so, it highlights the need for additional research in this area.

Effects of Obstructive Sleep Apnea on Airway Immunity and Susceptibility to Respiratory Infections   219

Samuel Epstein, Dale Jun, Jane C. Deng, and Michelle Zeidler

> Obstructive sleep apnea is a prevalent sleep disorder characterized by recurrent episodes of partial or complete upper airway collapse during sleep, leading to disrupted breathing patterns and intermittent hypoxia. OSA results in systemic inflammation but also directly affects the upper and lower airways leading to upregulation of inflammatory pathways and alterations of the local microbiome. These changes result in increased susceptibility to respiratory infections such as influenza, COVID-19, and bacterial pneumonia. This relationship is more complex and bidirectional in individuals with chronic lung disease such as chronic obstructive lung disease, interstitial lung disease and bronchiectasis.

Hypoxic and Autonomic Mechanisms from Sleep-Disordered Breathing Leading to Cardiopulmonary Dysfunction   229

Avantika Nathani, Amy Attaway, and Reena Mehra

> Obstructive sleep apnea (OSA) is a common sleep-related breathing disorder. Its prevalence has increased due to increasing obesity and improved screening and diagnostic strategies. OSA overlaps with cardiopulmonary diseases to promote intermittent hypoxia and autonomic dysfunction. Intermittent hypoxia increases the risk for oxidative stress and inflammation, which promotes endothelial dysfunction and predisposes to atherosclerosis and other cardiovascular complications. OSA is associated with an increased sympathetic nervous system drive resulting in autonomic dysfunction leading to worsening of cardiopulmonary diseases. Cardiovascular diseases are observed in 40% to 80% of OSA patients. Therefore, it is essential to screen and treat cardiovascular diseases.

Subjects with interstitial lung disease (ILD) often suffer from nocturnal cough, insomnia, and poor sleep quality. Subjects with ILD and obstructive sleep apnea (OSA) seem to have relatively mild symptoms from sleep fragmentation compared to subjects with only ILD. The overlap of ILD, OSA, and sleeping hypoxemia may be associated with poor outcome, even though there is no agreement on which sleep parameter is mostly associated with worsening ILD prognosis. Randomized controlled trials are needed to understand when positive airway pressure (PAP) treatment is required in subjects with ILD and OSA and the impact of PAP treatment on ILD progression.

Obstructive sleep apnea (OSA) is very prevalent in sarcoidosis patients. Sarcoidosis of the upper respiratory tract may affect upper airway patency and increase the risk of OSA. Weight gain due to steroid use, upper airway myopathy due to steroids and sarcoidosis itself, and interstitial lung disease with decreased upper airway patency are other reasons for the higher OSA prevalence seen in sarcoidosis. Several clinical manifestations such as fatigue, hypersomnolence, cognitive deficits, and pulmonary hypertension are common to both OSA and sarcoidosis. Therefore, early screening and treatment for OSA can improve symptoms and overall patient quality of life.

The pathophysiological interplay between sleep-disordered breathing (SDB) and pulmonary hypertension (PH) is complex and can involve a variety of mechanisms by which SDB can worsen PH. These mechanistic pathways include wide swings in intrathoracic pressure while breathing against an occluded upper airway, intermittent and/or sustained hypoxemia, acute and/or chronic hypercapnia, and obesity. In this review, we discuss how the downstream consequences of SDB can adversely impact PH, the challenges in accurately diagnosing and classifying PH in the severely obese, and review the limited literature assessing the effect of treating obesity, obstructive sleep apnea, and obesity hypoventilation syndrome on PH.

In a variety of physiologic and pathologic states, people may experience both chronic sustained hypoxemia and intermittent hypoxemia ("combined" or "overlap" hypoxemia). In general, hypoxemia in such instances predicts a variety of maladaptive outcomes, including excess cardiovascular disease or mortality. However, hypoxemia may be one of the myriad phenotypic effects in such states, making it difficult to ascertain whether adverse outcomes are primarily driven by hypoxemia, and if so, whether these effects are due to intermittent versus sustained hypoxemia.

An emerging body of literature describes the prevalence and consequences of hypercapnic respiratory failure. While device qualifications, documentation practices, and previously performed clinical studies often encourage conceptualizing patients as having a single "cause" of hypercapnia, many patients encountered in practice have several contributing conditions. Physiologic and epidemiologic data suggest that sleep-disordered breathing—particularly obstructive sleep apnea (OSA)—often contributes to the development of hypercapnia. In this review, the authors summarize the frequency of contributing conditions to hypercapnic respiratory failure among patients identified in critical care, emergency, and inpatient settings with an aim toward understanding the contribution of OSA to the development of hypercapnia.

Hypoventilation is a complication that is not uncommon in chronic obstructive pulmonary disease and calls for both medical treatment of the underlying disease and, frequently, noninvasive ventilation either during exacerbations requiring hospitalization or in a chronic state in the patient at home. Obesity hypoventilation syndrome by definition is associated with ventilatory failure and hypercapnia. It may or may not be accompanied by obstructive sleep apnea, which when detected becomes an additional target for positive airway pressure treatment. Intensive research has not completely resolved the best choice of treatment, and the simplest modality, continuous positive airway pressure, may still be entertained.

Obstructive sleep apnea (OSA) has emerged as a significant and prevalent comorbidity associated with chronic lung diseases, including chronic obstructive pulmonary disease, asthma, and interstitial lung diseases. These overlap syndromes are associated with worse patient-reported outcomes (sleep quality, quality of life measures, mental health) than each condition independently. Observational studies suggest that patients with overlap syndrome who are adherent to positive airway pressure therapy report improved quality of life, sleep quality, depression, and daytime symptoms. Screening for and management of OSA in patients with overlap syndrome should emphasize the interconnected nature of these 2 conditions and the positive impact that OSA management can have on patients' well-being and overall health.

Preface

How Important Is it to Address Sleep-Disordered Breathing in Patients with Chronic Lung Disease?

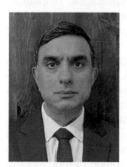

Krishna M. Sundar, MD

Editor

The human airway is a remarkably versatile structure with different portions of the airway undertaking differing functions. The nasal passages serve as the initial conduit for air performing tasks of filtration, olfaction, and humidification. The muscular upper airway starting from the velopharynx performs additional functions of swallowing and speaking, and to undertake these volitional activities, the upper airway is endowed with skeletal musculature which relaxes during sleep, making it vulnerable to collapse during each breath. Evolutionary changes that allowed humans the facility of complex speech (the basis of the Great Leap Forward) resulted in long muscular upper airways, that increased its propensity to collapse during sleep. The breath-dependent collapsibility of the upper airway during sleep, which increases with age and increasing body mass index, has led to the recognition of obstructive sleep apnea (OSA) as one of the most prevalent disorders affecting adults in the last few decades.

Despite the enormous body of literature on the effects of OSA on a multitude of organ systems, its effects on the contiguous lower airways and lung parenchyma have not been fully understood. This issue of the *Sleep Medicine Clinics* is focused upon expanding the understanding of this interaction between OSA and chronic lung diseases. The issue starts with mechanical interactions between the upper and lower airways, focusing on the effects of tracheal caudal traction and end-expiratory lung volume on the tendency to upper airway collapse during sleep. Subsequent articles explore the immediate downstream effects of recurrent decreases in airflow during sleep with the most evident effect being the fluctuations in oxygen tensions in the blood—intermittent hypoxia. Patients with OSA however experience, much larger fluctuations in oxygen tensions at the level of bronchial and alveolar epithelia during obstructive apneas and hypopneas as compared to the fluctuations seen in their blood oxygen levels. How these wide fluctuations in partial pressures of oxygen within the airways affect airway immunity, the susceptibility to respiratory infections (both viral and bacterial), and acute exacerbations of asthma and chronic obstructive pulmonary disease (COPD) are discussed in multiple articles, but much remains to be understood. Additional mechanical effects of intrathoracic pressure fluctuations on the distensible lung parenchyma may predispose to recurrent tractional injury and the long-term mechanical effects of OSA on the pulmonary interstitium are unknown.

Virtually every chronic respiratory disease, from chronic cough, to airway diseases such as asthma, COPD, bronchiectasis, and cystic fibrosis, to interstitial lung diseases has a close interaction with OSA due to the effects from dynamic airflow changes during sleep. While these interactions

Sleep Med Clin 19 (2024) xiii–xiv
https://doi.org/10.1016/j.jsmc.2024.02.015
1556-407X/24/Published by Elsevier Inc.

have common mechanistic pathways by which OSA affects the occurrence and progression of each pulmonary disorder, further research is needed to understand the myriad pathways by which OSA affects airway, interstitial, and vascular disorders of the lung. A consistent theme in the approach to understanding the relationship between OSA and chronic lung disease is the need to factor in the high prevalence of OSA, which makes the possibility of a chance association significant. Another aspect that is peculiar to the relationship of lung disorders and OSA is that of bidirectional relationships, which is not typically seen with other chronic diseases—besides the overlap syndrome seen between COPD and OSA, other chronic disorders, like asthma, sarcoidosis etc. represent "alternative overlap" syndromes when they cooccur with OSA. With patients living longer and the obesity pandemic, there is a greater likelihood of OSA worsening hypoxemia and hypercapnia, adding to the pulmonary hypertension stemming from underlying lung disease. Additional autonomic and cardiac effects from OSA increase morbidity and worsen symptom expression, quality of life, and disease outcomes. Beyond inflammatory and mechanical effects, epigenetic alterations, prothrombotic effects, and circadian interactions on lung parenchyma can add to the injury resulting from untreated OSA.

The superimposition of OSA on chronic lung disease makes the expression of hypoxemia and hypercapnia more complex. There is increasing understanding of the differing effects of *intermittent hypoxia* typical of OSA versus *sustained hypoxia* occurring from chronic lung disease, but when these two cooccur, the net effects are unclear. With increasingly available technologies to continuously monitor carbon dioxide tensions during sleep, there is also increasing appreciation of the role of hypercapnia in independently affecting outcomes. Beyond obesity hypoventilation syndrome, OSA appears to contribute to hypercapnic respiratory failure in a wide variety of settings, and further understanding is critical to optimal management of these patients.

Given the health care burden from lung disease, the superimposition of OSA not only worsens underlying chronic lung disease but also increases health care utilization. Despite the limited availability of sleep clinics and sleep-certified professionals, it is incumbent upon pulmonologists and respiratory providers to enable their patients to realize the full benefits of treating comorbid OSA on the course of their underlying chronic lung disease.

Krishna M. Sundar, MD, ATSF, FCCP, FAASM
Clinical Professor
Division of Pulmonary and Critical Care Medicine
Medical Director, Sleep-Wake Center
University of Utah, Salt Lake City, USA

E-mail address:
krishna.sundar@hsc.utah.edu

Mechanical Interactions Between the Upper Airway and the Lungs that Affect the Propensity to Obstructive Sleep Apnea in Health and Chronic Lung Disease

Bernie Y. Sunwoo, MBBS*, Atul Malhotra, MD[1]

KEYWORDS

- Obstructive sleep apnea • Chronic lung disease • Overlap syndrome
- Pharyngeal critical closing pressure • End-expiratory lung volume

KEY POINTS

- Obstructive sleep apnea (OSA) is caused by multiple anatomic and nonanatomic factors, but end-expiratory lung volume (EELV) is an important contributor. Increased EELV can stabilize the upper airway via caudal traction forces, and as such, mechanical interactions between the lungs and upper airway can impact the propensity to OSA.
- The pharyngeal critical closing pressure (P_{CRIT}) is a measure of upper airway collapsibility and there is a continuum of P_{CRIT} associated with increasing levels of sleep-related airflow obstruction. P_{CRIT} is normally negative but in patients with OSA, P_{CRIT} is positive inducing collapse and occlusion of the upper airways during sleep. P_{CRIT} is affected by lung volumes.
- There is a complex relationship between sleep stages, weight, and body position on EELV and consequently OSA risk.
- In obstructive lung diseases, like chronic obstructive pulmonary disease, air trapping and hyperinflation can reduce upper airway collapsibility due to tracheal traction, and be potentially protective against OSA. There are even less data on the mechanical interactions between the upper airways and restrictive lung diseases, highlighting the need for research in this area.

INTRODUCTION

Obstructive sleep apnea (OSA) is a common disorder characterized by repetitive narrowing and collapse of the upper airways during sleep. The precise pathophysiological mechanisms leading to the airway obstruction remain unknown but are likely multifactorial due to anatomic and nonanatomic factors, including ineffective upper airway dilator muscles, low arousal threshold, and an overly sensitive ventilatory control system (also referred to as high loop gain).[1] End-expiratory lung volume (EELV) is also an important factor as increased EELV can stabilize the upper airway via caudal traction forces. That is, mechanical interactions between the upper airways and the lungs can affect the propensity for OSA, both in health and chronic lung disease. This article reviews these mechanical interactions, understanding there is little research specific to this topic.

Department of Medicine, Division of Pulmonary, Critical Care and Sleep Medicine, University of California San Diego, San Diego, CA, USA
[1] Present address: 9500 Gilman Drive, La Jolla, CA 92093.
* Corresponding author. 4520 Executive Drive, Suite P2, San Diego, CA 92121.
E-mail address: besunwoo@health.ucsd.edu

Sleep Med Clin 19 (2024) 211–218
https://doi.org/10.1016/j.jsmc.2024.02.001
1556-407X/24/© 2024 Elsevier Inc. All rights reserved.

Pharyngeal Critical Closing Pressure and Upper Airway Collapsibility

The upper airway can be viewed as a tube with a collapsible segment. By applying the principles of the Starling resistor, pressure-flow relationships of the pharyngeal airways and the factors contributing to airflow obstruction can be better understood (**Fig. 1**).[2,3] The collapsible segment sits within a sealed box flanked by relatively rigid segments, the upstream nasal and the downstream tracheal airways, and patency depends on transmural pressure (pressure inside minus pressure outside the pharyngeal airway). The pharyngeal critical closing pressure (P_{CRIT}) is a measure of upper airway collapsibility.[4] It is measured while participants are on continuous positive airway pressure (CPAP) to minimize pharyngeal dilator muscle activity, and is the estimated nasal pressure at which the 'passive' upper airway collapses and airflow ceases. Using the described model, it can be thought of as the surrounding pressure that equals the pressure within the collapsible segment at the moment of collapse. Flow cannot occur until the pressure upstream of the collapsible segment exceeds Pcrit. When upstream pressure (P_{US}) is lower than P_{CRIT}, complete occlusion of the tube occurs. When downstream pressure (P_{DS}) is decreased below P_{CRIT}, inspiratory flow limitation occurs. Under these circumstances, the level of maximal inspiratory airflow (Vimax) is determined by upstream and critical closing pressures and the upstream nasal resistance (Rus), that is, Vimax = $(P_{US}-P_{CRIT})/R_{US}$. Pressures downstream from P_{CRIT} do not influence flow as long as P_{DS} is less than P_{CRIT}.

P_{CRIT} or pharyngeal collapsibility has been studied during sleep in normal subjects, snorers, and patients with OSA, and there is a continuum of P_{CRIT} associated with increasing levels of sleep-related airflow obstruction.[2,4–7] When P_{CRIT} is positive relative to atmospheric nasal pressure, the airway occludes and airflow becomes zero. Conversely, the more negative P_{CRIT} becomes, the lower the tendency toward pharyngeal collapse. In normal subjects, P_{CRIT} is negative and the upper airway is patent. Schwartz and colleagues[7] showed a P_{CRIT} of -13.3 ± 3.2 cm H_2O and a normal inspiratory airflow during sleep in healthy individuals with a P_{CRIT} of below -8 cm H_2O. As P_{CRIT} increased above -8 cm H_2O, airway pressures fell below P_{CRIT} during inspiration leading to pharyngeal collapse and flow limitation. Conversely, in patients with OSA, P_{CRIT} has been shown to be positive, inducing collapse and occlusion of the upper airways during sleep. Studies looking at the effects of sleep stage on P_{CRIT} have been mixed, likely in part due to challenges in accurate P_{CRIT} measurements, but a larger study by Carberry and colleagues[8] showed P_{CRIT} to be higher (more collapsible) during rapid eye movement (REM) sleep versus slow-wave and N2 sleep.[8–10] This study also showed a reduction in genioglossus activity from wakefulness off CPAP to on CPAP and from slow-wave sleep to N2 to REM sleep.

Relationship Between Critical Closing Pressure and End-Expiratory Lung Volume

The etiology for the increased P_{CRIT} seen in OSA is again likely due to structural factors but P_{CRIT} is affected by lung volumes, thereby potentially predisposing or protecting patients with chronic lung disease from OSA. EELVs have been shown to affect P_{CRIT} independently, both in healthy individuals and in OSA.[11–16] Squier and colleagues[15] studied the relationship between changes in absolute EELV and pharyngeal collapsibility using P_{CRIT}

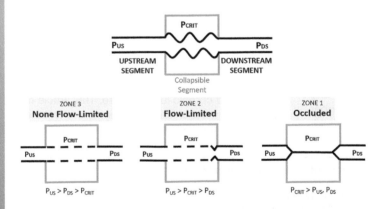

Fig. 1. Using the Starling resistor model, a collapsible segment is interposed within a sealed box, bound by a rigid upstream and downstream segment with corresponding upstream and downstream pressures (P_{US} and P_{DS}) and resistances. When there is no flow limitation (open airway), the critical opening pressure is the most negative with $P_{US} > P_{DS} > P_{CRIT}$, as in zone 3 of the Starling resistor model. When flow is present but slowed, as in an obstructive hypopnea, the downstream pressure is less than P_{CRIT} because of partial closure of the airway, and $P_{US} > P_{CRIT} > P_{DS}$ as seen in zone 2. When flow is completely occluded, as in an obstructive apnea, $P_{CRIT} > P_{US} > P_{DS}$ as seen in zone 1. (Susheel P. Patil et al., Adult Obstructive Sleep Apnea: Pathophysiology and Diagnosis, Chest, 132 (1), 2007, 325-337, https://doi.org/10.1378/chest.07-0040.)

in 18 healthy subjects. P_{CRIT} varied inversely with absolute EELV. Similarly, Stanchina and colleagues[14] sought to investigate systematically the isolated effects of lung volume changes on pharyngeal collapsibility in 19 healthy adults. Using a rigid head-out shell, adapted with a vacuum/blower allowing manipulations of extrathoracic pressure and thus lung volumes, they also demonstrated increased pharyngeal collapsibility with reduced lung volumes during non-REM sleep. Studies have also shown lung volumes influence P_{CRIT} measurements in OSA. Owens and colleagues[13] looked at EELV in 15 OSA patients and 7 controls and found passive P_{CRIT} decreased substantially with increased lung volumes, although by a similar amount in OSA and control subjects, concluding a role for lung volumes in the pathogenesis of OSA and consideration of lung volumes during the assessment of pharyngeal mechanics. Others have demonstrated greater reductions in EELV in patients with moderate OSA than those without OSA. Stadler and colleagues[17] measured expiratory diaphragmatic activity (eEMGdia) and EELV in 8 obese men with OSA and 8 healthy-weight men without OSA in the supine position using intraesophageal catheters and magnetometer coils. OSA patients experienced a greater fall in eEMGdia and EELV (61 mL in OSA vs 34 mL in controls) following sleep onset with greater falls at transitions accompanied by respiratory events, again suggesting a role for decreasing lung volumes to increased propensity for upper airway collapse in OSA. Tagaito and colleagues[16] examined the static mechanical properties of the passive pharynx before and during lung inflation by applying negative extrathoracic pressure in 8 anesthetized and paralyzed patients with OSA. Application of -50 cm H_2O negative extrathoracic pressure produced an increase in lung volume of approximately 0.72 L, and resulted in a significant reduction of velopharyngeal closing pressure.

Studies on CPAP further support the role of lung volumes in OSA. CPAP acts as a pneumatic splint to increase upper airway transmural pressure but is also known to increase EELV to counteract airway collapse. The apnea-hypopnea index (AHI) was shown to decrease from 62.3 ± 10.2 events/hr off CPAP to $37.2 + 5.0$ events/hr on CPAP and $31.2 + 6.7$ events/hr on 500 mL above the treating CPAP volume in 12 subjects with OSA where lung volumes were increased using the rigid head-out shell described earlier.[12] The same group sought to determine the influence of lung volumes on the level of CPAP required to prevent flow limitation in 17 adults with OSA during non-REM selep.[11] When lung volumes were increased

by 1035 ± 22 mL, the CPAP level could be decreased from 11.9 ± 0.7 to 4.8 ± 0.7 cm H_2O without flow limitation, while when lung volumes were reduced by 732 ± 74 mL, the CPAP level had to be increased from 11.9 ± 0.7 to 17.1 ± 1.0 cm H_2O to prevent flow limitation, suggesting even small changes in lung volumes have an important effect on upper airway patency in OSA.

End-Expiratory Lung Volume, Tracheal Traction, and Upper Airway Collapse

Animal and human models suggest the mechanisms by which lung volumes influence airway size and collapsibility are through caudal traction forces whereby the pharyngeal airway is stiffened with increasing lung volume. Various animal models have explored the effects of tracheal traction on upper airway patency.[18–21] The effects of airway elongation and dilation was explored in a feline model by displacing the trachea caudally and the tongue anteriorly, respectively, under complete neuromuscular blockade.[19] With caudal-tracheal displacement, P_{CRIT} fell progressively, while anterior-tongue displacement decreased P_{CRIT} when the trachea had been caudally displaced but not with the trachea in the neutral position, suggesting longitudinal tension within the airway mucosa modulates both P_{CRIT} and the response in P_{CRIT} to dilating forces. In another animal study using anesthetized, tracheostomized dogs, both mediastinal traction and the force generated by changes in intrathoracic pressure were shown to explain thoracic traction on the trachea.[21] Consequently lung volumes again play a central role. Hillman and colleagues[22] used phrenic nerve–stimulated diaphragmatic contraction to evaluate the effects of selective diaphragm contraction on upper airway collapsibility and the extent with which any of the observed change was attributable to lung volume-related changes in pressure gradients or to diaphragm descent–related mediastinal traction in 9 anesthetized healthy subjects. Peak inspiratory flow only increased when diaphragmatic contraction was associated with an increase in lung volumes suggesting lung volume–induced changes in transthoracic pressure gradients and not mediastinal caudal traction was the primary mediator of upper airway stabilization. Kairaitis and colleagues[18] hypothesized a threshold lung volume for optimal mechanical effects on upper airflow dynamics using and anesthetized rabbit model. Lung volume change, airflow, pharyngeal pressure, upper airway extraluminal tissue pressures laterally and anteriorly, tracheal displacement, and sternohyoid muscle activity were measured with extrathoracic pressure changes. Increasing lung volume displaced the trachea caudally, reduced extraluminal tissue pressures, and abolished flow limitation but had little effect on resistance or conductance.

EELV falls at sleep onset increasing susceptibility to upper airway collapse.[23] EELV are further decreased during REM sleep, when there is reduced tone of upper airway and chest wall and neck muscles.[24,25] Additionally, obesity and body position influence functional residual capacity (FRC) and lung volumes. The relationship between obesity, body position, and lung volumes is complex. Central obesity increases transdiaphragmatic pressure, reducing lung volumes and subsequently causing caudal tracheal traction to increase upper airway collapsibility.[26] However, body position and assuming the recumbent position are also associated with cephalad displacement of the diaphragm and decreases in lung volumes. Even in normal individuals with normal body mass index (BMI), FRC falls moving from the lateral to supine position. Teasing out the differential effects of sleep, obesity, and body position on lung volumes is challenging and weight may mediate positional changes, possibly by increased tonic diaphragm muscle activity.[17] Obese individuals have been shown to have smaller decreases in FRC and EELV going from the seated to supine position compared to nonobese individuals.[27–30]

Positional effects in OSA have been clearly shown and can be used to improve OSA. Neill and colleagues[31] measured upper airway closing pressure and upper airway opening pressure in 8 patients with OSA in the supine, 30° elevation, and lateral positions using a specially adapted nasal CPAP mask. The elevated posture resulted in a less collapsible airway compared with both the supine and lateral positions. In contrast, studies exploring pharyngeal cross-sectional size have not consistently shown significant changes between the lateral and supine position in OSA, although studied when awake.[32–34] Joosten and colleagues[34] studied airway cross-sectional area and shape using 4-dimensional computed tomography (CT) scanning of the upper airways and FRC, in the seated, supine, and lateral decubitus positions, in patients with supine OSA (more than twice the number of respiratory events in supine when compared with non-supine position), patients with REM-predominant OSA and patients without OSA, matched for age, gender, and BMI. Patients with supine OSA demonstrated a significant decrease in FRC of 340 mL when moving from the lateral to supine position compared to controls with no OSA and REM-predominant OSA. There was no significant difference in upper airway size

and shape, but all groups showed a significant change in airway shape with the velopharyngeal airway adopting a more elliptical shape (long axis laterally orientated) with reduced anteroposterior diameter in the supine airway, which may be of relevance in patients with airways disease as discussed in the following sections.

Chronic Lung Disease

These normal mechanical interactions between the upper airway and the lungs can further impact the propensity for OSA in patients with chronic lung disease, but few studies have explored mechanisms causing upper airway collapse in the various chronic lung diseases.

Chronic obstructive pulmonary disease (COPD) is a heterogeneous lung condition characterized by chronic respiratory symptoms due to abnormalities of the airways (bronchitis, bronchiolitis) and/or alveoli (emphysema) that cause persistent, often progressive, airflow obstruction. Expiratory flow limitation results in gas trapping or hyperinflation, reduces dynamic pulmonary compliance, and imposes increased load on respiratory muscles. Based on BOLD (Burden of Obstructive Lung Disease) and other large scale epidemiologic studies, it is estimated that the global prevalence of COPD is 10.3%.[35,36] Given the high prevalence of both OSA and COPD, the 2 diseases can coexist. The coexistence of OSA and COPD was coined by David Flenley in 1985 as the overlap syndrome and is associated with worse outcomes including mortality than either condition alone.[37]

Despite the potential mechanical risk factors for OSA in COPD, epidemiologic studies have not consistently supported that having 1 disorder increases risk for the other.[38] Studies, however, are largely restricted to cohorts with mild COPD, and studies including more severe COPD suggest a possible increased risk of OSA.[39] In a study of adult males with more moderate to severe COPD (forced expiratory volume in the first second [FEV_1] mean[standard deviation] of 42.8[19.8]%, FEV_1/FVC 42.3[13.1]), 52% had OSA as defined by an AHI greater than 5 events/hr.[40] Differences in prevalence may also be explained by heterogeneity of COPD clinical phenotypes that vary in predisposition to upper airway obstruction. Studies have suggested a protective mechanism for OSA with the 'pink puffer' phenotype versus the 'blue bloater' phenotype of COPD, due to the described effects of lung volumes on upper airways.

Expiratory flow limitation and increases in lung volumes seen in COPD can affect upper airway patency and compensatory responses to inspiratory flow limitation during sleep. Biselli and colleagues[41] completed sleep studies and quantified P_{CRIT} and respiratory timing responses to experimentally induced inspiratory flow limitation in 18 patients with COPD and 18 controls matched by age, BMI, sex, and OSA severity. COPD patients had lower passive P_{CRIT} (less collapsible airway) than their matched controls and a greater compensatory timing response during airway obstruction. Krachman and colleagues[42] investigated lung inflation using spirometry and volumetric chest CT in 51 smokers in the COPDGene project with emphysema and FEV_1 58 ± 14% predicted who underwent polysomnography for suspected OSA. 57% had OSA and there was an inverse correlation between the AHI and CT-derived measures of emphysema and air trapping, both for the entire study group and when just those patients with OSA were evaluated (r = −0.43 [P = .04] and r = −0.49 [p+.03], respectively). Multiple linear regression revealed that, in addition to CT-derived percent emphysema and CT-derived percent gas trapping, sex and BMI were important in determining the AHI in these patients. The Sleep Heart Health Study cohort also suggested a possible protective mechanism of hyperinflation in OSA.[43] For every 200 mL decrease in FEV_1, all-cause mortality increased by 11.0% in those without OSA (hazard ratio [HR] 1.11; 95% confidence interval, 1.08–1.13) but by only 6.0% in participants with OSA (HR 1.06; 95% confidence interval, 1.04–1.09), and the incremental influence of lung function on all-cause mortality was less with increasing severity of OSA.

Dynamic hyperinflation in COPD may reduce upper airway collapsibility due to tracheal traction, but airflow obstruction is also associated with significant changes in tracheal morphology that may further modify risk of upper airways collapse. In COPD, the tracheal index, the ratio between coronal and sagittal diameter of the trachea at the same level, is significantly reduced and shown to correlate with severity of emphysema.[44,45] At its more extreme, the saber-sheath trachea, which consists of marked coronal narrowing associated with sagittal widening, is a specific radiographic parameter for COPD linked to the functional severity of airway obstruction.[46] The propensity to airway collapse is related to airway size and shape. According to Laplace's law, a more rounded airway is inherently more stable than an elliptically shaped one as the transmural pressure gradient required to collapse the airway varies inversely with the radius of curvature. It is possible that in obstructive lung disease the reduced tracheal index offers some protection against the normal reductions in antero-posterior diameter that occur with supine positioning described earlier.

Table 1
Potential factors influencing upper airway collapsibility in chronic lung disease[67]

Promotion of airway collapse	Promotion of airway patency
• Negative pressure on inspiration	• Pharyngeal dilator muscle contraction (genioglossus)
• Extraluminal positive pressure	• End-expiratory lung volume through caudal traction forces
Fat deposition	
Small mandible	
Rostral fluid shifts	

Reprinted with permission from Elsevier. The Lancet, Jul 20 2002;360(9328):237-45.

In contrast to the pink puffers, 'blue bloaters' may be at increased risk for upper airways obstruction due to rostral fluid shifts when supine. Changes in leg fluid volume and neck circumference were measured in 23 non-obese healthy men referred for sleep studies for suspected OSA, from the beginning to the end of the night and the time spent sitting during the previous day.[47] Overnight changes in leg fluid volume and neck circumference correlated strongly with the AHI, together explaining 68% of the variability in AHI. In blue bloaters with cor pulmonale, rostral shift of peripheral edema when supine could in theory lead to fluid accumulation in the neck, contributing to pharyngeal narrowing and increased risk of OSA.

There are even fewer studies studying OSA in fibrotic lung disease. The relationship between interstitial lung disease (ILD) and OSA remains unclear, but a possible association has been suggested.[48–50] Cross-sectional analyses of 1690 adults in the Multi-Ethnic Study of Atherosclerosis cohort who underwent both chest CT and polysomnography found an association between moderate to severe OSA and subclinical ILD.[48] An obstructive AHI ≥ 15 events/hr was associated with a 35% increased odds (95% CI 13%–61%, P=.001) of interstitial lung abnormalities on CT, although the association varied by BMI with the strongest association seen among normal-weight individuals. Theoretically, in contrast to obstructive lung diseases, small lung volumes in ILD can reduce caudal traction in the upper airways, increasing the collapsibility and risk of OSA. However, Pereira and colleagues[51] determined potential predictive factors of OSA in 49 patients with fibrotic lung disease and BMI less than 30 kg/m^2. AHI showed a statistically significant correlation with age, BMI, duration of immunosuppressant treatment, and FEV_1 but only BMI remained an independent predictor of OSA in a multivariate correlation model adjusted for the other statistically meaningful variables, and additional studies are needed investigating the relationship between ILDs and OSA.

SUMMARY

Of note, there is generally a lack of rigorous research regarding upper airway mechanics in the context of chronic lung disease. A number of possible links exist (Table 1). First, as stated, caudal traction forces may affect upper airway patency in patients with lung disease.[11,12,20,21,52,53] Hyperinflation in emphysema may thus have a protective effective on the upper airway. However, an argument could be made that loss of elastic recoil in emphysema could reduce caudal traction and thus may not have the same mechanical benefit as compared to increased EELV in patients with normal lung parenchyma. Similarly, increased lung elastic recoil in pulmonary fibrosis may, in theory, have benefits despite low EELVs due to increased caudal traction forces. Second, the role of airway inflammation has been debated in the pathogenesis of OSA. In theory, inflamed airways may attenuate upper airway protective reflexes contributing to OSA risk.[54–56] Third, changes in body weight are common in chronic lung disease. Cachexia is seen in late COPD which in theory could be protective of OSA risk.[57] In contrast, glucocorticoid therapy can increase body fat and risk for OSA.[58,59] Fourth, as stated, rostral fluid shifts have been hypothesized to contribute to pharyngeal collapsibility.[60] The importance of this mechanism in chronic lung disease is unclear, but, given recent observations in asthma, may be a topic for future investigation.[61] Fifth, a sedentary lifestyle is common in patients with chronic lung disease who are limited by dyspnea. Exercise can clearly be helpful in reducing obesity, but exercise per se has also been associated with reduced OSA risk, independent of body weight.[62] Increased motor output to the diaphragm during exercise is also associated with increased output to the upper airway dilator muscles which may be helpful in mitigating OSA risk. Sixth, hypoxemia is common in chronic lung disease which has complex effects on control of breathing. Hypoxia can increase respiratory drive which may be destabilizing as seen in periodic breathing at high altitude.[63–65] On the other hand, chronic lung disease may reduce the efficiency of carbon dioxide excretion (so called plant gain) which may actually stabilize breathing.[66] In aggregate, the impact of COPD on overall ventilatory control instability is variable and thus its impact on OSA risk is unclear. In summary, the relationships between chronic lung diseases and OSA pathogenesis are complex and likely extend beyond direct mechanical and/or neuromuscular effects. Only by further rigorous research studies in this area are new therapeutic targets likely to emerge.

CLINICS CARE POINTS

- Animal and human models suggest lung volumes influence airway size and collapsibility through caudal traction forces whereby the pharyngeal airway is stiffened with increasing lung volume.

- Expiratory flow limitation and dynamic hyperinflation in COPD may reduce upper airway collapsibility due to tracheal traction, but airflow obstruction is also associated with significant changes in tracheal morphology that may further modify risk of upper airways collapse.

- CPAP acts as a pneumatic splint to increase upper airway transmural pressure but is also known to increase EELV to counteract airway collapse.

REFERENCES

1. Eckert DJ, White DP, Jordan AS, et al. Defining phenotypic causes of obstructive sleep apnea. Identification of novel therapeutic targets. Am J Respir Crit Care Med 2013;188(8):996–1004.
2. Gold AR, Schwartz AR. The pharyngeal critical pressure. The whys and hows of using nasal continuous positive airway pressure diagnostically. Chest 1996; 110(4):1077–88.
3. Patil SP, Schneider H, Schwartz AR, et al. Adult obstructive sleep apnea: pathophysiology and diagnosis. Chest 2007;132(1):325–37.
4. Smith PL, Wise RA, Gold AR, et al. Upper airway pressure-flow relationships in obstructive sleep apnea. J Appl Physiol (1985) 1988;64(2):789–95.
5. Gleadhill IC, Schwartz AR, Schubert N, et al. Upper airway collapsibility in snorers and in patients with obstructive hypopnea and apnea. Am Rev Respir Dis 1991;143(6):1300–3.
6. Issa FG, Sullivan CE. Upper airway closing pressures in obstructive sleep apnea. J Appl Physiol Respir Environ Exerc Physiol 1984;57(2):520–7.
7. Schwartz AR, Smith PL, Wise RA, et al. Induction of upper airway occlusion in sleeping individuals with subatmospheric nasal pressure. J Appl Physiol (1985) 1988;64(2):535–42.
8. Carberry JC, Jordan AS, White DP, et al. Upper airway collapsibility (Pcrit) and pharyngeal dilator muscle activity are sleep stage dependent. Sleep 2016;39(3):511–21.

9. Ong JS, Touyz G, Tanner S, et al. Variability of human upper airway collapsibility during sleep and the influence of body posture and sleep stage. J Sleep Res 2011;20(4):533–7.

10. Penzel T, Moller M, Becker HF, et al. Effect of sleep position and sleep stage on the collapsibility of the upper airways in patients with sleep apnea. Sleep 2001;24(1):90–5.

11. Heinzer RC, Stanchina ML, Malhotra A, et al. Lung volume and continuous positive airway pressure requirements in obstructive sleep apnea. Am J Respir Crit Care Med 2005;172(1):114–7.

12. Heinzer RC, Stanchina ML, Malhotra A, et al. Effect of increased lung volume on sleep disordered breathing in patients with sleep apnoea. Thorax 2006;61(5):435–9.

13. Owens RL, Malhotra A, Eckert DJ, et al. The influence of end-expiratory lung volume on measurements of pharyngeal collapsibility. J Appl Physiol (1985) 2010;108(2):445–51.

14. Stanchina ML, Malhotra A, Fogel RB, et al. The influence of lung volume on pharyngeal mechanics, collapsibility, and genioglossus muscle activation during sleep. Sleep 2003;26(7):851–6.

15. Squier SB, Patil SP, Schneider H, et al. Effect of end-expiratory lung volume on upper airway collapsibility in sleeping men and women. J Appl Physiol (1985) 2010;109(4):977–85.

16. Tagaito Y, Isono S, Remmers JE, et al. Lung volume and collapsibility of the passive pharynx in patients with sleep-disordered breathing. J Appl Physiol (1985) 2007;103(4):1379–85.

17. Stadler DL, McEvoy RD, Bradley J, et al. Changes in lung volume and diaphragm muscle activity at sleep onset in obese obstructive sleep apnea patients vs. healthy-weight controls. J Appl Physiol (1985) 2010;109(4):1027–36.

18. Kairaitis K, Verma M, Amatoury J, et al. A threshold lung volume for optimal mechanical effects on upper airway airflow dynamics: studies in an anesthetized rabbit model. J Appl Physiol (1985) 2012;112(7):1197–205.

19. Schwartz AR, Rowley JA, Thut DC, et al. Structural basis for alterations in upper airway collapsibility. Sleep 1996;19(10 Suppl):S184–8.

20. Van de Graaff WB. Thoracic influence on upper airway patency. J Appl Physiol (1985) 1988;65(5):2124–31.

21. Van de Graaff WB. Thoracic traction on the trachea: mechanisms and magnitude. J Appl Physiol (1985) 1991;70(3):1328–36.

22. Hillman DR, Walsh JH, Maddison KJ, et al. The effect of diaphragm contraction on upper airway collapsibility. J Appl Physiol (1985) 2013;115(3):337–45.

23. Hudgel DW, Devadatta P. Decrease in functional residual capacity during sleep in normal humans. J Appl Physiol Respir Environ Exerc Physiol 1984;57(5):1319–22.

24. Koo P, Gartman EJ, Sethi JM, et al. Change in end-expiratory lung volume during sleep in patients at risk for obstructive sleep apnea. J Clin Sleep Med 2017;13(8):941–7.

25. Koo P, Gartman EJ, Sethi JM, et al. End-expiratory lung volume decreases during REM sleep despite continuous positive airway pressure. Sleep Breath 2020;24(1):119–25.

26. Stadler DL, McEvoy RD, Sprecher KE, et al. Abdominal compression increases upper airway collapsibility during sleep in obese male obstructive sleep apnea patients. Sleep 2009;32(12):1579–87.

27. Bae J, Ting EY, Giuffrida JG. The effect of changes in the body position obsese patients on pulmonary volume and ventilatory function. Bull N Y Acad Med 1976;52(7):830–7.

28. Steier J, Lunt A, Hart N, et al. Observational study of the effect of obesity on lung volumes. Thorax 2014;69(8):752–9.

29. Watson RA, Pride NB. Postural changes in lung volumes and respiratory resistance in subjects with obesity. J Appl Physiol (1985) 2005;98(2):512–7.

30. Yap JC, Watson RA, Gilbey S, et al. Effects of posture on respiratory mechanics in obesity. J Appl Physiol (1985) 1995;79(4):1199–205.

31. Neill AM, Angus SM, Sajkov D, McEvoy RD. Effects of sleep posture on upper airway stability in patients with obstructive sleep apnea. Am J Respir Crit Care Med 1997;155(1):199–204.

32. Martin SE, Marshall I, Douglas NJ. The effect of posture on airway caliber with the sleep-apnea/hypopnea syndrome. Am J Respir Crit Care Med 1995;152(2):721–4.

33. Pevernagie DA, Stanson AW, Sheedy PF 2nd, et al. Effects of body position on the upper airway of patients with obstructive sleep apnea. Am J Respir Crit Care Med 1995;152(1):179–85.

34. Joosten SA, Sands SA, Edwards BA, et al. Evaluation of the role of lung volume and airway size and shape in supine-predominant obstructive sleep apnoea patients. Respirology 2015;20(5):819–27.

35. Adeloye D, Chua S, Lee C, et al. Global and regional estimates of COPD prevalence: systematic review and meta-analysis. J Glob Health 2015;5(2):020415. https://doi.org/10.7189/jogh.05-020415.

36. Adeloye D, Song P, Zhu Y, et al. Global, regional, and national prevalence of, and risk factors for, chronic obstructive pulmonary disease (COPD) in 2019: a systematic review and modelling analysis. Lancet Respir Med 2022;10(5):447–58.

37. Flenley DC. Sleep in chronic obstructive lung disease. Clin Chest Med 1985;6(4):651–61.

38. Malhotra A, Schwartz AR, Schneider H, et al. Research priorities in pathophysiology for sleep-disordered breathing in patients with chronic obstructive pulmonary disease. An official American

thoracic society research statement. Am J Respir Crit Care Med 2018;197(3):289–99.

39. Orr JE, Schmickl CN, Edwards BA, et al. Pathogenesis of obstructive sleep apnea in individuals with the COPD + OSA Overlap syndrome versus OSA alone. Physiol Rep 2020;8(3):e14371.

40. Soler X, Gaio E, Powell FL, et al. High prevalence of obstructive sleep apnea in patients with moderate to severe chronic obstructive pulmonary disease. Ann Am Thorac Soc 2015;12(8):1219–25.

41. Biselli P, Grossman PR, Kirkness JP, et al. The effect of increased lung volume in chronic obstructive pulmonary disease on upper airway obstruction during sleep. J Appl Physiol (1985) 2015;119(3):266–71.

42. Krachman SL, Tiwari R, Vega ME, et al. Effect of emphysema severity on the apnea-hypopnea index in smokers with obstructive sleep apnea. Ann Am Thorac Soc 2016;13(7):1129–35.

43. Putcha N, Crainiceanu C, Norato G, et al. Influence of lung function and sleep-disordered breathing on all-cause mortality. A community-based study. Am J Respir Crit Care Med 2016;194(8):1007–14.

44. Lee HJ, Seo JB, Chae EJ, et al. Tracheal morphology and collapse in COPD: correlation with CT indices and pulmonary function test. Eur J Radiol 2011;80(3):e531–5.

45. Tsao TC, Shieh WB. Intrathoracic tracheal dimensions and shape changes in chronic obstructive pulmonary disease. J Formos Med Assoc 1994;93(1):30–4.

46. Ciccarese F, Poerio A, Stagni S, et al. Saber-sheath trachea as a marker of severe airflow obstruction in chronic obstructive pulmonary disease. Radiol Med 2014;119(2):90–6.

47. Redolfi S, Yumino D, Ruttanaumpawan P, et al. Relationship between overnight rostral fluid shift and Obstructive Sleep Apnea in nonobese men. Am J Respir Crit Care Med 2009;179(3):241–6.

48. Kim JS, Podolanczuk AJ, Borker P, et al. Obstructive sleep apnea and subclinical interstitial lung disease in the multi-ethnic study of atherosclerosis (MESA). Ann Am Thorac Soc 2017;14(12):1786–95.

49. Lancaster LH, Mason WR, Parnell JA, et al. Obstructive sleep apnea is common in idiopathic pulmonary fibrosis. Chest 2009;136(3):772–8.

50. Mermigkis C, Bouloukaki I, Schiza SE. Obstructive sleep apnea in patients with interstitial lung diseases: past and future. Sleep Breath 2013;17(4):1127–8.

51. Pereira N, Cardoso AV, Mota PC, et al. Predictive factors of obstructive sleep apnoea in patients with fibrotic lung diseases. Sleep Med 2019;56:123–7.

52. van de Borne P, Mark AL, Montano N, et al. Effects of alcohol on sympathetic activity, hemodynamics, and chemoreflex sensitivity. Hypertension 1997;29(6):1278–83.

53. Heinzer R, White DP, Malhotra A, et al. Effect of expiratory positive airway pressure on sleep disordered breathing. Sleep 2008;31(3):429–32.

54. Nguyen AT, Jobin V, Payne R, et al. Laryngeal and velopharyngeal sensory impairment in obstructive sleep apnea. Sleep 2005;28(5):585–93.

55. Kimoff R, Sforza E, Champagne V, et al. Upper airway sensation in snoring and obstructive sleep apnea. Am J Respir Crit Care Med 2001;160:250–5.

56. Kimoff RJ. Upper airway myopathy is important in the pathophysiology of obstructive sleep apnea. J Clin Sleep Med 2007;3(6):567–9.

57. Foster GD, Borradaile KE, Sanders MH, et al. A randomized study on the effect of weight loss on obstructive sleep apnea among obese patients with type 2 diabetes: the Sleep AHEAD study. Arch Intern Med 2009;169(17):1619–26.

58. Gokosmanoglu F, Guzel A, Kan EK, et al. Increased prevalence of obstructive sleep apnea in patients with Cushing's syndrome compared with weight- and age-matched controls. Eur J Endocrinol 2017;176(3):267–72.

59. Wang LU, Wang TY, Bai YM, et al. Risk of obstructive sleep apnea among patients with Cushing's syndrome: a nationwide longitudinal study. Sleep Med 2017;36:44–7.

60. Lyons OD, Inami T, Perger E, et al. The effect of fluid overload on sleep apnoea severity in haemodialysis patients. Eur Respir J 2017;49(4). https://doi.org/10.1183/13993003.01789-2016.

61. Bhatawadekar SA, Inman MD, Fredberg JJ, et al. Contribution of rostral fluid shift to intrathoracic airway narrowing in asthma. J Appl Physiol (1985) 2017;122(4):809–16.

62. Awad KM, Malhotra A, Barnet JH, et al. Exercise is associated with a reduced incidence of sleep-disordered breathing. Am J Med 2012;125(5):485–90.

63. West JB. Man at extreme altitude. J Appl Physiol Respir Environ Exerc Physiol 1982;52(6):1393–9.

64. Simonson TS. Altitude adaptation: a glimpse through various lenses. High Alt Med Biol 2015;16(2):125–37.

65. Simonson TS, McClain DA, Jorde LB, et al. Genetic determinants of Tibetan high-altitude adaptation. Hum Genet 2012;131(4):527–33.

66. Salloum A, Rowley JA, Mateika JH, et al. Increased propensity for central apnea in patients with obstructive sleep apnea: effect of nasal continuous positive airway pressure. Am J Respir Crit Care Med 2010;181(2):189–93.

67. Malhotra A, White DP. Obstructive sleep apnoea. Lancet 2002;360(9328):237–45.

Effects of Obstructive Sleep Apnea on Airway Immunity and Susceptibility to Respiratory Infections

Samuel Epstein, MD[a,b], Dale Jun, MD[a,b], Jane C. Deng, MD[c,d], Michelle Zeidler, MD, MS[a,b],*

KEYWORDS

- Obstructive sleep apnea • Airway immunity • Airway inflammation • Upper airway • Lower airway
- Respiratory infection • Intermittent hypoxia

KEY POINTS

- OSA results in upper and lower airway inflammation through mechanical airways collapse, gastroesophageal reflux, intermittent hypoxia, oxidative stress, and sympathetic activation.
- OSA significantly alters the upper and lower airway microbiomes.
- Patients with OSA have higher rates of pulmonary infections including influenza, COVID-19, and bacterial pneumonia and may have more severe disease than patients without OSA.
- In patients with OSA and lung disease the inflammation from each disorder results in a bidirectional effect resulting in impaired airway immunity, changes in the local microbiome and increased susceptibility to respiratory infections, as well as exacerbations of lung disease such as asthma, COPD, and ILD.

INTRODUCTION

Obstructive sleep apnea (OSA) is a common disorder affecting up to one-third of the population between 30 to 70 years of age, with many patients remaining undiagnosed.[1–3] The prevalence of OSA continues to rise due, in part, to rising rates of obesity.[4] OSA is characterized by recurrent pharyngeal airway collapse during sleep resulting in cessation of breathing termed apneas, and reduction in breathing, called hypopneas leading to intermittent hypoxia (IH). OSA results in systemic inflammation associated with multiple comorbidities including cardiovascular disease, glucose intolerance, arrhythmias and cognitive impairment, among others.[5]

In addition to systemic inflammation, local upper and lower airway inflammation is also described. This upregulated inflammation along with changes in the local airway microbiome increases susceptibility to respiratory infectious diseases in patients with OSA. In patients with OSA and lung disease the inflammation from each disorder results in a bidirectional relationship resulting in impaired airway immunity, changes in the local microbiome and increased susceptibility to respiratory infections, all contributing to disease exacerbation. This has been evaluated in diseases such as tobacco related chronic obstructive pulmonary disease, asthma, interstitial lung disease, as well as non-cystic fibrosis bronchiectasis and cystic fibrosis.

[a] Division of Pulmonary, Critical Care and Sleep Medicine, David Geffen School of Medicine, UCLA, 10833 Le Conte Ave, Los Angeles, CA 90095, USA; [b] Division of Pulmonary, Critical Care and Sleep Medicine, Greater Los Angeles VA Healthcare System, 11301 Wilshire Boulevard 111Q, Los Angeles, CA 90073, USA; [c] Pulmonary Medicine, VA Ann Arbor Healthcare System, 2215 Fuller Road, Ann Arbor, MI 48105, USA; [d] Division of Pulmonary and Critical Care Medicine, University of Michigan Medical School, 1500 E. Medical Center Drive, Ann Arbor, MI 48109, USA
* Corresponding author. Division of Pulmonary, Critical Care and Sleep Medicine, Greater Los Angeles VA Healthcare System, 11301 Wilshire Blvd. 111Q, Los Angeles, CA 90073.
E-mail address: mzeidler@mednet.ucla.edu

Sleep Med Clin 19 (2024) 219–228
https://doi.org/10.1016/j.jsmc.2024.02.002
1556-407X/24/Published by Elsevier Inc.

EFFECT OF OBSTRUCTIVE SLEEP APNEA ON AIRWAY IMMUNE PATHWAYS
Overview of Local and Systemic Immunity

To understand how the immune system is impacted by a systemic process such as obstructive sleep apnea, one must consider the multiple components of immunity involved in host defense against pathogens.[6] At the forefront are physical barriers on the inner and outer surfaces of the body, including the respiratory mucosal epithelium, which are further protected by mucous, cilia, antimicrobial peptides, and complement. Pathogen invasion past these physical barriers triggers the activation of resident macrophages, dendritic cells, and epithelial cells through engagement of pattern recognition receptors (PRRs), which in turn activates a cascade of inflammatory signaling pathways via NF-κB, leading to the induction of which induces pro-inflammatory cytokines such as interleukin-1 (IL-1), interleukin-6 (IL-6), and tumor necrosis factor.[7] These acute phase cytokines prompt an enhanced local response via recruitment of other innate immune cell populations as well as a response at the systemic level. Following the initial phase of pulmonary host defense, adaptive immunity provides antigen-specific responses, through antigen presenting cells (APCs) such as dendritic cells that engage naïve T-cell populations to differentiate into effector T-cells. These cells then activate macrophages and B-cells, which along with CD8+ T cells, eliminate the pathogen. Memory B and T-cells can persist after the initial exposure to provide prolonged secondary immune response. More recently, there has been increased recognition of immune regulation through checkpoint molecules such as programmed cell death protein 1 (PD-1) which is expressed by cytotoxic T-cells, B cells and myeloid cells. The binding of the ligand, PD-L1, to its receptor inhibits activation of IL-2 production, T-cell proliferation, enhancement of myeloid-derived suppressor cell (MDSC) proliferation which are involved in inhibiting innate and adaptive immune responses.[8] Although PD-1 and PD-L1 are best known for their role in tumor biology and currently targeted in various cancer treatments, they are increasingly being recognized to have important immunoregulatory functions during autoimmune diseases and chronic infections.

Systemic Immune Effects of Obstructive Sleep Apnea via Intermittent Hypoxia and Sleep Fragmentation

Though the effects of sleep disordered breathing on our immune system are multifactorial, the most influential role is linked with intermittent hypoxia (IH), a hallmark of OSA caused by recurrent episodes of partial or complete upper airway obstruction during sleep (**Fig. 1**). Repeated episodes of hypoxia promote the propagation of pro-inflammatory cytokines including TNF and IL-6 via the transcription factor, NF-κB [9,10] with measurable increases in inflammatory markers in various study groups with sleep apnea.[11,12] Furthermore, oxidative stress caused by the hypoxic episodes create reactive oxygen species (ROS) which contribute to endothelial dysfunction.[13] The downstream effects of OSA-induced systemic inflammation include arterial atherosclerosis,[13,14] metabolic syndrome,[13–15] and insulin resistance,[16] among others, which reflects the association of these diseases with sleep apnea risk factors.

Sleep Fragmentation (SF), a common feature of patients with OSA due to repeated end-apneic arousals, also plays a role in the systemic inflammatory response. In murine models simulating SF, there was increased TNF expression in the central nervous system and other tissues suggesting increased activation of inflammatory pathways.[17] Additionally, chronic sleep deprivation as result of sleep fragmentation promotes pro-inflammatory cytokines[18] with a reduction in CD4 and CD8 cells.[19] These findings suggest a complex interaction of the immune response with the central nervous system in sleep apnea.

Effect of Obstructive Sleep Apnea and Intermittent Hypoxia on Susceptibility to Respiratory Infection

Regulation of the immune system response is also affected by intermittent hypoxia and can affect susceptibility to airway viral and bacterial infections. Recent studies have highlighted the role of activator and inhibitor pathways modulating T-cell activity, primarily via the role of the PD-L1/PD1 mediated pathway. Hypoxia-induced factor (HIF)-1α, a transcription factor that responds to decreases in oxygen levels in the cellular environment, binds to a hypoxia response element of the PD-L1 promoter, and activates PD-L1 transcription.[20] Cubillos-Zapata et al. showed a severity-dependent overexpression of PD-L1 and PD-1 in-vitro in human subjects with OSA as well as murine models in a severity-dependent manner.[21] The overexpression of PD-L1 and PD-1 suppressed T-cell proliferation and activation and reduced the cytotoxic capacity of CD8+ T-cells. T cell dysregulation is shown to increase highly virulent influenza in a mouse model providing a potential pathway for increased susceptibility of infection in patients with OSA.[22] In addition, HIF-1α upregulates platelet-activating factor receptor (PAFR) on airway epithelial cells. The PAFR receptor is utilized by

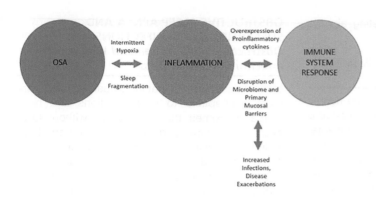

Fig. 1. Overview of the bidirectional relationships between OSA, inflammation, and immune system response. The hallmark features of OSA include intermittent hypoxia and sleep fragmentation. This, in addition to the changes from gastroesophageal reflux, promotes inflammation through oxidative stress and increased sympathetic activities. Inflammation occurs at both systemic and local (upper and lower airways) level causing disruption of physical barriers and changes to the microbiome which increases risk for infections and disease exacerbations. Along with overexpression of proinflammatory cytokines, these events trigger an immune system response via cellular pathways.

PAFR-dependent bacteria including Haemophilus influenzae, Pseudomonas aeruginosa, and Streptococcus pneumoniae, to cause pulmonary infections.[23]

Local Immune Effects of Obstructive Sleep Apnea on the Lower and Upper Airway Systems

In addition to causing systemic effects, OSA also results in significant local lower and upper airway inflammation. At the lower airway level, the inflammatory cascade mediated by cytokines can cause airway damage, altering respiratory structural integrity and function. In an in-vitro airway cell model, IH induced upregulation of matrix metalloproteinase (MMP)-9 and MMP-2 and pro-MMP-9 activation as well as increased levels of IL-8, platelet-derived growth factor and vascular endothelial growth factor.[23] Neutrophil chemotaxis was also enhanced with IH.[24] In a mouse model, intermittent hypoxia, compared to normoxia, over 4 weeks led to pulmonary damage through increased oxidative stress, increased inflammation (increase in CD68+lung macrophages), and dysregulation of the protease and antiprotease system with increased desmosine levels, a byproduct of elastin degradation.[25] Clinically, neutrophilia is noted in induced sputa of children and adults with OSA compared to those without, suggesting that OSA-induced neutrophilic inflammation may contribute to lower airway immune pathology.[26–28] Lower airway inflammation in OSA may also occur in conjunction with gastroesophageal reflux disorders (GERD) which has overall a high prevalence in patients with OSA. While the exact nature of their relationship is unclear, OSA is thought to contribute to GERD via increased intrathoracic pressure during apneic events. Microaspiration of gastric contents can increase lower airways

inflammation as well as the likelihood of respiratory tract infections and exacerbation of various chronic respiratory conditions.[29,30]

Local inflammation also occurs at the level of the upper airways resulting in narrowing and edema of critical structures that contribute to pharyngeal collapse. There is rostral accumulation of interstitial fluid at night compounded by increased fat deposition in pharyngeal fat pads and muscles seen in metabolic syndromes.[31] In patients with OSA, pharyngeal lavage showed higher levels of CD4+ T-cells, IL-6 and IL-8 when compared with snorers or healthy controls.[12] Examination of excised tissues from subjects who underwent uvulopalatopharyngoplasty for OSA show increased inflammatory cell infiltration (mainly T-cells) and subepithelial edema not present in healthy controls.[32] GERD can further increase laryngeal inflammation and edema, leading to alteration of the local biome and further worsening of OSA.[29]

OBSTRUCTIVE SLEEP APNEA AND ALTERNATIONS OF THE UPPER AND LOWER AIRWAY MICROBIOME

The microbiome of the upper and lower airway is a complex environment which regulates the host immune system. Disruption of the normal microbiome, or dysbiosis, can result in increased systemic and local inflammation and increased susceptibility to infectious disease. Processes such as dietary choices, smoking, and disruptions to circadian rhythm have been shown to disrupt the human microbiome. OSA is known to alter the microbiome with most reports focusing on the gut microbiome.[33] However, data suggests that OSA also causes alterations in the upper and lower airway microbiome leading to worsening inflammation, increased susceptibility to airways infections, as well as to exacerbations of existing airways diseases.[34]

Obstructive Sleep Apnea and the Nasal Microbiome

Typical normal organisms comprising the human nasal airway microbiome include Staphylococcus species, Propionibacterium, and Corynebacterium.[35] Patients with severe OSA are noted to have alterations in the nasal microbiome. Utilizing nasal lavage, Wu and colleagues found increased levels of Streptococcus, Prevotella, and Veillonella in individuals with OSA compared with controls. This alteration in nasal flora was associated with increased levels of IL-6 and IL-8 as well as increased neutrophils on nasal lavage compared with non OSA controls.[36]

Obstructive Sleep Apnea and the Oral Microbiome

In the human oral cavity normal flora include Abiotrophia, Gemella, Granulicatella, Neisseria, Prevotella, Rothia, and Streptococcus.[37] Using an oral swab Xu and colleagues evaluated the oral microbiome in 30 pediatric patients with OSA and 30 controls noting differences within the groups. Children with OSA had higher levels of *Actinobacteria, Bacteroidetes, Firmicutes, Fusobacteria*, and *Proteobacteria* within their oral cavity.[38] Similarly, the oral microbiome was significantly different in a study of middle-aged men with and without OSA. The OSA group was noted to have less biodiversity, with Neisseria slightly higher in individuals with moderate and severe OSA. Decreased microbiome diversity is seen in other disease processes as well such as COPD, obesity, and inflammatory lung disease.[39]

Obstructive Sleep Apnea and the Lung Microbiome

The lower airway microbiome is also altered in individuals with OSA. Using bronchoalveolar lavage in patients with and without OSA, Proteobacteria and Fusobacteria were noted to be higher in patients with OSA, while Firmicutes was markedly lower in patients with OSA.[40,41] Although causal relationships between specific taxonomic composition and immune phenotypes are difficult to establish in human patient populations, microbial composition is considered to play a critical role in appropriate regulation of immune "tone" particularly during childhood, with dysbiosis being associated with allergic airway diseases. Furthermore, during adulthood, interactions between resident microbes and the host immune system are increasingly being recognized to contribute to the pathogenesis of chronic lung diseases.[42]

OBSTRUCTIVE SLEEP APNEA AND SUSCEPTIBILITY TO INFECTIONS

Obstructive Sleep Apnea and Viral Airway Infections - Clinical Data

Clinical data suggest that individuals with OSA are more susceptible to viral infections and have worse outcomes than individuals without OSA even after correcting for other comorbidities including obesity. In a cross sectional study of 15,057 US adults, individuals with a diagnosis of OSA were significantly more likely to contract and be hospitalized for COVID-19 compared with individuals without OSA. Individuals with OSA who received COVID-19 vaccination were still more likely to contract COVID-19 compared to those without OSA.[43] Similar results were found in international studies spanning multiple countries[44] with one study showing a two fold risk of severe COVID-19 in patients with OSA.[45] In a study assessing the effect of OSA on influenza diagnosis and severity, researchers in Taiwan reviewed a database of over a million patients and identified 6508 individuals with OSA and 26,032 controls. After controlling for age, gender, comorbidities, income status and urbanization, individuals with OSA were significantly more likely to both contract influenza and also develop severe respiratory infection from influenza compared to the control group.[46,47] A retrospective study evaluated influenza infection in OSA patients who were compliant versus those non-compliant with positive airway pressure. Non-compliant patients or patients who had never started positive airway pressure were much more likely to be hospitalized for influenza (OR 4.5).[48] A study of first and second grade school children in Japan revealed that both children who frequently snored and those who were diagnosed with OSA were more likely to develop upper respiratory tract infections. Children with an apnea-hypopnea index $\geq$ 2.0/h had an OR of 2.65 for developing more than 3 upper respiratory infections in 6 months when compared to their counterparts with an apnea-hypopnea index less than 1.0/h.[49] Although the reasons for this increased susceptibility are unclear and likely multifactorial, one likely factor is that decreased sleep is associated with suboptimal antibody responses following vaccination.[50,51]

Obstructive Sleep Apnea and Bacterial Pneumonia - Clinical Data

Emerging data indicates that obstructive sleep apnea is also associated with higher rates of bacterial pneumonia. Review of a pediatric population in southern Israel showed that there was a significant increase in community-acquired alveolar pneumonia in children diagnosed with OSA in the prior 12 months when compared with non OSA controls.[52] Increased risk for bacterial pneumonia is noted in adult OSA patients admitted to the hospital.[53] Using the 2004 National Hospital Discharge Survey 371,000 individuals were identified with a diagnosis of sleep apnea using ICD coding. Pneumonia was the fifth most common admission diagnosis for this group.[54] A recent analysis of the Atherosclerosis Risk in Communities study reviewed 253 hospitalizations over a 20-year period. Individuals with severe OSA were 1.62 times more likely to be admitted with a diagnosis of pneumonia compared to non-OSA controls after adjusting for BMI, asthma and COPD.[55] Finally, in a retrospective case control study in Finland, Keto and colleagues showed increased risk of pneumonia in patients 1 year before and 1 year after their diagnosis of OSA when compared to matched controls.[56]

BIDIRECTIONAL RELATIONSHIP OF OBSTRUCTIVE SLEEP APNEA AND AIRWAY IMMUNITY IN CHRONIC LUNG DISEASE

Both OSA and airways diseases result in upregulation of airway inflammatory pathways with a bidirectional effect on each other. OSA impacts airway disorders most dramatically during acute apneic episodes when neurohormonal surges and changes in intrathoracic pressure disrupt normal physiology. The resulting chronic intermittent hypoxia from apneic episodes also upregulates inflammation and contributes to airways disease progression. The mechanisms through which airways inflammation impact OSA are more variable.

ASTHMA

Symptoms of asthma are worse at night likely due to circadian modulation of inflammation and altered hormonal activity.[40,57] Symptoms of nocturnal asthma include shortness of breath, gasping, and disrupted sleep. These symptoms can be difficult to differentiate from OSA and increasingly data suggests these two diseases increase the likelihood of one another and likely affect each other through upregulated inflammation.[58]

Asthma Effect on Obstructive Sleep Apnea

Asthma increases the risk of developing OSA.[59] Beyond shared risk factors, alterations in respiratory mechanics in asthma may promote the development of OSA. Bronchoconstriction in asthma reduces airway cross-sectional area and results in narrowing of the oropharynx and glottis.[59,60] Sleep deprivation and specifically sleep fragmentation caused by symptoms of asthma increases airway collapsibility.[61,62]

Obstructive Sleep Apnea Effect on Asthma

Both acute and chronic effects of hypoxia from OSA can affect asthma. The acute hypoxia associated with apneic episodes can increase bronchial reactivity.[63] The effect of chronic intermittent hypoxia is associated with an increase in inflammatory cytokines and metalloproteinases which may lead to a decrease in the reticular basal membrane, increased neutrophilia, and airway remodeling which result in asthma which is more treatment resistant.[64,65] Patients with asthma and OSA have been shown to have worse asthma control, increased frequency of exacerbations, and worse symptoms, particularly at night.[66]

CHRONIC OBSTRUCTIVE PULMONARY DISEASE

Hypoxia plays a central role in the pathogenesis of OSA and chronic obstructive pulmonary disease (COPD). Though there are differences between the sustained hypoxia associated with COPD and the intermittent hypoxia of OSA, it does appear that both mechanisms traverse similar pathways including upregulation of TNF alpha, IL-6, and IL-8.[67]

COPD Effect on Obstructive Sleep Apnea

COPD is a heterogeneous condition with a phenotypic spectrum ranging from emphysema to chronic bronchitis. Patients with the chronic bronchitis phenotype tend to have a higher BMI, which is an independent risk factor for the development of OSA.[5] Additionally, this phenotype is more at risk for right sided heart failure and fluid retention which increases airway obstruction through an edematous airway.[68] Patients with a primary emphysema phenotype can desaturate with even subtle increases in airway resistance due to alterations of the oxygen-hemoglobin desaturation curve from chronic hypoxia.[68,69] Hyperinflation is associated with a low arousal threshold in COPD which plays a critical role in developing OSA in this population.[70] COPD is also associated with skeletal muscle myopathy which can increase the likelihood of airway collapse. Additionally, cigarette smoking, a shared risk factor in COPD and OSA, has well documented associations with impairment in airway dilator muscles and reflexes.[71,72]

Obstructive Sleep Apnea Effect on COPD

In cases of OSA and COPD overlap, chronic nocturnal hypoxia attributable to COPD may be potentiated by intermittent hypoxia from OSA. In animal models, intermittent hypoxia was noted to induce lung damage through inflammatory mediators and reactive oxygen species.[73] Individuals with overlap syndrome have increased COPD exacerbations as well as increased overall mortality as compared to patients with COPD alone.[74,75]

INTERSTITIAL LUNG DISEASE

Interstitial lung disease (ILD) refers to a group of disorders characterized by inflammation and scarring of lung tissue, leading to impaired lung function, and breathing difficulties. The pathophysiology of these conditions is highly variable however there does seem to be some shared disease characteristics that predispose ILD patients to OSA and vice versa.

Interstitial Lung Disease Effect on Obstructive Sleep Apnea

As opposed to the theorized protective effects of hyperinflation on OSA associated with COPD, ILD is a restrictive lung disease with low lung volumes which may contribute to the increased prevalence of OSA in the ILD population. Lower lung volumes decrease upper airway stability leading to increased likelihood of airway collapse and apnea.[69]

Obstructive Sleep Apnea Effect on Interstitial Lung Disease

Patients with ILD are more likely to have OSA than the general population[76] and the development of OSA further exacerbates lower airways inflammation in ILD. Mortality is higher in patients with concomitant ILD and OSA, compared to ILD alone.[77] In patients with idiopathic pulmonary fibrosis, it is theorized that apneic episodes from OSA may expedite fibrosis. Intrathoracic pressure swings cause tractional alveolar injury which in turn damages alveolar cells and results in inflammation and progression of fibrosis.[78] Chronic intermittent hypoxia from apneic episodes serves as a potent stimulus for oxidative stress and subsequent pulmonary fibrosis.[79]

Cystic Fibrosis

Cystic fibrosis (CF) is a genetic disorder that affects the respiratory system causing the production of thick mucus and poor clearance of secretions leading to chronic lung infections and digestive problems. Although this disease is progressive, even early stage CF patients are at increased risk of OSA.[80] Patients with CF and OSA have been shown to have worse clinical outcomes.[81]

Cystic Fibrosis Effect on Obstructive Sleep Apnea

Due to impaired respiratory mechanics at night, patients with CF have increased nocturnal hypoxia and hypercapnia which may precede daytime respiratory abnormalities.[82] In a mechanism similar to that of COPD, this may predispose patients to arousals from desaturations related to airway obstruction and increase likelihood of developing OSA. Patients with CF, particularly children, are noted to have airway inflammation related to poor clearance of secretions. Both mechanical obstruction from secretions and narrowing from associated inflammation are proposed mechanisms that may lead to upper airway obstruction in CF patients.[82–84] Furthermore, chronic sinus congestion may promote mouth breathing which decreases oropharyngeal humidification, thickening secretions and promoting airway collapsibility.[71,85]

Obstructive Sleep Apnea Effect on Cystic Fibrosis

Effects of chronic intermittent hypoxia are the most likely mechanisms by which OSA affects CF. Inflammation caused by CIH damages sensitive lung tissue and increases colonization with harmful organisms like *Pseudomonas aeruginosa*, which is associated with increased mortality in CF patients.[86]

NON-CYSTIC FIBROSIS BRONCHIECTASIS

Non-cystic fibrosis bronchiectasis (NCFB) is a chronic respiratory condition characterized by the irreversible dilation and damage of bronchi. In this condition, there is infiltration of inflammatory cells in the walls of small airways resulting in airway obstruction, as well as proteases released by neutrophils which damage the large airways resulting in airway dilation.[87] This results in impaired mucociliary clearance, increased retained airway secretions, and an increased risk of airways infections with bacterial and non-tuberculous mycobacterial species.[88]

Bronchiectasis Effect on Obstructive Sleep Apnea

Data evaluating OSA in the NCFB population is limited, but there does seem to be an increased prevalence of OSA in these patients.[89] Impaired clearance of airway secretions and airway dilation may result in obstructed airflow which can increase risk of OSA and can potentiate airways inflammation.[90] Additionally, patients with NCFB have higher rates of hypoxia and hypercapnia which can increase arousals during sleep from even mild airway collapse.[89] In addition, chronic infections that may represent the etiology of bronchiectasis can be associated with airway inflammation and edema which increases airway collapsibility.[91]

Obstructive Sleep Apnea Effect on Bronchiectasis

Repetitive airway collapse and dramatic swings in intrathoracic pressure, as seen in OSA, are hypothesized to contribute to permanent airway dilation seen in bronchiectasis likely due to upregulation of inflammatory pathways.[91,92] Patients with bronchiectasis and concomitant OSA are at higher risk for respiratory infections. NCFB patients with OSA were noted to have a significantly higher prevalence of colonization with Pseudomonas aeruginosa, a predictor of NCFB severity.[89]

FUTURE DIRECTIONS FOR RESEARCH

OSA is a potent modulator of the immune response system. Future directions in research and clinical care include personalizing OSA phenotypes inclusive of biomarkers in order to develop patient tailored care and identify effective response to therapy. Long term clinical outcomes include prevalence of airway inflammation, rate of infection, and exacerbation of chronic lung disease.

CLINICS CARE POINTS

- Patients with OSA have altered upper and lower airway microbiomes likely resulting in increased susceptibility to airway infection.
- Patients with OSA may be more susceptible to pulmonary infections even when immunized.
- Patients with OSA are more likely to be hospitalized with pulmonary infection compared to individuals without OSA. This is more pronounced in untreated OSA.
- OSA induced local inflammation exacerbates established pulmonary disease such as COPD and asthma.

DISCLOSURE

The authors have no disclosures.

REFERENCES

1. Benjafield AV, Ayas NT, Eastwood PR, et al. Estimation of the global prevalence and burden of obstructive sleep apnoea: a literature-based analysis. Lancet Respir Med 2019;7(8):687–98.
2. Peppard PE, Young T, Barnet JH, et al. Increased prevalence of sleep-disordered breathing in adults. Am J Epidemiol 2013;177(9):1006–14.
3. Heinzer R, Vat S, Marques-Vidal P, et al. Prevalence of sleep-disordered breathing in the general population: the HypnoLaus study. Lancet Respir Med 2015;3(4):310–8.
4. Peppard PE, Young T, Palta M, et al. Longitudinal study of moderate weight change and sleep-disordered breathing. JAMA 2000;284(23):3015–21.
5. Gleeson M, McNicholas WT. Bidirectional relationships of comorbidity with obstructive sleep apnoea. Eur Respir Rev 2022;31(164). https://doi.org/10.1183/16000617.0256-2021.
6. Besedovsky L, Lange T, Haack M. The sleep-immune crosstalk in Health and disease. Physiol Rev 2019;99(3):1325–80.
7. Liu T, Zhang L, Joo D, et al. NF-κB signaling in inflammation. Signal Transduct Target Ther 2017;2:17023.
8. Francisco LM, Sage PT, Sharpe AH. The PD-1 pathway in tolerance and autoimmunity. Immunol Rev 2010;236:219–42.
9. Kheirandish-Gozal L, Gozal D. Obstructive sleep apnea and inflammation: Proof of Concept based on two Illustrative cytokines. Int J Mol Sci 2019;20(3). https://doi.org/10.3390/ijms20030459.
10. Ryan S, McNicholas WT. Intermittent hypoxia and activation of inflammatory molecular pathways in OSAS. Arch Physiol Biochem 2008;114(4):261–6.
11. Bouloukaki I, Mermigkis C, Tzanakis N, et al. Evaluation of inflammatory markers in a large Sample of obstructive sleep apnea patients without comorbidities. Mediators Inflamm 2017;2017:4573756.
12. Vicente E, Marin JM, Carrizo SJ, et al. Upper airway and systemic inflammation in obstructive sleep apnoea. Eur Respir J 2016;48(4):1108–17.
13. Oyama JI, Yamamoto H, Maeda T, et al. Continuous positive airway pressure therapy improves vascular dysfunction and decreases oxidative stress in patients with the metabolic syndrome and obstructive sleep apnea syndrome. Clin Cardiol 2012;35(4):231–6.
14. Jiang YQ, Xue JS, Xu J, et al. Efficacy of continuous positive airway pressure treatment in treating obstructive sleep apnea hypopnea syndrome associated with carotid arteriosclerosis. Exp Ther Med 2017;14(6):6176–82.
15. Hirotsu C, Albuquerque RG, Nogueira H, et al. The relationship between sleep apnea, metabolic dysfunction and inflammation: the gender influence. Brain Behav Immun 2017;59:211–8.
16. Leon-Cabrera S, Arana-Lechuga Y, Esqueda-León E, et al. Reduced systemic levels of IL-10 are associated with the severity of obstructive sleep apnea and insulin resistance in morbidly obese humans. Mediators Inflamm 2015;2015:493409.

17. Kaushal N, Ramesh V, Gozal D. TNF-α and temporal changes in sleep architecture in mice exposed to sleep fragmentation. PLoS One 2012;7(9):e45610.

18. Vgontzas AN, Zoumakis E, Lin HM, et al. Marked decrease in sleepiness in patients with sleep apnea by etanercept, a tumor necrosis factor-alpha antagonist. J Clin Endocrinol Metab 2004;89(9):4409–13.

19. Savard J, Laroche L, Simard S, et al. Chronic insomnia and immune functioning. Psychosom Med 2003;65(2):211–21.

20. Noman MZ, Desantis G, Janji B, et al. PD-L1 is a novel direct target of HIF-1α, and its blockade under hypoxia enhanced MDSC-mediated T cell activation. J Exp Med 2014;211(5):781–90.

21. Cubillos-Zapata C, Avendaño-Ortiz J, Hernandez-Jimenez E, et al. Hypoxia-induced PD-L1/PD-1 cross-talk impairs T-cell function in sleep apnoea. Eur Respir J 2017;50(4). https://doi.org/10.1183/13993003.008 33-2017.

22. Rutigliano JA, Sharma S, Morris MY, et al. Highly pathological influenza A virus infection is associated with augmented expression of PD-1 by functionally compromised virus-specific CD8+ T cells. J Virol 2014;88(3):1636–51.

23. Shukla SD, Walters EH, Simpson JL, et al. Hypoxia-inducible factor and bacterial infections in chronic obstructive pulmonary disease. Respirology 2020; 25(1):53–63.

24. Philippe C, Boussadia Y, Prulière-Escabasse V, et al. Airway cell involvement in intermittent hypoxia-induced airway inflammation. Sleep Breath 2015; 19(1):297–306.

25. Tuleta I, Stöckigt F, Juergens UR, et al. Intermittent hypoxia contributes to the lung damage by increased oxidative stress, inflammation, and Disbalance in protease/antiprotease system. Lung 2016; 194(6):1015–20.

26. Carpagnano GE, Kharitonov SA, Resta O, et al. Increased 8-isoprostane and interleukin-6 in breath condensate of obstructive sleep apnea patients. Chest 2002;122(4):1162–7.

27. Li AM, Hung E, Tsang T, et al. Induced sputum inflammatory measures correlate with disease severity in children with obstructive sleep apnoea. Thorax 2007;62(1):75–9.

28. Salerno FG, Carpagnano E, Guido P, et al. Airway inflammation in patients affected by obstructive sleep apnea syndrome. Respir Med 2004;98(1): 25–8.

29. Zanation AM, Senior BA. The relationship between extraesophageal reflux (EER) and obstructive sleep apnea (OSA). Sleep Med Rev 2005;9(6):453–8.

30. Sweet MP, Patti MG, Hoopes C, et al. Gastro-oesophageal reflux and aspiration in patients with advanced lung disease. Thorax 2009;64(2):167–73.

31. Perger E, Jutant EM, Redolfi S. Targeting volume overload and overnight rostral fluid shift: a new perspective to treat sleep apnea. Sleep Med Rev 2018;42:160–70.

32. Paulsen FP, Steven P, Tsokos M, et al. Upper airway epithelial structural changes in obstructive sleep-disordered breathing. Am J Respir Crit Care Med 2002;166(4):501–9.

33. Farré N, Farré R, Gozal D. Sleep apnea Morbidity: a Consequence of microbial-immune cross-Talk? Chest 2018;154(4):754–9.

34. Elgamal Z, Singh P, Geraghty P. The upper airway microbiota, environmental exposures, inflammation, and disease. Medicina 2021;57(8). https://doi.org/10.3390/medicina57080823.

35. Human Microbiome Project Consortium. Structure, function and diversity of the healthy human microbiome. Nature 2012;486(7402):207–14.

36. Wu BG, Sulaiman I, Wang J, et al. Severe obstructive sleep apnea is associated with alterations in the nasal microbiome and an increase in inflammation. Am J Respir Crit Care Med 2019;199(1):99–109.

37. Bik EM, Long CD, Armitage GC, et al. Bacterial diversity in the oral cavity of 10 healthy individuals. ISME J 2010;4(8):962–74.

38. Xu H, Li X, Zheng X, et al. Pediatric obstructive sleep apnea is associated with changes in the oral microbiome and Urinary Metabolomics Profile: a Pilot study. J Clin Sleep Med 2018;14(9):1559–67.

39. Yang W, Shao L, Heizhati M, et al. Oropharyngeal microbiome in obstructive sleep apnea: decreased diversity and Abundance. J Clin Sleep Med 2019; 15(12):1777–88.

40. Segal LN, Rom WN, Weiden MD. Lung microbiome for clinicians. New discoveries about bugs in healthy and diseased lungs. Ann Am Thorac Soc 2014; 11(1):108–16.

41. Lu D, Yao X, Abulimiti A, et al. Profiling of lung microbiota in the patients with obstructive sleep apnea. Medicine 2018;97(26):e11175.

42. Ubags NDJ, Marsland BJ. Mechanistic insight into the function of the microbiome in lung diseases. Eur Respir J 2017;50(3). https://doi.org/10.1183/13993003.02467-2016.

43. Quan SF, Weaver MD, Czeisler MÉ, et al. Associations between obstructive sleep apnea and COVID-19 infection and hospitalization among US adults. J Clin Sleep Med 2023;19(7):1303–11.

44. Chung F, Waseem R, Pham C, et al. The association between high risk of sleep apnea, comorbidities, and risk of COVID-19: a population-based international harmonized study. Sleep Breath 2021;25(2): 849–60.

45. Rögnvaldsson KG, Eyþórsson ES, Emilsson ÖI, et al. Obstructive sleep apnea is an independent risk factor for severe COVID-19: a population-based study. Sleep 2022;45(3). https://doi.org/10.1093/sleep/zsab272.

46. Chen TYT, Chang R, Chiu LT, et al. Obstructive sleep apnea and influenza infection: a nationwide

population-based cohort study. Sleep Med 2021; 81:202–9.

47. Tsai MS, Chen HC, Li HY, et al. Sleep apnea and risk of influenza-associated severe acute respiratory infection: Real-World Evidence. Nat Sci Sleep 2022;14:901–9.

48. Mok EM, Greenough G, Pollack CC. Untreated obstructive sleep apnea is associated with increased hospitalization from influenza infection. J Clin Sleep Med 2020;16(12):2003–7.

49. Kitazawa T, Wada H, Onuki K, et al. Snoring, obstructive sleep apnea, and upper respiratory tract infection in elementary school children in Japan. Sleep Breath 2023. https://doi.org/10.1007/s11325-023-02932-y.

50. Spiegel K, Sheridan JF, Van Cauter E. Effect of sleep deprivation on response to immunization. JAMA 2002;288(12):1471–2.

51. Brown R, Pang G, Husband AJ, et al. Suppression of immunity to influenza virus infection in the respiratory tract following sleep disturbance. Reg Immunol 1989;2(5):321–5.

52. Goldbart AD, Tal A, Givon-Lavi N, et al. Sleep-disordered breathing is a risk factor for community-acquired alveolar pneumonia in early childhood. Chest 2012;141(5):1210–5.

53. Chiner E, Llombart M, Valls J, et al. Association between obstructive sleep apnea and community-acquired pneumonia. PLoS One 2016;11(4): e0152749.

54. Spurr KF, Graven MA, Gilbert RW. Prevalence of unspecified sleep apnea and the use of continuous positive airway pressure in hospitalized patients, 2004 National Hospital Discharge Survey. Sleep Breath 2008;12(3):229–34.

55. Lutsey PL, Zineldin I, Misialek JR, et al. OSA and subsequent risk of hospitalization with pneumonia, respiratory infection, and Total infection: the atherosclerosis risk in Communities study. Chest 2023; 163(4):942–52.

56. Keto J, Feuth T, Linna M, et al. Lower respiratory tract infections among newly diagnosed sleep apnea patients. BMC Pulm Med 2023;23(1):332.

57. Skloot GS. Nocturnal asthma: mechanisms and management. Mt Sinai J Med 2002;69(3):140–7.

58. Teodorescu M, Broytman O, Curran-Everett D, et al. Obstructive sleep apnea risk, asthma burden, and lower airway inflammation in adults in the severe asthma research Program (SARP) II. J Allergy Clin Immunol Pract 2015;3(4):566–75.e1.

59. Kong DL, Qin Z, Shen H, et al. Association of obstructive sleep apnea with asthma: a Meta-analysis. Sci Rep 2017;7(1):4088.

60. Ioachimescu OC, Teodorescu M. Integrating the overlap of obstructive lung disease and obstructive sleep apnoea: OLDOSA syndrome. Respirology 2013;18(3):421–31.

61. Sériès F, Roy N, Marc I. Effects of sleep deprivation and sleep fragmentation on upper airway collapsibility in normal subjects. Am J Respir Crit Care Med 1994;150(2):481–5.

62. Wang R, Mihaicuta S, Tiotiu A, et al. Asthma and obstructive sleep apnoea in adults and children - an up-to-date review. Sleep Med Rev 2022;61: 101564.

63. Dagg KD, Thomson LJ, Clayton RA, et al. Effect of acute alterations in inspired oxygen tension on methacholine induced bronchoconstriction in patients with asthma. Thorax 1997;52(5):453–7.

64. Everson CA, Thalacker CD, Hogg N. Phagocyte migration and cellular stress induced in liver, lung, and intestine during sleep loss and sleep recovery. Am J Physiol Regul Integr Comp Physiol 2008; 295(6):R2067–74.

65. Liang L, Gu X, Shen HJ, et al. Chronic intermittent hypoxia reduces the effects of Glucosteroid in asthma via activating the p38 MAPK signaling pathway. Front Physiol 2021;12:703281.

66. Dixit R. Asthma and obstructive sleep apnea: more than an association. Lung India 2018;35(3):191–2.

67. Kendzerska T, Leung RS, Aaron SD, et al. Cardiovascular outcomes and all-cause mortality in patients with obstructive sleep apnea and chronic obstructive pulmonary disease (overlap syndrome). Ann Am Thorac Soc 2019;16(1):71–81.

68. White LH, Bradley TD. Role of nocturnal rostral fluid shift in the pathogenesis of obstructive and central sleep apnoea. J Physiol 2013;591(5):1179–93.

69. Locke BW, Lee JJ, Sundar KM. OSA and chronic respiratory disease: mechanisms and Epidemiology. Int J Environ Res Public Health 2022;19(9). https://doi.org/10.3390/ijerph19095473.

70. Antonaglia C, Passuti G, Giudici F, et al. Low arousal threshold: a common pathophysiological trait in patients with obstructive sleep apnea syndrome and asthma. Sleep Breath 2023;27(3):933–41.

71. Jagpal SK, Jobanputra AM, Ahmed OH, et al. Sleep-disordered breathing in cystic fibrosis. Pediatr Pulmonol 2021;56(Suppl 1):S23–31.

72. Renner B, Mueller CA, Shephard A. Environmental and non-infectious factors in the aetiology of pharyngitis (sore throat). Inflamm Res 2012;61(10):1041–52.

73. Spina G, Spruit MA, Alison J, et al. Analysis of nocturnal actigraphic sleep measures in patients with COPD and their association with daytime physical activity. Thorax 2017;72(8):694–701.

74. Marin JM, Soriano JB, Carrizo SJ, et al. Outcomes in patients with chronic obstructive pulmonary disease and obstructive sleep apnea: the overlap syndrome. Am J Respir Crit Care Med 2010;182(3):325–31.

75. Machado MCL, Vollmer WM, Togeiro SM, et al. CPAP and survival in moderate-to-severe obstructive sleep apnoea syndrome and hypoxaemic COPD. Eur Respir J 2010;35(1):132–7.

76. Pihtili A, Bingol Z, Kiyan E, et al. Obstructive sleep apnea is common in patients with interstitial lung disease. Sleep Breath 2013;17(4):1281–8.

77. Bosi M, Milioli G, Fanfulla F, et al. OSA and prolonged oxygen desaturation during sleep are Strong predictors of poor outcome in IPF. Lung 2017; 195(5):643–51.

78. Leslie KO. Idiopathic pulmonary fibrosis may be a disease of recurrent, tractional injury to the periphery of the aging lung: a unifying hypothesis regarding etiology and pathogenesis. Arch Pathol Lab Med 2012;136(6):591–600.

79. Mermigkis C, Bouloukaki I, Schiza SE. Sleep as a new target for Improving outcomes in idiopathic pulmonary fibrosis. Chest 2017;152(6):1327–38.

80. Shakkottai A, O'Brien LM, Nasr SZ, et al. Sleep disturbances and their impact in pediatric cystic fibrosis. Sleep Med Rev 2018;42:100–10.

81. Milross MA, Piper AJ, Dobbin CJ, et al. Sleep disordered breathing in cystic fibrosis. Sleep Med Rev 2004;8(4):295–308.

82. Isaiah A, Daher A, Sharma PB, et al. Predictors of sleep hypoxemia in children with cystic fibrosis. Pediatr Pulmonol 2019;54(3):273–9.

83. Deniz M, Gultekin E, Ciftci Z, et al. Nasal mucociliary clearance in obstructive sleep apnea syndrome patients. Am J Rhinol Allergy 2014;28(5):178–80.

84. Villa MP, Pagani J, Lucidi V, et al. Nocturnal oximetry in infants with cystic fibrosis. Arch Dis Child 2001; 84(1):50–4.

85. Mahdavinia M, Hui JW, Zitun M, et al. Patients with chronic rhinosinusitis and obstructive sleep apnea have increased paroxysmal limb movement. Am J Rhinol Allergy 2018;32(2):94–7.

86. Urquhart DS, Montgomery H, Jaffé A. Assessment of hypoxia in children with cystic fibrosis. Arch Dis Child 2005;90(11):1138–43.

87. King P. Pathogenesis of bronchiectasis. Paediatr Respir Rev 2011;12(2):104–10.

88. Radovanovic D, Santus P, Blasi F, et al. A comprehensive approach to lung function in bronchiectasis. Respir Med 2018;145:120–9.

89. Faria Júnior NS, Urbano JJ, Santos IR, et al. Evaluation of obstructive sleep apnea in non-cystic fibrosis bronchiectasis: a cross-sectional study. PLoS One 2017;12(10):e0185413.

90. Faria Júnior NS, Oliveira LVF, Perez EA, et al. Observational study of sleep, respiratory mechanics and quality of life in patients with non-cystic fibrosis bronchiectasis: a protocol study. BMJ Open 2015;5(7): e008183.

91. Cole PJ. Inflammation: a two-edged sword–the model of bronchiectasis. Eur J Respir Dis Suppl 1986;147:6–15.

92. Faverio P, Zanini U, Monzani A, et al. Sleep-disordered breathing and chronic respiratory infections: a Narrative review in adult and pediatric population. Int J Mol Sci 2023;24(6). https://doi.org/10.3390/ijms24065504.

Hypoxic and Autonomic Mechanisms from Sleep-Disordered Breathing Leading to Cardiopulmonary Dysfunction

Avantika Nathani, MD[a],*, Amy Attaway, MD[a], Reena Mehra, MD, MS[a,b,c]

KEYWORDS

- Obstructive sleep apnea • Autonomic dysfunction • Cardiovascular disease
- Pulmonary hypertension • Chronic obstructive pulmonary disease • Overlap syndrome

KEY POINTS

- Obstructive sleep apnea (OSA) is a common disease that can overlap with other cardiopulmonary diseases like chronic obstructive pulmonary disease, pulmonary hypertension, and other cardiovascular diseases including heart failure and stroke. Overlapping syndromes increase the risk for intermittent hypoxia and autonomic dysfunction through shared pathophysiologic mechanisms.
- Outcomes of overlapping diseases tend to be worse than with OSA alone.
- Intermittent hypoxia increases the risk for oxidative stress and inflammation, which promotes endothelial dysfunction and predisposes to atherosclerosis and other cardiovascular complications.
- OSA is associated with an increased sympathetic nervous system drive resulting in autonomic dysfunction leading to worsening of cardiopulmonary diseases.
- In patients with OSA, cardiovascular disease is observed in the vast majority of patients, that is, 40% to 80%. Therefore, screening and treatment of cardiovascular diseases are essential.

INTRODUCTION

Obstructive sleep apnea (OSA) is a common sleep-related breathing disorder. It has increased in prevalence over the previous decades due to the rising obesity epidemic as well as improved screening and diagnostic strategies yet remains underrecognized and underdiagnosed.[1] When accompanied by other cardiopulmonary dysfunctions like chronic obstructive pulmonary disease (COPD), pulmonary hypertension (PH), or cardiovascular disease (CVD), OSA is associated with increased health care burden, morbidity, and mortality.[2–4]

OSA causes intermittent hypoxia due to repetitive episodes of apneas and hypopneas leading to recurrent desaturation episodes. Episodes of intermittent hypoxia can be short but occur often and with high frequency.[5] Low oxygen tension due to OSA causes the release of inflammatory mediators like C-reactive protein (CRP),[6–8] tumor necrosis factor-α,[9–12] and interleukin (IL)-8,[13,14] as well as prothrombotic factors like plasminogen activator inhibitor-1 and fibrinogen.[15] Some of these proinflammatory and prothrombotic biomarkers have diurnal alterations such that morning levels more so than evening levels are elevated likely reflecting overnight sleep apnea–related

[a] Respiratory Institute, Cleveland Clinic, 9500 Euclid Avenue A90, Cleveland, OH 44195, USA; [b] Heart, Vascular and Thoracic Institute, Cleveland Clinic, Cleveland, OH, USA; [c] Neurological Institute, Cleveland Clinic, Cleveland, OH, USA
* Corresponding author.
E-mail address: avantika.nathani@gmail.com

Sleep Med Clin 19 (2024) 229–237
https://doi.org/10.1016/j.jsmc.2024.02.003

physiologic stresses. The resultant proinflammatory milieu leads to a state of systemic inflammation.[16] Hypoxia is also a stimulus for an increase in hypoxia-inducible factor 1α, a transcription factor with many downstream effects that can lead to an increase in reactive oxygen species (ROS) generation.[17] Intermittent hypoxia also directly activates the sympathetic nervous system by dysregulation of the chemoreceptor and baroreceptor reflexes leading to an increase in sympathetic tone, which has many downstream consequences including increased heart rate and blood pressure.[16,18]

In this literature review, we will focus on the underlying pathophysiology by which OSA leads to hypoxic and autonomic dysfunction in patients with cardiopulmonary disorders, and emphasize important areas of future research.

CHRONIC OBSTRUCTIVE PULMONARY DISEASE AND OBSTRUCTIVE SLEEP APNEA

The concurrent presentation of OSA with COPD was first recognized by David Flenley in 1985, who referred to it as overlap syndrome.[19] In the general population, the prevalence is between 1% and 3.6% but it increases in populations already diagnosed with COPD (2.9%–65%) or OSA (7.6%–55.7%).[20] This wide range in prevalence is attributed in part to the heterogeneity of study designs as well as the definitions of COPD and OSA utilized. Nevertheless, the concurrent presence of the 2 diseases is associated with significantly greater adverse outcomes than the presence of one alone.[21,22] Overlapping pathophysiological mechanisms of the 2 diseases may play a synergistic role in contributing to adverse health care outcomes.

Hypoxic and Autonomic Pathophysiologic Mechanisms of Obstructive Sleep Apnea that Affect Chronic Obstructive Pulmonary Disease

Even without the presence of sleep-disordered breathing, it is well-recognized that COPD patients are prone to nocturnal oxygen desaturations.[23,24] There are multiple reasons that nocturnal hypoxemia is common in COPD, which include the following:

1. A drop in alveolar ventilation during sleep, commonly occurring in rapid eye movement (REM) sleep. This is due to changes in brain signaling which cause loss of tone of the skeletal muscles, except the diaphragm.
2. There is a blunting of hypoxic and hypercapnic responses during sleep, most pronounced during REM sleep in patients with OSA[25] leading to

a lower increase in tidal volume, respiratory rate, and minute ventilation.
3. In COPD, the contractility of the diaphragm is impaired due to hyperinflation causing stretching of the diaphragm and disturbances in length-tension ratio. This leads to significant hypoventilation during sleep.
4. Ventilation/perfusion in COPD patients worsens during sleep due to decreased functional residual capacity (related to atonia of the inspiratory muscles).
5. During REM sleep, cholinergic activity is increased and this leads to worsening bronchoconstriction in the airways particularly in the latter portion of the sleep cycle when REM sleep predominates.
6. Loss of cough reflex, which can lead to increased volume and inspissation of mucus in the airways of COPD patients.

Thus, nocturnal hypoxemia is common in COPD and can take the form of a persistent, mild-to-moderate–level desaturation that can last throughout the duration of sleep. When combined with the intermittent desaturation that occurs in patients with OSA, COPD patients with OSA overlap have increased episodes of intermittent hypoxemia without recovery of oxygen levels in between episodes. These patients tend to have worse nocturnal oxygen desaturations and a higher degree of the resultant autonomic effects.

Patients with COPD-OSA overlap syndrome have an increased risk of COPD exacerbation. Moreover, the treatment of the underlying OSA component with noninvasive ventilation (NIV) reduced hospitalizations in COPD patients.[26] While the underlying pathophysiology remains to be determined, it has been postulated that the increase in exacerbations is caused by a greater systemic inflammatory state due to hypoxia.

A common risk factor for adverse outcomes in both COPD and OSA is active tobacco smoking.[27,28] Active smoking increases upper airway inflammation that can adversely impact OSA, and contributes to lung injury as manifested by chronic bronchitis or emphysema. A recent study showed that smokers with OSA tend to have a higher severity of OSA as well as an increased prevalence of COPD.[29]

Hypoxia and Cardiovascular Impact in Chronic Obstructive Pulmonary Disease

The cardiovascular impact of overlap syndrome is complex (**Fig. 1**). The hypoxia resulting from nocturnal oxygen desaturation causes an inflammatory state that leads to an increased risk of cardiovascular events in COPD and OSA.[30] There is a

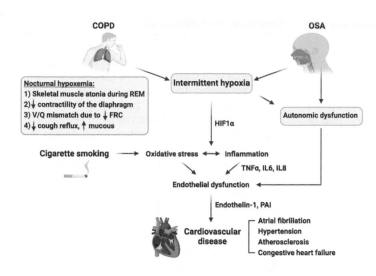

Fig. 1. Mechanisms of development of cardiovascular disease in chronic obstructive pulmonary disease (COPD)-obstructive sleep apnea (OSA) overlap syndrome. FRC, functional residual capacity; HIF 1 α, hypoxia-inducible factor 1 alpha; IL-6, interleukin 6; IL-8, interleukin 8; PAI, plasminogen activator inhibitor; REM, rapid eye movement; TNF-α, tumor necrosis factor-alpha; V/Q, ventilation/perfusion. (Created with BioRender.com.)

significant increase in the prevalence of PH and right heart dysfunction in patients with overlap syndrome than with COPD alone.[31,32] The risk of developing new-onset atrial fibrillation (AF) is also much higher with overlap syndrome than with COPD or OSA alone.[33] The overall risk of hospitalization and death is higher in patients with overlap syndrome than isolated COPD,[26,34] with a significant impact attributed to cardiopulmonary effects.

Screening and Diagnosis of Chronic Obstructive Pulmonary Disease-Obstructive Sleep Apnea Overlap

A strong index of suspicion is needed to diagnose COPD-OSA overlap syndrome. The American Thoracic Society recommends screening COPD patients with chronic stable hypercapnia for overlap syndrome with the STOP-BANG questionnaire (snoring, tiredness, observed apneas, high blood pressure, body mass index [BMI], age, neck circumference, gender) before initiating NIV for the chronic hypercapnic respiratory failure.[35] Preliminary data suggest the utilization of a COPD-specific OSA questionnaire to screen for overlap syndrome.[36] However, the gold standard for diagnosing sleep-disordered breathing in COPD patients remains polysomnography which also offers the ability to conduct surrogate arterial carbon dioxide (CO_2) monitoring with transcutaneous or end-tidal CO_2 to assess for possible concomitant sleep-related hypoventilation.

Treatment of Chronic Obstructive Pulmonary Disease-Obstructive Sleep Apnea Overlap

Once diagnosed, treatment with positive airway pressure in the form of continuous positive airway pressure (CPAP) or bilevel positive airway pressure (bilevel PAP, a form of NIV) is recommended.

The choice between the 2 is based on the predominant underlying pathophysiology. In patients with mild COPD and severe OSA, treatment with CPAP alone may be sufficient to correct the underlying hypoxemia.[37] In COPD patients with associated phenotypes such as higher BMI and chronic bronchitis, bilevel PAP therapy may be optimal. COPD patients with an emphysema-predominant phenotype may benefit from CPAP therapy to counteract dynamic hyperinflation.[37] Finally, in those with sleep-related hypoventilation observed during diagnostic sleep testing with surrogate CO_2 monitoring, bilevel PAP therapy can be initiated using protocols involving maximization of pressure support to target optimization of treatment of hypoventilation.

In general, treatment with NIV in COPD-OSA overlap syndrome has been shown to improve nocturnal hypoxemia[38] and inflammatory markers[37] as well as reduce COPD exacerbations and health care costs.[39]

PULMONARY HYPERTENSION AND SLEEP APNEA

The sixth World Symposium on Pulmonary Hypertension defines PH as a mean pulmonary artery (mPA) pressure of more than 20 mm Hg.[40] In the majority of cases, OSA is associated with PH related to left heart disease (group 2), or with COPD which is associated with PH related to chronic lung disease (group 3).[41] Data suggest that in the absence of comorbidities, OSA is an independent risk factor for the development of PH (group 3), albeit with a mild-to-moderate elevation in mPA pressures.[42] OSA associated with obesity hypoventilation syndrome is associated with higher mPA pressures than OSA alone.[43]

Hypoxic and Autonomic Pathophysiologic Mechanisms of Sleep Apnea Affecting Pulmonary Hypertension

OSA has both immediate and permanent effects on pulmonary hemodynamics.[44] The immediate consequences are related to periods of apnea and hypopnea that lead to inspiratory efforts against an obstructed upper airway. This leads to hypoxia, hypercapnia, as well as swings in intra-thoracic pressure which affect the systemic venous return and left ventricular afterload. Post-apneic arousal is associated with a surge in sympathetic activity which further increases heart rate and stroke volume causing elevation of mPA pressures.[45] The long-term permanent effects are related to intermittent hypoxia, endothelial dysfunction, increased sympathetic activity, and oxidative stress. A unique property of pulmonary vasculature is its ability to vasoconstrict in response to alveolar hypoxia. This is a protective mechanism that allows blood to be shunted to well-oxygenated segments of the lungs and improves ventilation-perfusion mismatch and allowing for optimal oxygen delivery.[46] Chronic intermittent hypoxia leads to hypoxic pulmonary vasoconstriction causing an increase in pulmonary vascular resistance (PVR). This occurs due to the release of several inflammatory and proliferative cytokines driven by hypoxia that cause vascular remodeling and the development of PH. Hypoxia is a potent stimulant for the production of nicotin-amide adenine dinucleotide phosphate oxidase which leads to superoxide production. Elevated superoxide levels cause vasoconstriction and vascular proliferation.[47] Patients with OSA also demonstrate lower levels of endothelial nitric ox-ide[48] and an increased expression and respon-siveness to endothelin-1.[49] This imbalance leads to an overall increased vascular tone and elevated pulmonary pressures due to increased PVR. The elevation in pulmonary artery pressure is closely related to the degree of hypoxia or the time spent at a saturation of less than 90% (T90).[50,51]

Recent data from the Pulmonary Vascular Disease Phenomics Study Group, a National Institute of Health initiative of a richly phenotyped multi-center prospective cohort, suggest that the overall presence of OSA is highest amongst the group 2 PH patients (secondary to left heart disease).[52] In patients with group 1 pulmonary arterial hypertension (PAH) and coexisting OSA, the presence of sleep-related hypoxia (T90) was strongly associated with measures of right ventricular dysfunction, death, or transplantation in patients with PAH. A 10% increase in T90 was associated with a 17% increase in transplantation or death.[53]

Screening and Diagnosis

OSA and PH share a close relationship and screening should be considered bidirectionally. In patients with diagnosed PH, guidelines recommend screening for OSA in patients with suspected sleep-disordered breathing.[54] This can be performed by overnight oximetry or polysomnography. A small prospective study found that the STOP-BANG questionnaire had 81% sensitivity and 43% specificity for predicting sleep apnea in PH and may be a good screening tool.[55] Conversely, while there are no formal guidelines to screen for PH in OSA patients, smaller studies have found that screening with echocardiography can diagnose PH in up to 34% of patients.[42,56,57] The historical gold standard for the diagnosis of OSA is polysomnography, while the gold standard for the diagnosis of PH is right heart catheterization.

Treatment

Treatment of OSA with CPAP has been shown to reduce both mPA pressures as well as right ventricular systolic pressures and thus improve pulmonary hemodynamics.[44] The effect on lowering these pressures is of low magnitude and is seen particularly in patients that have elevated mPA pressures (ie, PH) at baseline.[58,59] The improvement was attributed to the correction of oxygenation and thus reducing PVR.[60]

CARDIOVASCULAR DISEASE (HEART FAILURE, HYPERTENSION, ATRIAL FIBRILLATION STROKE) AND OBSTRUCTIVE SLEEP APNEA

OSA has been associated with several cardiovascular complications including hypertension, stroke, heart failure, coronary artery disease, and AF.[61,62] The prevalence of OSA in CVD is estimated to be as high as 40% to 80%.[62] The pathophysiological mechanisms by which these complications develop in OSA share several common pathways. In this section, we will review the hypoxic and autonomic mechanisms that cause cardiovascular complications in OSA.

Hypoxic and Autonomic Pathophysiologic Mechanisms of Sleep Apnea Affecting Cardiovascular Disease

There are multiple mechanisms by which OSA results in CVDs, including

1. *Increased sympathetic drive.* Apneic and hypopneic episodes in sleep apnea are followed by episodes of arousal and sympathetic overdrive. This results in an elevation of heart rate and

blood pressure. Repetitive arousals have been associated with hypertension in patients with OSA.[63]

2. *Atherosclerosis.* Atherosclerosis is a common pathologic link between most of the cardiovascular comorbidities associated with OSA like hypertension, heart failure, and stroke.[64] The pathophysiology of developing atherosclerosis is complex and involves interplay between many factors (**Fig. 2**):

a. *Intermittent hypoxia and endothelial dysfunction.* The intermittent hypoxia associated with OSA leads to the production of ROS which causes oxidative stress and endothelial damage.[17,65] As mentioned earlier, there are increases in vasoconstrictor molecules like endothelin-1 and decreases in vasodilator molecules like endothelial nitric oxide. This leads to endothelial dysfunction predisposing to atherosclerosis.

b. *Inflammation.* Intermittent hypoxia and the resultant oxidative stress that occurs in OSA cause the release of multiple proinflammatory cytokines and chemokines like IL-6) and IL-8[66],[11] as well as elevation of CRP.[7] This inflammatory milieu leads to the formation, progression, and rupture of atherosclerotic plaques.[64]

c. *Autonomic dysfunction.* The within-night repetitive increased sympathetic nervous system activation over time results in vascular remodeling with daytime increases in blood pressure and development of systemic hypertension. This in turn causes oxidative and shearing stress to the endothelium resulting in atherogenesis.[67]

d. *Mechanical stress.* Heavy snoring has been implicated in the development of atherosclerosis, particularly carotid artery atherosclerosis.[68] This is likely due to vibrations from the pharyngeal tissues that cause carotid artery endothelial dysfunction due to mechanical stress.[69,70]

e. *Platelet dysfunction.* OSA has been associated with an increase in prothrombotic factors like fibrinogen[71] and plasminogen activation inhibitor.[72] This results in platelet activation which promotes the formation of atherosclerotic plaques.[73]

3. *Increased myocardial oxygen demand.* The respiratory efforts made against a collapsed upper airway lead to an increase in the negative intrathoracic pressure during OSA. As a result, the transmural pressure across the left ventricle increases (measured as intracardiac pressure minus intrathoracic pressure).[74] There is an increase in right ventricular preload and left ventricular afterload.[75] The increased stress on the myocardium results in increased oxygen demand and over time leads to mechanical stresses and influences on the thin-walled atrial as well as left ventricular dysfunction and heart failure.[74]

Screening and Diagnosis

Screening for OSA in high-risk patients with CVD is important because it improves patient-centered outcomes and mood,[76] although it has not been shown to prevent cardiovascular events. Guidelines recommend screening for OSA with questionnaires like STOP-BANG in patients with CVD.[77] In those who screen positive with significant CVD (such as heart failure, congenital heart disease, or complicated valvular disease) or stroke, a polysomnogram should be used to diagnose sleep apnea.[77]

Treatment

Treatment of OSA is geared toward reducing blood pressure and atherosclerosis, the primary

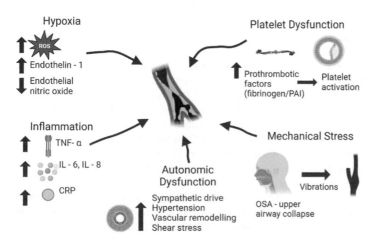

Fig. 2. Mechanisms of development of atherosclerosis in obstructive sleep apnea (OSA). CRP, C-reactive protein; IL-6, interleukin 6; IL-8, interleukin 8; PAI, plasminogen activator inhibitor; ROS, reactive oxygen species; TNF-α, tumor necrosis factor-alpha. (Created with BioRender.com.)

mechanisms by which OSA causes CVD. CPAP therapy, when adhered to, has been shown to reduce diastolic blood pressure in patients with hypertension.[78,79] The reduction in blood pressure is similar to the use of mandibular advancement devices, although both modalities do not demonstrate a drastic reduction in blood pressure with the range of drop between 2 and 4 mm Hg.[80] However, even this modest reduction in blood pressure has been shown to mitigate adverse cardiovascular outcomes such as stroke. CPAP has also been shown to decrease endothelial dysfunction[81] and atherosclerotic plaques.[82] The American Heart Association recommends treating all patients with OSA with behavioral modifications and weight loss in addition to oral appliances for mild-to-moderate OSA and CPAP for those with a severe degree of OSA.[62]

CLINICS CARE POINTS

- OSA commonly overlaps with other pulmonary disorders like COPD to promote intermittent hypoxia and autonomic dysfunction through shared pathophysiologic mechanisms. Intermittent hypoxia causes inflammation, oxidative stress, and the development of endothelial dysfunction.

- Endothelial dysfunction promotes atherosclerosis and predisposes to cardiovascular complications.

- It is critical to screen for and treat CVDs in OSA patients, particularly if they have comorbid COPD.

REFERENCES

1. Recognition of sleep apnea is increasing. Analysis of trends in two large, representative databases of outpatient practice | annals of the American thoracic society. https://www-atsjournals-org.ccmain.ohionet.org/doi/10.1513/AnnalsATS.201603-152OC. [Accessed 15 December 2023].
2. Hong YD, Onukwugha E, Slejko JF. The economic burden of comorbid obstructive sleep apnea among patients with chronic obstructive pulmonary disease. J Manag Care Spec Pharm 2020;26(10). https://doi.org/10.18553/jmcp.2020.26.10.1353.
3. Tang M, Wang Y, Wang M, et al. Risk for cardiovascular disease and one-year mortality in patients with chronic obstructive pulmonary disease and obstructive sleep apnea syndrome overlap syndrome. Front Pharmacol 2021;12. https://www.

frontiersin.org/articles/10.3389/fphar.2021.767982. [Accessed 15 December 2023].
4. Marrone O, Lo Bue A, Salvaggio A, et al. Comorbidities and survival in obstructive sleep apnoea beyond the age of 50. Eur J Clin Invest 2013;43(1): 27–33.
5. Dewan NA, Nieto FJ, Somers VK. Intermittent hypoxemia and OSA: implications for comorbidities. Chest 2015;147(1):266–74.
6. Shamsuzzaman ASM, Winnicki M, Lanfranchi P, et al. Elevated C-reactive protein in patients with obstructive sleep apnea. Circulation 2002;105(21): 2462–4.
7. Yi M, Zhao W, Tan Y, et al. The causal relationships between obstructive sleep apnea and elevated CRP and TNF-α protein levels. Ann Med 2022; 54(1):1578–89.
8. Kokturk O, Ciftci TU, Mollarecep E, et al. Elevated C-reactive protein levels and increased cardiovascular risk in patients with obstructive sleep apnea syndrome. Int Heart J 2005;46(5):801–9.
9. Ryan S, Taylor CT, McNicholas WT. Predictors of elevated nuclear factor-kappaB-dependent genes in obstructive sleep apnea syndrome. Am J Respir Crit Care Med 2006;174(7):824–30.
10. Minoguchi K, Tazaki T, Yokoe T, et al. Elevated production of tumor necrosis factor-alpha by monocytes in patients with obstructive sleep apnea syndrome. Chest 2004;126(5):1473–9.
11. Cao Y, Song Y, Ning P, et al. Association between tumor necrosis factor alpha and obstructive sleep apnea in adults: a meta-analysis update. BMC Pulm Med 2020;20(1):215.
12. Reyad E, Abdelaty N, Prince ME, et al. Plasma levels of TNF in obstructive sleep apnea syndrome (OSA) before and after surgical intervention. Eur Respir J 2012; 40(Suppl 56). https://erj.ersjournals.com/content/40/Suppl_56/P3824. [Accessed 8 December 2023].
13. Li X, Hu R, Ren X, et al. Interleukin-8 concentrations in obstructive sleep apnea syndrome: a systematic review and meta-analysis. Bioengineered 2021; 12(2):10650–65.
14. Ke D, Kitamura Y, Lejtenyi D, et al. Enhanced interleukin-8 production in mononuclear cells in severe pediatric obstructive sleep apnea. Allergy Asthma Clin Immunol 2019;15(1):23.
15. Mehra R, Xu F, Babineau DC, et al. Sleep-disordered breathing and prothrombotic biomarkers: cross-sectional results of the Cleveland Family Study. Am J Respir Crit Care Med 2010;182(6):826–33.
16. May AM, Mehra R. Obstructive sleep apnea: role of intermittent hypoxia and inflammation. Semin Respir Crit Care Med 2014;35(5):531–44.
17. Prabhakar NR, Peng YJ, Nanduri J. Hypoxia-inducible factors and obstructive sleep apnea. J Clin Invest 2020;130(10):5042–51. https://doi.org/10.1172/JCI137560.

18. Kumar GK, Rai V, Sharma SD, et al. Chronic intermittent hypoxia induces hypoxia-evoked catecholamine efflux in adult rat adrenal medulla via oxidative stress. J Physiol 2006;575(Pt 1):229–39.

19. Flenley DC. Sleep in chronic obstructive lung disease. Clin Chest Med 1985;6(4):651–61.

20. Shawon MSR, Perret JL, Senaratna CV, et al. Current evidence on prevalence and clinical outcomes of co-morbid obstructive sleep apnea and chronic obstructive pulmonary disease: a systematic review. Sleep Med Rev 2017;32:58–68.

21. Tondo P, Scioscia G, Sabato R, et al. Mortality in obstructive sleep apnea syndrome (OSAS) and overlap syndrome (OS): the role of nocturnal hypoxemia and CPAP compliance. Sleep Med 2023;112:96–103.

22. Zhang P, Chen B, Lou H, et al. Predictors and outcomes of obstructive sleep apnea in patients with chronic obstructive pulmonary disease in China. BMC Pulm Med 2022;22(1):16.

23. Lewis CA, Fergusson W, Eaton T, et al. Isolated nocturnal desaturation in COPD: prevalence and impact on quality of life and sleep. Thorax 2009;64(2):133–8.

24. Yoshizaki A, Nagano T, Izumi S, et al. Characteristics of the nocturnal desaturation waveform pattern of SpO2 in COPD patients: an observational study. Respir Res 2021;22(1):276.

25. Yuan H, Pinto SJ, Huang J, et al. Ventilatory responses to hypercapnia during wakefulness and sleep in obese adolescents with and without obstructive sleep apnea syndrome. Sleep 2012;35(9):1257–67.

26. Marin JM, Soriano JB, Carrizo SJ, et al. Outcomes in patients with chronic obstructive pulmonary disease and obstructive sleep apnea. Am J Respir Crit Care Med 2010;182(3):325–31.

27. Jang YS, Nerobkova N, Hurh K, et al. Association between smoking and obstructive sleep apnea based on the STOP-Bang index. Sci Rep 2023;13(1):9085.

28. Zeng X, Ren Y, Wu K, et al. Association between smoking behavior and obstructive sleep apnea: a systematic review and meta-analysis. Nicotine Tob Res 2023;25(3):364–71.

29. Oțelea MR, Trenchea M, Rașcu A, et al. Smoking obstructive sleep apnea: arguments for a distinctive phenotype and a personalized intervention. J Personalized Med 2022;12(2):293.

30. Fletcher EC, Schaaf JW, Miller J, et al. Long-term cardiopulmonary sequelae in patients with sleep apnea and chronic lung disease. Am Rev Respir Dis 1987;135(3):525–33.

31. Hawryłkiewicz I, Sliwiński P, Górecka D, et al. Pulmonary haemodynamics in patients with OSAS or an overlap syndrome. Monaldi Arch Chest Dis Arch Monaldi Mal Torace 2004;61(3):148–52.

32. Chaouat A, Weitzenblum E, Krieger J, et al. Association of chronic obstructive pulmonary disease and sleep apnea syndrome. Am J Respir Crit Care Med 1995;151(1):82–6.

33. Ganga HV, Nair SU, Puppala VK, et al. Risk of new-onset atrial fibrillation in elderly patients with the overlap syndrome: a retrospective cohort study. J Geriatr Cardiol JGC 2013;10(2):129–34.

34. Du W, Liu J, Zhou J, et al. Obstructive sleep apnea, COPD, the overlap syndrome, and mortality: results from the 2005-2008 National Health and Nutrition Examination Survey. Int J Chronic Obstr Pulm Dis 2018;13:665–74.

35. Macrea M, Oczkowski S, Rochwerg B, et al. Long-Term Noninvasive Ventilation in Chronic Stable Hypercapnic Chronic Obstructive Pulmonary Disease. An Official American Thoracic Society Clinical Practice Guideline. Am J Respir Crit Care Med 2020;202(4):e74–87.

36. Soler X, Liao SY, Ries AL, et al. A screening tool to predict obstructive sleep apnea in patients with chronic obstructive pulmonary disease: a pilot study of the UCSD COPD-OSA questionnaire. In: C66. "WALK this way" - update on exercise tests and pulmonary rehabilitation. American thoracic society international conference abstracts. American Thoracic Society; 2016. p. A5745. https://doi.org/10.1164/ajrccm-conference.2016.193.1_MeetingAbstracts.A5745.

37. Suri TM, Suri JC. A review of therapies for the overlap syndrome of obstructive sleep apnea and chronic obstructive pulmonary disease. FASEB BioAdvances 2021;3(9):683–93.

38. Ozsancak A, D'Ambrosio C, Hill NS. Nocturnal noninvasive ventilation. Chest 2008;133(5):1275–86.

39. Sterling KL, Pépin JL, Linde-Zwirble W, et al. Impact of positive airway pressure therapy adherence on outcomes in patients with obstructive sleep apnea and chronic obstructive pulmonary disease. Am J Respir Crit Care Med 2022;206(2):197–205.

40. Condon DF, Nickel NP, Anderson R, et al. The 6th world symposium on pulmonary hypertension: what's old is new. F1000Research 2019;8:F1000. Faculty Rev-888.

41. Chaouat A, Weitzenblum E, Krieger J, et al. Pulmonary hemodynamics in the obstructive sleep apnea syndrome. results in 220 consecutive patients. Chest 1996;109(2):380–6.

42. Sajkov D, McEvoy RD. Obstructive sleep apnea and pulmonary hypertension. Prog Cardiovasc Dis 2009;51(5):363–70.

43. Kessler R, Chaouat A, Schinkewitch P, et al. The obesity-hypoventilation syndrome revisited: a prospective study of 34 consecutive cases. Chest 2001;120(2):369–76.

44. Adir Y, Humbert M, Chaouat A. Sleep-related breathing disorders and pulmonary hypertension. Eur Respir J 2021;57(1):2002258.

45. Marrone O, Bonsignore MR. Pulmonary haemodynamics in obstructive sleep apnoea. Sleep Med Rev 2002;6(3):175–93.

46. Dunham-Snary KJ, Wu D, Sykes EA, et al. Hypoxic pulmonary vasoconstriction. Chest 2017;151(1):181–92.

47. Li JM, Shah AM. Endothelial cell superoxide generation: regulation and relevance for cardiovascular pathophysiology. Am J Physiol Regul Integr Comp Physiol 2004;287(5):R1014–30.

48. Wang B, Yan B, Song D, et al. Chronic intermittent hypoxia down-regulates endothelial nitric oxide synthase expression by an NF-κB-dependent mechanism. Sleep Med 2013;14(2):165–71.

49. Wang Z, Li AY, Guo QH, et al. Effects of cyclic intermittent hypoxia on ET-1 responsiveness and endothelial dysfunction of pulmonary arteries in rats. PloS One 2013;8(3):e58078.

50. Samhouri B, Venkatasaburamini M, Paz Y Mar H, et al. Pulmonary artery hemodynamics are associated with duration of nocturnal desaturation but not apnea-hypopnea index. J Clin Sleep Med 2020;16(8):1231–9.

51. Huang Z, Duan A, Hu M, et al. Implication of prolonged nocturnal hypoxemia and obstructive sleep apnea for pulmonary hemodynamics in patients being evaluated for pulmonary hypertension: a retrospective study. J Clin Sleep Med 2023;19(2):213–23.

52. Musco K, Wang L, Hill N, et al. 0834 Association of sleep disordered breathing and hemodynamics of world symposium on pulmonary hypertension groups in PVDOMICS cohort. Sleep 2023;46(Supplement_1):A367–8.

53. Lowery MM, Hill NS, Wang L, et al. Sleep-related hypoxia, right ventricular dysfunction, and survival in patients with group 1 pulmonary arterial hypertension. J Am Coll Cardiol 2023;82(21):1989–2005.

54. Humbert M, Kovacs G, Hoeper MM, et al. 2022 ESC/ERS Guidelines for the diagnosis and treatment of pulmonary hypertension. Eur Heart J 2022;43(38):3618–731.

55. Fox TH, LaNasa M, Saketkoo LA, et al. STOP-Bang for OSA screening in patients with pulmonary hypertension. Respir Med 2023;217:107339.

56. Bady E, Achkar A, Pascal S, et al. Pulmonary arterial hypertension in patients with sleep apnoea syndrome. Thorax 2000;55(11):934–9.

57. Hetzel M, Kochs M, Marx N, et al. Pulmonary hemodynamics in obstructive sleep apnea: frequency and causes of pulmonary hypertension. Lung 2003;181(3):157–66.

58. Sun X, Luo J, Xiao Y. Continuous positive airway pressure is associated with a decrease in pulmonary artery pressure in patients with obstructive sleep apnoea: a meta-analysis. Respirol Carlton Vic 2014;19(5):670–4.

59. Imran TF, Ghazipura M, Liu S, et al. Effect of continuous positive airway pressure treatment on pulmonary artery pressure in patients with isolated obstructive sleep apnea: a meta-analysis. Heart Fail Rev 2016;21(5):591–8.

60. Sajkov D, Wang T, Saunders NA, et al. Continuous positive airway pressure treatment improves pulmonary hemodynamics in patients with obstructive sleep apnea. Am J Respir Crit Care Med 2002;165(2):152–8.

61. Shahar E, Whitney CW, Redline S, et al. Sleep-disordered breathing and cardiovascular disease: cross-sectional results of the Sleep Heart Health Study. Am J Respir Crit Care Med 2001;163(1):19–25.

62. Yeghiazarians Y, Jneid H, Tietjens JR, et al. Obstructive sleep apnea and cardiovascular disease: a scientific statement from the american heart association. Circulation 2021;144(3):e56–67.

63. Ren R, Zhang Y, Yang L, et al. Association between arousals during sleep and hypertension among patients with obstructive sleep apnea. J Am Heart Assoc 2022;11(1):e022141.

64. Lui MMS, Sau-Man M. OSA and atherosclerosis. J Thorac Dis 2012;4(2):164–72.

65. Dyugovskaya L, Lavie P, Lavie L. Increased adhesion molecules expression and production of reactive oxygen species in leukocytes of sleep apnea patients. Am J Respir Crit Care Med 2002;165(7):934–9.

66. Yi M, Zhao W, Fei Q, et al. Causal analysis between altered levels of interleukins and obstructive sleep apnea. Front Immunol 2022;13:888644.

67. Schulz E, Gori T, Münzel T. Oxidative stress and endothelial dysfunction in hypertension. Hypertens Res 2011;34(6):665–73.

68. Lee SA, Amis TC, Byth K, et al. Heavy snoring as a cause of carotid artery atherosclerosis. Sleep 2008;31(9):1207–13. https://www.ncbi.nlm.nih.gov/pmc/articles/PMC2542975/. [Accessed 17 December 2023].

69. The frequency and energy of snoring sounds are associated with common carotid artery intima-media thickness in obstructive sleep apnea patients | scientific reports. https://www.nature.com/articles/srep30559. [Accessed 17 December 2023].

70. Cho JG, Witting PK, Verma M, et al. Tissue vibration induces carotid artery endothelial dysfunction: a mechanism linking snoring and carotid atherosclerosis? Sleep 2011;34(6):751–7.

71. Deokar K, Meshram S, Chawla G, et al. Obstructive sleep apnea, intermittent hypoxemia and prothrombotic biomarkers. Sleep Sci 2020;13(4):230–4.

72. Qiu Y, Li X, Zhang X, et al. Prothrombotic factors in obstructive sleep apnea: a systematic review with meta-analysis. Ear Nose Throat J 2022;101(9):NP412–21.

73. Krieger AC, Anand R, Hernandez-Rosa E, et al. Increased platelet activation in Sleep Apnea

subjects with intermittent hypoxemia. Sleep Breath Schlaf Atm 2020;24(4):1537–47.

74. Kasai T, Bradley TD. Obstructive sleep apnea and heart failure: pathophysiologic and therapeutic implications. J Am Coll Cardiol 2011;57(2):119–27.

75. Naughton MT. The link between obstructive sleep apnea and heart failure: underappreciated opportunity for treatment. Curr Heart Fail Rep 2006;3(4): 183–8.

76. McEvoy RD, Antic NA, Heeley E, et al. CPAP for prevention of cardiovascular events in obstructive sleep apnea. N Engl J Med 2016;375(10):919–31.

77. Tan JWC. Asian pacific society of cardiology consensus statements on the diagnosis and management of obstructive sleep apnoea in patients with cardiovascular disease. 2022. https://www.ecrjournal.com/articles/asian-pacific-society-cardiology-consensus-statements-diagnosis-and-management-obstructive. [Accessed 17 December 2023].

78. Martínez-García MA, Capote F, Campos-Rodríguez F, et al. Effect of CPAP on blood pressure in patients with obstructive sleep apnea and resistant hypertension: the HIPARCO randomized clinical trial. JAMA 2013;310(22):2407–15.

79. Long-term effect of continuous positive airway pressure therapy on blood pressure in patients with obstructive sleep apnea | Scientific Reports. https://www.nature.com/articles/s41598-021-98553-0. [Accessed 17 December 2023].

80. Bratton DJ, Gaisl T, Wons AM, et al. CPAP vs mandibular advancement devices and blood pressure in patients with obstructive sleep apnea: a systematic review and meta-analysis. JAMA 2015; 314(21):2280–93.

81. Schwarz EI, Puhan MA, Schlatzer C, et al. Effect of CPAP therapy on endothelial function in obstructive sleep apnoea: a systematic review and meta-analysis. Respirol Carlton Vic 2015;20(6):889–95.

82. Dohi T, Kasai T, Endo H, et al. CPAP effects on atherosclerotic plaques in patients with sleep-disordered breathing and coronary artery disease: the ENTERPRISE trial. J Cardiol 2019;73(1):89–93.

Chronic Cough and Obstructive Sleep Apnea

Krishna M. Sundar, MD, FCCP, ATSF, FAASM[a,*], Amanda Carole Stark, PhD[b], Peter Dicpinigaitis, MD, FCCP[c]

KEYWORDS

- Cough • Sleep apnea • Obstructive • Gastroesophageal reflux • Cough hypersensitivity syndrome

KEY POINTS

- Both chronic cough and obstructive sleep apnea (OSA) are highly prevalent conditions. OSA is more commonly associated with chronic cough than can be explained by the occurrence of 2 common disorders.
- Despite guideline-directed treatment for chronic cough, a substantial proportion of patients persist with their cough, and it is in these treatment-refractory patients that therapy of comorbid OSA has been pursued with improvements in chronic cough.
- Refractory chronic cough (RCC) occurs due to alterations in the cough reflex leading to a state of cough hypersensitivity, characterized by allotussia, urge-to-cough sensations centered over the throat often accompanied by paroxysms of coughing, frequent throat clearing, and other features of irritable larynx syndrome.
- The mechanistic pathways through which OSA is related to chronic cough include OSA-driven gastroesophageal reflux, and upper and lower airway inflammation. The dominant phenotype of laryngeal hypersensitivity in patients with RCC has shown pathophysiological relationships with OSA.
- The use of continuous positive airway pressure in patients with comorbid OSA can favorably impact the course of chronic cough.

INTRODUCTION

Of the many symptoms such as dyspnea, cough, and chest pain encountered in pulmonary practices, the relationship of cough to sleep-disordered breathing is the most studied. Chronic cough is one of the commonest problems encountered within specialty and subspecialty clinics. Its interaction with obstructive sleep apnea (OSA), another highly prevalent disorder, is therefore not surprising. Beyond the frequent overlap of these 2 common conditions, this review examines pathophysiological relationships between these 2 common disorders and the basis for improvement of chronic cough that is frequently noted following the treatment of sleep-disordered breathing. To understand these relationships, a description of the current understanding of the basis of chronic cough, the clinical entity of refractory chronic cough (RCC) and its relationship to cough hypersensitivity, and the mechanisms of how treatment of OSA leads to improvement in chronic cough are discussed.

CHRONIC COUGH

Current categorizations of cough are based upon cough durations with chronic cough defined as a cough lasting for more than 8 weeks.[1] The 2006 American College of Chest Physicians' guidelines

[a] Division of Pulmonary & Critical Care Medicine, 30 N, Mario Capecchi Drive, 2nd floor North, University of Utah, Salt Lake City, UT 84112, USA; [b] Voice Disorders Center, University of Utah, 729 Arapeen Drive, Salt Lake City, UT 84106, USA; [c] Department of Medicine, Albert Einstein College of Medicine and Montefiore Medical Center, 1825 Eastchester Road, Bronx, NY 10461, USA
* Corresponding author. Division of Pulmonary & Critical Care Medicine, 30 N, Mario Capecchi Drive, 2nd floor North, University of Utah, Salt Lake City, UT 84112.
E-mail address: krishna.sundar@hsc.utah.edu

Sleep Med Clin 19 (2024) 239–251
https://doi.org/10.1016/j.jsmc.2024.02.004
1556-407X/24/Published by Elsevier Inc.

proposed algorithms for the diagnosis and management for acute, subacute, and chronic cough[1] that were reviewed a decade later to reestablish their usefulness in the management of cough.[2] Chronic cough lasting more than 2 months can occur due to a number of pulmonary and extrapulmonary conditions. Evaluation of chronic cough is initiated with a detailed history and examination followed by chest radiology. In those with relatively normal chest radiology and pulmonary function, 1 or more of these commonest causes of chronic cough—gastroesophageal reflux disease (GERD), upper airway cough syndrome (UACS), asthma, non-asthmatic eosinophilic bronchitis—are diagnosed and treated empirically.[3] The basis for treating these common conditions of GERD, UACS, or asthma is that these disorders involve structures (upper and lower airways, esophagus) that are innervated by vagal afferents which mediate the cough reflex.[4]

Over the last few decades, a number of studies have shown that despite the application of guideline-based approaches, cough persists in a substantial proportion of patients (~40%).[5] Such treatment-refractory patients often seek evaluation from multiple specialists and experience significant impairments in quality of life and health care costs from their chronic cough.[6,7] Given that RCC is commonly encountered in both the primary care and subspecialist setting, there is a tremendous need to understand the basis of cough and reasons for its persistence. Amongst different conditions implicated in the persistence of chronic cough, OSA has emerged as an important association whose treatment often impacts the course of RCC.[8] In order to understand this association between OSA and cough, it is important to understand the alterations of cough reflex seen in RCC before discussion of different aspects of the relationship between RCC and OSA.

COUGH REFLEX AND COUGH HYPERSENSITIVITY

Cough is a triphasic reflex designed to protect the lower airways and lungs from noxious stimuli. It helps with the clearance of particulate matter and the absence of the cough reflex can have dire consequences.[9] The finding that vagotomy abolishes coughing led to the identification of chemically and mechanically sensitive vagal afferent nerves from airways that trigger the cough reflex.[10] Amongst different bronchopulmonary vagal afferents, unmyelinated C-fibers with transient receptor vanilloid receptor-1 receptors with cell bodies in nodose ganglia and myelinated fibers that subserve rapidly adaptive mechanoreceptors to punctate stimuli (and also to pH and hypotonic solutions) with cell bodies in jugular ganglia are involved in cough initiation to different stimuli.[9,10] The proximal projections of neurons in vagal ganglia project to the nucleus tractus solitarius in the medulla before relay to the brainstem respiratory medullary group which produces the distinct cough motor pattern.[10] This brainstem respiratory network includes neuronal groups that also generate breathing[10] and produce a characteristic cough response comprising of an initial inspiratory phase to generate lung volume for effective cough, a compression phase with increasing intrathoracic pressure followed by rapid exhalation phase that results from glottic opening.[11] Ascending projections from the medulla mediate the sensory perception of coughing to cortex and particularly the urge-to-cough sensations that are relayed to the thalamus and somatosensory cortex.[12] Descending pathways from primary and accessory motor cortices provide volitional control of coughing including cough suppression.[12]

Alterations in the neural cough pathways have been proposed to explain the sensitized cough reflex underlying cough hypersensitivity, the mechanistic basis for RCC.[13] This neuropathic basis of cough hypersensitivity is yet to be understood in terms of changes in cough pathways at the peripheral level,[14] midbrain and cortical processing[15] and descending modulation of cough.[15] Despite considerable work needed at understanding the neural substrate(s) for RCC, a clinical phenotype characterized by the finding of allotussia (coughing in response to stimuli that typically do not lead to coughing such as talking, changes in position or ambient temperature, strong perfumes, and so forth), abnormal throat sensations triggering cough, and paroxysmal coughing is demonstrable in the majority of patients with RCC.[16] Why such a "laryngeal hypersensitivity" phenotype is the most prevalent pattern in RCC remains to be understood,[17] although it is increasingly clear that the complex roles played by the laryngeal musculature in breathing, airway protection, speech, and swallowing along with larynx's high innervation predisposes it to a constellation of functional disorders including chronic cough.[18]

RELATIONSHIP OF CHRONIC COUGH AND OBSTRUCTIVE SLEEP APNEA

Current prevalence estimates for chronic cough range from 5% to 10% of the adult population, which is comparable to that of asthma and COPD.[19,20] Patients with RCC are often middle aged (mean age 55 years) with highest prevalence in the age group 60 to 69 years with a female to male ratio of 2 to 3:1.[19–21] Comparable to chronic cough, prevalence rates for OSA are even higher with OSA being present in 9% to 38% of the general population.[22] The prevalence of OSA increases with age[22] and while OSA is more common in males, its prevalence increases in females following menopause and with obesity.[23] Interestingly the 2 important factors that drive the increasing prevalence of OSA—increasing age and body mass index (BMI)—both increase the likelihood of chronic cough as well. Chronic cough is most prevalent in elderly and this association has been demonstrated in studies from different regions across the world.[21,24–27] While studies focusing on populations from cough clinics have shown female predominance,[21] other population-based studies show equivalent gender distribution or even a slightly higher male predominance.[25–27] Like increasing age, there is an increasing prevalence of chronic cough with increasing obesity.[28–30] Even though GERD has been consistently implicated as the driver for chronic cough due to obesity, OSA has not been implicated in the causation of cough with increasing BMI despite an almost linear relationship between BMI and the apnea-hypopnea index (AHI), a measure of the severity of OSA.[31]

Given such a high prevalence of OSA in the general population and particularly in those with chronic cough (see the following paragraphs), studies have looked at the prevalence of chronic cough in OSA (**Table 1**). An initial study evaluating 108 consecutive patients with sleep-disordered breathing, out of which 53 patients were excluded, showed that 33% of the remaining 55 patients with OSA experienced chronic cough[32] (see **Table 1**). A subsequent study examined 131 patients and compared the presence of chronic cough in those with and without OSA. This study demonstrated a much higher prevalence of chronic cough in those with OSA (39.4% compared with 12.5% without OSA) (see **Table 1**). In contrast to these 2 studies, another looked at 233 patients undergoing testing for OSA (out of which OSA was diagnosed in 171 patients) and failed to show a significant difference in prevalence of chronic cough in those with and without OSA (11.7% vs 19.3%).[34]

Given the higher prevalence of OSA as compared to chronic cough, most studies have looked at the effect of treating comorbid OSA in patients with chronic cough (**Table 2**). In addition, they have looked at potential mechanistic pathways particularly GERD that can be easily

Table 1
Studies looking at chronic cough in patients being evaluated for obstructive sleep apnea

Publication or Abstract	Place of Study	Number of Patients and Demographics	Findings
Chan et al,[32] 2010	Sleep disorders clinic, Concord General Hospital, Sydney, Australia	53/108 patients excluded; out of 55 patients, 67% male and 18/55 patients had chronic cough. 11/18 female	33% of patients with sleep-disordered breathing had chronic cough with 61% of these patients being female and more likely to have GERD and rhinitis.
Wang et al,[33] 2013	Chang Gung Memorial Hospital, Taoyuan City, Taiwan	131 (75% male); 99 OSA patients (mean age 52.2 y, BMI of 28.9 with 75% male) and 32 non-OSA patients (mean age 48.3 y and BMI 24.9 with 53% male)	Incidence of chronic cough higher in OSA group vs non-OSA group (39.4% vs 12.5%). Resolution of cough more in patients on CPAP (95%) vs that were not (67%). Higher proportion of OSA patients had GERD, UACS, and asthma
Rybka et al,[34] 2018	Medical University of Warsaw, Poland	233 patients referred for evaluation of OSA. OSA diagnosed in 171 (126 males, median age 58 y, BMI 32.3).	Prevalence of chronic cough comparable in those with and without OSA (11.7% vs 19.3%). Patients with chronic cough and OSA also had HTN, allergies, rhinitis, asthma, and COPD

Abbreviations: BMI, body mass index; COPD, chronic obstructive pulmonary disease; CPAP, continuous positive airway pressure; GERD, gastroesophageal reflux disease; HTN, hypertension; OSA, obstructive sleep apnea; UACS, upper airway cough syndrome; y, year.

Table 2
Studies looking at the impact of treating obstructive sleep apnea on the course of chronic cough

Study or Case Series	Place of Study	Number of Patients, Demographics	Findings
Birring et al,[35] 2007	Concord Hospital, Sydney, Australia	4 patients ranging in ages from 46-73 y (2 female, 2 male) with BMI range from 32-37 and cough durations 6–48 mo	All patients had significant improvements in cough. The improvement was noted as early as 2–5 d after CPAP therapy with patients experiencing complete resolution of cough in 6 wk to months.
Sundar et al,[36] 2010	Utah Valley Pulmonary Clinic, Provo, Utah, USA	Retrospective study on 75 patients with chronic cough with 38/75 patients undergoing testing for OSA. 27/38 patients started on CPAP with 93% improving their cough.	44/75 patients had other etiologies for cough with 31/44 patients being treated for multiple etiologies of cough.
Sundar et al,[37] 2013	Utah Valley Pulmonary Clinic, Provo, Utah, USA	Out of 37 patients, 22/28 underwent testing for OSA. 19/28 found to have OSA and followed prospectively with CPAP intervention.	Significant improvement in LCQ scores following CPAP therapy in 19 patients with OSA and chronic cough. 13/19 patients were female with mean BMI of 34.9.
Good et al,[38] 2018	National Jewish Medical Center, Denver, USA	Out of 99 patients (73% female), 76/99 patients had follow-up available (mean age—60.9 y and mean BMI—28.9). 71/76 patients resolved cough. Apart from OSA found in 54/64 evaluated for OSA, TBM was found in 32/42 patients.	Cough duration did not help determine etiology. <1 y—100% OSA, 1–10 y—84% OSA and >10 y—78% with OSA. 54/99 had documented OSA. Not clear how CPAP related to overall improvement in cough although it was discussed as an important etiology.
Sundar et al,[38] 2020[38]	University of Utah clinics, Salt Lake City, Utah, USA	9 patients each randomized to CPAP vs sham CPAP.	Improvements in LCQ after 6 wk significantly greater in CPAP as compared to sham CPAP.
Su et al,[40] 2022	First Affiliated Hospital of Zhengzhou University	86 patients with OSA and concomitant GERD divided into 2 groups—treatment group with CPAP with 46 patients and control group with lifestyle measures and antireflux treatment with 40 patients	Both groups had younger patients (mean ages 37 y), predominant male and had lower BMIs 27–28. Improvements in GERD-Q, VAS, daytime and night cough symptom scores at 3 mo higher in the CPAP-treated group. Correlations between AHI and VAS, and AHI and weak acid reflux noted.

Abbreviations: AHI, apnea-hypopnea index; BMI, body mass index; CPAP, continuous positive airway pressure; GERD, gastroesophageal reflux disease; LCQ, Leicester Cough Questionnaire; GERD Q, GERD Questionnaire; OSA, obstructive sleep apnea; TBM, tracheobronchomalacia; VAS, visual analog scale (cough); y, year.

measured in these patients, to establish relationships between these 2 disorders. The first case series highlighting the relationship of chronic cough and OSA was reported by Birring and colleagues[35] which detailed 4 patients (ages 46–73 years) with chronic cough lasting 6 to 48 months whose cough resolved completely after the treatment of OSA (see **Table 2**). The first community-based study of OSA intervention in chronic cough was performed in 75 patients with chronic cough out of which 51% underwent specific testing for OSA with the majority of these patients showing improvement in cough following treatment with continuous positive airway pressure (CPAP).[36] Subsequent to this, Sundar and colleagues[37] conducted a prospective study on 37 patients with chronic cough out of which 28 patients compliant with follow-up visits underwent testing for OSA; 68% of these patients were found to have OSA and improved their cough as based upon change in the Leicester Cough Questionnaire (LCQ) before and following CPAP therapy (see **Table 2**). Improvement in cough occurred not only in overall LCQ score but also in the psychological and social domains within the LCQ.[37] Another series of RCC patients segregated patients based on the duration of cough and looked at etiologies for chronic cough.[38] Interestingly, testing for OSA was carried out in 100% of patients with cough duration of less than 1 year as compared to 84% in those with cough duration of 1 to 10 years, and 77.8% in those with cough more than 10 years.[38] To date, only 1 randomized study has been conducted in patients with chronic cough that evaluated change in the score of the cough quality of life questionnaire—LCQ—after 6 weeks of CPAP versus sham-CPAP therapy. There was a significant improvement in LCQ score after CPAP that was significantly greater than in the sham-CPAP group.[39] This study also looked at changes in exhaled breath condensate markers of airway inflammation and even though there were improvements following CPAP, these were not significant when compared to the sham CPAP group.[39] A recent study specifically examined patients with chronic cough who had OSA and GERD (based upon screening GERD questionnaire and 24-h esophageal pH monitoring) and divided them into 2 groups, one of which received CPAP treatment whereas the other received antireflux treatment with lifestyle modifications.[40] While GERD questionnaire scores improved only at 3 months in both groups (being significantly greater in CPAP group), cough symptom scores improved significantly at 1 week in CPAP group as compared to the control group and were improved further at 3 months.[40]

Over the last decade, it has become increasingly apparent that untreated OSA can lead to myriad airway manifestations and larger population-based studies have shown a significant impact of high-risk OSA determined based upon the STOP-BANG score [snoring history, tired during the day, observed stop of breathing while sleeping, high blood pressure, BMI>35 kg/m2 (or 30 kg/m2), age>50 years, neck circumference>40 cm, and male gender] on chronic cough[41] and the reduction of chronic cough following CPAP therapy for 2 years.[42] Although a reduction in GERD was proposed for the reduction in cough after 2 years of OSA treatment,[42] the frequent finding of the association of OSA with different airway diseases necessitates a much greater understanding of mechanistic pathways by which OSA can both initiate and perpetuate chronic cough.

Multiple mechanistic pathways are implicated in the causation of chronic cough from OSA (**Fig. 1**). A detailed discussion of the each of different processes that can explain the occurrence of chronic cough from OSA follows.

Gastroesophageal Reflux Disease

Of the major causes of chronic cough, GERD has been the most studied in terms of its relationship to chronic cough.[43] While the proportion of GERD accounting for cough has varied with studies, it is consistently treated in patients with chronic cough with an anticipation of improvement in chronic cough.[44] GERD is largely driven by transient lower esophageal sphincter relaxations although hypotensive lower esophageal sphincter (LES), ineffective esophageal motility, and the presence of hiatal hernia can all contribute to GERD.[45] OSA increases GERD[46] with the severity of reflux increasing with worsening OSA severity[46] with obesity playing a key role in the worsening of reflux.[47] While only 10% of obstructive apneas-hypopneas may be solely associated with reflux, multiple mechanisms have been proposed to explain the increased GERD in OSA.[48] These include reflux associated with arousals from sleep during apneas and hypopneas,[49,50] effect on LES during an obstructive event (although it is less likely that an intact LES dilates during an apnea given that there is increase in LES tone during an obstructive event), effects of coexisting obesity on the occurrence of hiatal hernia, and changes in transabdominal pressures during obstructive apneas-hypopneas.[51] Yet to be fully understood is the effect of OSA on weakly acidic or non-acidic reflux that is present in the later part of the night[52] and often present in patients on proton-pump inhibitors.[53] Despite the lack of full understanding of why GERD is worse with OSA,

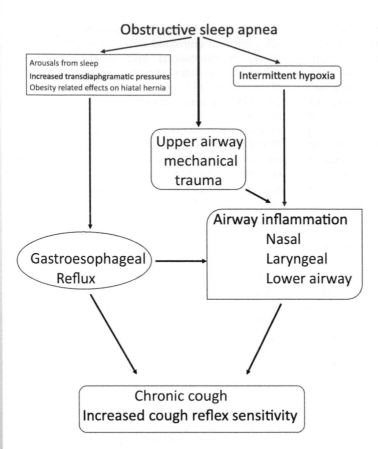

Fig. 1. Mechanistic pathways by which obstructive sleep apnea leads to chronic cough.

multiple studies have shown that CPAP therapy improves GERD as based on changes in GERD-related symptom scores, number of reflux events, and duration of acid contact time measured by esophageal pH monitoring.[50,54] This improvement in GERD following CPAP therapy has been purported to be the main reason for resolution of cough when objectively measured GERD has been tracked following CPAP therapy.[40,55] One case report showed that in a patient with chronic cough and severe OSA, there was improvement in cough early on with CPAP therapy although the cough reflex sensitivity measured using citric acid inhalation improved only after a year of CPAP therapy.[55] In the only study that measured change in severity of chronic cough with CPAP in patients with objectively established GERD and OSA, there were correlations between AHI and weak acid reflux at baseline with improvement in both GERD questionnaire scores and cough scores at 3 months that was greater in the CPAP-treated group as compared to the group treated with antireflux treatments.[40] Even in population studies tracking respiratory symptoms in CPAP users for up to 2 years, decrease in chronic cough has been attributed to decreases in GERD symptoms with long-term CPAP use.[42] While a number of questions remain in the relationship between OSA, GERD, and chronic cough, the benefit accorded by CPAP particularly in terms of the increases in LES tone[56] may have effects on both acid[48,51,54] and non-acid reflux with salutary effects on both GERD and laryngopharyngeal reflux (LPR).[57]

Upper and Lower Airway Inflammation

Like GERD, the mechanistic bases of relationships between chronic cough and its other causes such as UACS and asthma are not well understood.[58] While nasal C-fibers may contribute to cough reflex hypersensitivity,[59] the basis of symptoms such as post-nasal drip commonly reported by patients with chronic cough is unclear.[58] In patients with asthma, there is poor correlation between cough frequency[60] and airflow obstruction and in laboratory studies, pathways for bronchoconstriction and cough appear different.[61] Treating UACS and asthma is part of the empiric integrative approach for chronic cough and has been found to result in improvement in chronic cough.[3] OSA has been reported to cause both upper and lower airway inflammation. OSA is associated with nasal inflammation[62,63] and has a bidirectional relationship with asthma.[64] Particularly for lower airway inflammation, OSA has been associated with increased asthma exacerbations, increased asthma severity, and decreased asthma disease–specific quality of life.[64,65] Untreated OSA can lead to a shift to Th1-type inflammation, increases in neutrophils, and oxidative stress in airways that may be the result of a number of different processes seen with OSA—cyclic mechanical stresses, chronic intermittent hypoxia, and effects of comorbid obesity and GERD.[64,66] While there are no reports of association of OSA and cough-variant asthma, or consistent effects of OSA on bronchial hyperreactivity,[67] multiple studies have shown improvement in asthma disease course with CPAP therapy, particularly in those with moderate to severe OSA.[64,68]

Laryngeal Hypersensitivity

The larynx participates not only in breathing, speech, and swallowing but also in regulation of airflow and in airway protection through a number of protective reflexes such as the laryngeal adductor reflex, cough reflex, and expiration reflex.[69] Laryngeal dysfunction can manifest as exaggerated laryngeal protective responses resulting in laryngospasm, vocal cord dysfunction (VCD), or enhanced cough triggering to mechanical and chemical stimuli.[70] These abnormalities can result in a spectrum of manifestations often described as irritable larynx syndrome[71] or present individually as RCC, VCD, or muscle tension dysphonia (MTD).[72] These patients also experience abnormal throat sensations that range from tickle to dryness sensation to irritation or pain which can lead to frequent throat clearing or cough.[73,74] In addition to abnormal throat sensations, a significant proportion of patients with RCC may also complain of abnormal chest sensations that may lead to the cough or occur in relation to it.[16,73,74] The basis for laryngeal hypersensitivity is not well understood but given its occurrence following respiratory infections or with GERD, it is postulated that altered neural pathways may be responsible.[71] Whether changes that drive laryngeal hypersensitivity represent a different endotype or part of spectrum of alterations of neural pathways that drive RCC is not clear. Given the heterogeneity in cough, the neural bases of laryngeal hypersensitivity need to be understood as changes at the level of peripheral nerve endings in the larynx, or changes at the brainstem and cortical processing.[58,75] Over the last decade, there is increasing recognition that the laryngeal hypersensitivity phenotype may be the dominant pattern of symptoms expressed by patients with RCC.[16,17] While there are no clear-cut criteria defined for characterizing laryngeal hypersensitivity in RCC, the following manifestations are typical in these patients and overlap considerably with features described for cough hypersensitivity that underlies the basis for RCC.[13,76,77]

- Easy cough triggering as demonstrated by allotussia (coughing to stimuli that typically do not cause coughing such as talking, deep breathing, exercise, cold air, changes in temperature or position, perfumes) and/or hypertussia (excessive coughing to stimuli that lead to coughing such as outdoor irritants, air pollution, second-hand smoke)
- Abnormal throat or chest sensations that trigger coughing (urge-to-cough sensations)
- Paroxysmal coughing spells during which patients feel out of breath, dizzy, or nauseous. There is still understanding required as to why these patients are most prone to these coughing paroxysms which can include both coughing and expiration reflexes.[78]

Other features include throat clearing[16] and manifestations of other laryngeal functional disorders such as VCD or voice problems secondary to MTD.[16,72,75]

Several reports suggest laryngeal dysfunction with OSA, with patients often reporting symptoms of LPR.[79] LPR is characterized by throat clearing, persistent cough, sensation of something sticking or lump in the throat/globus sensation, and hoarseness.[80] Symptoms of LPR can be categorized based on the Reflux Symptom Index[81] and the degree of laryngeal and hypopharyngeal inflammation according to a standardized endoscopic scoring algorithm, Reflux Finding Score.[82] While there is still controversy about the specificity of these diagnostic attributes,[83] LPR represents the laryngeal and pharyngeal manifestations of reflux and therefore is considered distinct from GERD.[80] Like GERD, LPR is increased in patients with OSA[79,84,85] with correlation between degree of laryngeal inflammation and severity of OSA.[79] Additionally, this inflammation is also correlated with sensory laryngeal impairment[79] which is increasingly demonstrated in OSA.[86] Sensory laryngeal impairment in OSA has been purported to worsen OSA severity[86] and also predispose to cough[87–89] and VCD.[87] In fact, chronic laryngopharyngeal sensory neuropathy in the aftermath of viral infection or chronic LPR has been described as a potential driver for chronic cough[90] and compensatory hyperadduction resulting in VCD[91] even though OSA is yet to be implicated as the cause of this laryngeal sensory neuropathy and consequent functional disturbances. Additionally, this sensory impairment may be associated with increased laryngeal sensitivity to chemical stimuli such as ammonia vapor.[92] Improvement in both chemical laryngeal sensitivity[92] and sensory impairment over the palate[93,94] can occur with CPAP therapy and whether this accounts for improvements with CPAP in chronic cough is unclear. When specific evaluation for laryngeal-based symptoms is done in patients with OSA, a significant prevalence of chronic cough, daytime dyspnea, and dysphonia is found especially in women despite lower severity of OSA in women.[95] These laryngeal-based symptoms are fewer in those using nightly humidified CPAP who also report improved quality of life scores in relation to their laryngeal symptoms.[95] Besides mechanical trauma during apneas-hypopneas and LPR, additional mechanisms by which OSA can affect laryngeal mucosa include intermittent hypoxemia which has been shown to cause enhanced apneic responses to chemical stimulants in rats.[96] This apneic response in rats was mediated by capsaicin-sensitive superior laryngeal nerve fibers following inhalation of chemical stimulants and was increased following 14 days of intermittent hypoxia exposure which caused hypoxia-inducible factor 1-alpha–driven increases in oxidative stress through nicotinamide adenine dinucleotide phosphate oxidase (NADPH)–derived reactive oxygen species.[96]

Effects of Lung Inflation

During lung inflation, there is activation of slowly adapting receptors (SARs) and rapidly adapting receptors (RARs) that regulate inspiratory volumes and timing of inspiration and expiration.[10] This inspiratory lung volume affects subsequent expiratory airflows that are important during generation of effective cough.[11] While these SARs and RARs are not believed to be involved in initiating cough or regulating the duration of cough,[10] there is an effect of volume feedback on pattern of cough response.[97] Lung inflation in cats and rabbits makes expiration reflexes more frequent, but it has no effect on expiration reflexes occurring following vocal fold stimulation.[98] Understanding of lung inflation effects on cough is important given that CPAP therapy leads to increases in end-expiratory lung volumes.

The cough reflex is suppressed during the night when assessed by stimulating the larynx with mechanical stimuli in sleeping dogs, with suppression of coughing being more in rapid eye movement sleep as compared to slow-wave sleep.[99] Interestingly in this study, stimuli that did not lead to cough led to an apnea.[99] Similar effects were noted with tracheobronchial stimulation although arousal was required for coughing to occur with both mechanical and chemical stimuli.[100] Studies of lung inflation in sleeping dogs demonstrate apnea.[100] Similar apneas with lung inflation have also been shown in laryngectomized subjects who tolerated lung inflation of more than 3 liters without any apnea when awake, but showed apneas during electroencephalography-documented sleep with lung inflation of more than 1liter.[101] While these data do not clearly provide evidence for direct effects of CPAP-mediated lung stretch on cough, direct effects on cough reflex cannot be discounted and there have been reports of CPAP benefit in acute VCD attacks due to beneficial effects on larynx.[102] Additionally, during episodes of dynamic upper airway obstruction with OSA, there is increased phasic activity of vocal cord abductors that may impose increased stresses upon the larynx[103]—whether this contributes over long term to laryngeal dysfunction and chronic cough is unknown. How CPAP-related improvements in cough at night along with effects on lung inflation affect daytime cough reflex hypersensitivity needs to be better understood.

Other Factors

Neuropathic disorders such as chronic pain[104] and neurogenic bladder[105] have a bidirectional relationship with sleep with sleep disruption tending to worsen pain or bladder overactivity. While such bidirectional relationships between sleep and chronic cough have not yet been demonstrated, a significant proportion of patients with chronic cough experience decreases in sleep quality[106] that may contribute to their daytime symptoms of depression and anxiety. Mood disturbances are common in patients with chronic cough and add to the decreased quality of life that these patients often experience.[107] Improvement of factors causing sleep disruption such as OSA can result in consolidated sleep that may have restorative effects with improved recovery from inflammatory airway processes contributing to cough. Additionally, lack of sleep has been associated with increased risk of respiratory infections[108] that are the initiating events for many patients with chronic cough.[58] Further research is required to understand the myriad factors in relation to sleep that can affect the course of chronic cough and its resolution.

Based on the aforementioned interactions between RCC and OSA, a number of guidelines and reviews[75,109,110] have recommended evaluation for OSA in patients with RCC. Given the high prevalence of OSA in patients with chronic cough and the impact of CPAP treatment on factors driving cough such as GERD, earlier treatment of OSA should be considered given the other benefits accorded by the treatment of OSA.

FUTURE DIRECTIONS

Given the multiple pathways through which OSA can affect cough occurrence and its persistence, considerable work is needed to understand which patients with OSA are most susceptible to development of chronic cough and how interventions for OSA can be carried out in a timely manner in patients with RCC. Patients with chronic cough experience multiple comorbidities and understanding the impact of OSA on cough is often difficult to isolate when multiple interventions are undertaken. Of key importance is to appreciate the neuropathic effects of OSA on the upper airway that may predispose to the occurrence of laryngeal hypersensitivity, a key mechanism in the persistence of chronic cough.

CLINICS CARE POINTS

- Chronic cough and obstructive sleep apnea (OSA) are highly prevalent disorders in the adult population due to which there is considerable likelihood of overlap of these two conditions.
- OSA can contribute to the persistence of chronic cough through several mechanistic pathways – increase in gastroesophageal reflux, mechanical trauma to the upper airway (pharynx and larynx) during episodes of apneas and hypopneas during sleep, intermittent hypoxia resulting in laryngeal and lower airway inflammation and contribution to state of cough hypersensitivity that drives refractory chronic cough (RCC).
- Treatment of comorbid OSA in patients with chronic cough may improve chronic cough with many studies showing improvement in RCC when CPAP therapy is done in conjunction with other treatments for chronic cough.
- Further understanding of the myriad pathways by which OSA affects upper and lower airway inflammation and predisposes patients to chronic cough is needed.

DISCLOSURES

K.M. Sundar has served as consultant in the past for Merck Inc. He is a cofounder of Hypnoscure LLC (software for population management of sleep apnea) in conjuction with the University of Utah Technology Commercialization Office. A.C. Stark has no conflicts to disclose. P. Dicpinigaitis serves as a consultant to Bellus, Chiesi, GSK, Merck, Trevi.

REFERENCES

1. Irwin RS, Baumann MH, Bolser DC, et al. Diagnosis and management of cough executive summary: ACCP evidence-based clinical practice guidelines. CHEST 2006;129(1 suppl):1S–23S.
2. Irwin RS, French CL, Chang AB, et al, on behalf of the CHEST Expert Cough Panel. Classification of cough as a symptom in adults and management algorithms. CHEST Guideline and Expert Panel Report. CHEST 2017;153(1):196–209.
3. Pratter MR, Brightling CE, Boulet LP, et al. An empiric integrative approach to the management of cough. ACCP evidence-based clinical practice guidelines. CHEST 2006;129:222S–31S.
4. Irwin RS, Madison M. Anatomic diagnostic protocol in evaluating chronic cough with specific refernce to gastroesophageal reflux disease. Am J Med 2000;108(4A):126S–30S.
5. Haque RA, Usmani OS, Barnes PJ. Chronic idiopathic cough A discrete clinical entity? CHEST 2005;127:1710–3.
6. Zeiger RS, Schatz M, Butler RK, et al. Burden of specialist-diagnosed chronic cough in adults. J Allergy Clin Immunol 2020;8(5):1645–57.
7. McGarvey L, Morice AH, Martin A, et al. Burden of chronic cough in the UK: results from the 2018 national health and wellness survey. ERJ Open Res 2023;9:00157–2023.
8. Sundar KM, Daly SE. Chronic cough and OSA: a new association? J Clin Sleep Med 2011;7(6):669–77.
9. Canning BJ, Mori N, Mazzone SB. Vagal afferents regulating the cough reflex. Respir Physiol Neurobiol 2006;152:223–42.
10. Canning BJ, Chang AB, Bolser DC, et al. Anatomy and neurophysiology of cough: CHEST guideline and expert panel report. CHEST 2014;146(6):1633–48.
11. Lee KK, Davenport PW, Smith JA, et al. Global physiology and pathophysiology of cough Part 1: cough phenomenology – CHEST guideline and Expert panel report. CHEST 2021;159(1):282–93.
12. Mazzone SB, Farrell MJ. Heterogeneity of cough neurobiology: clinical implications. Pulm Pharmacol Ther 2019;55:62–6.
13. Morice AH, Millqvist e, Belvisi MG, et al. Expert opinion on the cough hypersensitivity syndrome in respiratory medicine. Eur Respir J 2014;10:1–17.

14. Shapiro CO, Proskocil BJ, Oppegard LJ, et al. Airway sensory nerve density is increased in chronic cough. Am J Respir Crit Care Med 2021; 203(3):348–55.

15. Ando A, Smallwood D, McMahon M, et al. Neural correlates of cough hypersensitivity in humans: evidence for central sensitisation and dysfunctional inhibitory control. Thorax 2016;71:323–9.

16. Sundar KM, Stark AC, Hu N, et al. Is laryngeal hypersensitivity the basis of unexplained or refractory chronic cough? ERJ Open Res 2021;7: 00793–2020.

17. Song W-J. Laryngeal dysfunction in chronic cough: a sign for a specific cough endotype. J Allergy Clin Immunol Pract 2018;6:2096–7.

18. Vertigan PE, Bone SL, Gibson PG. Laryngeal sensory dysfunction in laryngeal hypersensitivity syndrome. Respirol 2013;13:948–56.

19. Meltzer EO, Zeiger RS, Dicpinigaitis P, et al. Prevalence and burden of chronic cough in the United States. J Allergy Clin Immunol Pract 2021;9(11): 4037–44.

20. Song WJ, Change YS, Faruqi S, et al. The global epidemiology of chronic cough in adults: a systematic review and meta-analysis. Eur Respir J 2015; 45(5):1479–81.

21. Morice AH, James AD, Faruqui S, et al. A worldwide survey of chronic cough: a manifestation of enhanced somatosensory response. Eur Respir J 2014;44:1149–55.

22. Senaratna CV, Perret JL, Lodge CJ, et al. Prevalence of obstructive sleep apnea in the general population: a systematic review. Sleep Med Rev 2017;34:70–81.

23. Ralls FM, Grigg-Damberger M. Roles of gender, age, race/ethnicity, and residential socioeconomics in obstructive sleep apnea syndromes. Curr Opin Pulm Med 2012;18(6):568–73.

24. Abozid H, Baxter CA, Hartl S, et al. Distribution of chronic cough phenotypes in the general population: a cross-sectional analysis of the LEAD cohort in Austria. Respir Med 2022;192:106726.

25. Virchow JC, Li VW, Fonseca E, et al. Chronic cough in Germany: results from a general population survey. ERJ Open Res 2022;8:00420–2021.

26. Kang M-G, Song W-J, Kim H-J, et al. Point prevalence and epidemiological characteristics of chronic cough in the general adult population the Korean National Health and Nutrition Examination Survey 2010-2012. Medicine 2017;96: 13(e6486.

27. Satia I, Mayhew AJ, Sohel N, et al. Prevalence, incidence and characteristics of chronic cough among adults from the Canadian Longitudinal Study. ERJ Open Res 2021;7:00160–2021.

28. Arinze JT, deRoos EW, Karimi L, et al. Prevalence and incidence of, and risk factors for chronic cough in the adult population: the Rotterdam Study. ERJ Open Res 2020;6:00300–2019.

29. Guilleminault L. Chronic cough and obesity. Pulm Pharmacol Ther 2019;55:84–8.

30. Landt EM, Çolak Y, Nordestgaard BG, et al. Risk and impact of chronic cough in obese individuals from the general population. Thorax 2022;77: 223–30.

31. Fattal D, Hester S, Wendt L. Body weight and obstructive sleep apnea: a mathematical relationship between body mass index and apnea-hypopnea index in veterans. J Clin Sleep Med 2022;18(12):2723–9.

32. Chan KKY, Ing AJ, Laks L, et al. Chronic cough in patients with sleep-disordered breathing. Eur Respir J 2010;35:368–72.

33. Wang T-Y, Lo Y-L, Liu W-T, et al. Chornic cough and obstructive sleep apnoea in a sleep laboratory-based pulmonary practice. Cough 2013;9:24.

34. Rybka A, Wasik M, Grabczak E, et al. Chronic cough in patients with obstructive sleep apnea. Eur Respir J 2018;52. PA 2557.

35. Birring SS, Ing AJ, Chan K, et al. Obstructive sleep apnoea: a cause of chronic cough. Cough 2007;3:7.

36. Sundar KM, Daly SE, Pearce MJ, et al. Chronic cough and obstructive sleep apnoea in a community-based pulmonary practice. Cough 2010;6:2.

37. Sundar KM, Daly SE, Willis AM. A longitudinal study of CPAP therapy for patients with chronic cough and obstructive sleep apnoea. Cough 2013;9:19.

38. Good JT Jr, Rollins DR, Kolakowski CA, et al. New insights in the diagnosis of chronic refractory cough. Respir Med 2018;141:103–10.

39. Sundar KM, Willis AM, Smith S, et al. A randomized controlled study of CPAP for patients with chronic cough and obstructive sleep apnea. Lung 2020; 198(3):449–57.

40. Su J, Fang Y, Meng Y, et al. Effect of continuous positive airway pressure on chronic cough in patients with obstructive sleep apnea and concomitant gastroesophageal reflux. Nature Sci Sleep 2022;14:13–23.

41. Kim TH, Heo IR, Kim HC. Impact of high-risk of obstructive sleep apnea on chronic cough: data from the Korea National Health and Nutrition Examination Survey. BMC Pulm Med 2022;22:419.

42. Emilsson ÖI, Aspelund T, Janson C, et al. Positive airway pressure treatment affects respiratory symptoms and gastro-oesophageal reflux: the Icelandic Sleep Apnea Cohort Study. ERJ Open Res 2023;9:00387–2023.

43. Zhang L, Aierken A, Zhang M, et al. Pathogenesis and management of gastroesophageal reflux disease-associated cough: a narrative review. J Thoracic Dis 2023;15(4):2314–23.

44. Kahrilas P, Altman KW, Chang AB, et al. Chronic cough due to gastroesophageal reflux in adults CHEST Guideline and Expert Panel Report. Chest 2016;150(6):1341–60.

45. Boeckxstaens G, El-Serag HB, Smout AJP, et al. Symptomatic reflux disease: the present, the past and the future. Gut 2014;63:1185–93.

46. Shepherd KL, James AL, Musk AW, et al. Gastro-oesophageal reflux symptoms are related to the presence and severity of obstructive sleep apnea. J Sleep Res 2011;20(1 Pt 2):241–9.

47. Shepherd K, Orr W. Mechanism of gatroesophageal reflux in obstructive sleep apnea: airway obstruction or obesity? J Clin Sleep Med 2016; 12(1):87–94.

48. Ing AJ, Ngu MC, Breslin AB. Obstructive sleep apnea and gastroesophageal reflux. Am J Med 2000; 108(Suppl 4a):120S–5S.

49. Shepherd K, Ockelford J, Ganasan V, et al. Temporal relationship between night-time gastroesophageal reflux events and arousals from sleep. Am J Gastroenterol 2020;115(5):697–705.

50. Yang Y-X, Spencer G, Schutte-Rodin S, et al. Gastroesophageal reflux and sleep events in obstructive sleep apnea. Eur J Gastroenterol Hepatol 2013;25(9):1017–23.

51. Lim KG, Morgenthaler TI, Katzka DA. Sleep and nocturnal gastroesophageal reflux an update. Chest 2018;154(4):963–71.

52. Fornari F, Blondeau K, Mertens V, et al. Nocturnal gastroesophageal reflux revisited by impedance-pH monitoring. J Neurogastroenterol Motil 2011; 17(2):148–57.

53. Mainie I, Tutuian R, Shay S, et al. Acid and non-acid reflux in patients with persistent symptoms despite acid suppressive therapy: a multicentre study using combined ambulatory impedance-pH monitoring. Gut 2006;55(10):1398–402.

54. Tawk M, Goodrich S, Kinasewitz G, et al. Positive airway pressure treatment in obstructive sleep apnea patients with concomitant gastroesophageal reflux. Chest 2006;130:1003–8.

55. Faruqi A, Fahim A, Morice A. Chronic cough and obstructive sleep apnoea: reflux-associated cough hypersensitivity? Eur Respir J 2012;40: 1049–50.

56. Shepherd KL, Holloway RH, Hillman DR, et al. The impact of continuous positive airway pressure on the lower esophageal sphincter. Am J Physiol Gastrointest Liver Physiol 2007;292(5):G1200–5.

57. Magliulo G, Iannella G, Polimeni A, et al. Laryngopharyngeal reflux in obstructive sleep apnoea patients: literature review and meta-analysis. Am J Otolaryngol 2018;39(6):776–80.

58. Chung KF, McGarvey L, Song W-J, et al. Cough hypersensitivity and chronic cough. Nat Rev Dis Primers 2022;8(1):45.

59. Hennel M, Brozmanova M, Kollarik M. Cough reflex sensitization from the esophagus and nose. Pulm Pharmacol Ther 2015;35:117–21.

60. Marsden PA, Satia I, Ibrahim B, et al. Objective cough frequency, airway inflammation, and disease control in asthma. Chest 2016;149(6):1460–6.

61. Choudry NB, Fuller RW, Anderson N, et al. Separation of cough and reflex bronchoconstriction by inhaled local anaesthetics. Eur Respir J 1990;3: 579–83.

62. Rubinstein I. Nasal inflammation in patients with obstructive sleep apnea. Laryngoscope 1995; 105:175–7.

63. Olopade CO, Christon JA, Zakkar M, et al. Exhaled pentane and nitric oxide levels in patients with obstructive sleep apnea. Chest 1997;111:1500–4.

64. Prasad B, Nyenhuis SM, Imayama I, et al. Asthma and obstructive sleep apnea overlap: what has the evidence Taught Us? Am J Respir Crit Care Med 2020;201:1345–57.

65. Alkhalil M, Schulman E, Getsy J. Obstructive sleep apnea syndrome and asthma: what are the links? J Clin Sleep Med 2009;5(10):71–8.

66. Kong D-L, Qin Z, Shen H, et al. Association of obstructive sleep apnea with asthma: a meta-analysis. Sci Reports 2017;7:4088.

67. Holbrook JT, Sugar EA, Brown RH, et al. American Lung Association Airways Clinical Research Centers. Effect of continuous positive airway pressure on airway reactivity in asthma: a randomized, sham-controlled clinical trial. Ann Am Thorac Soc 2016;13:1940–50.

68. Serrano-Pariente J, Plaza V, Soriano JB, et al. CPASMA Trial Group. Asthma outcomes improve with continuous positive airway pressure for obstructive sleep apnea. Allergy 2017;72:802–12.

69. Ludlow CL. Laryngeal reflexes: physiology, technique and clinical use. J Clin Neurophysiol 2015; 32(4):284–93.

70. Hull JH, Backer V, Gibson PG, et al. Laryngeal dysfunction: Assessment and management for the clinician. Am J Respir Crit Care Med 2016;9: 1062–72.

71. Morrison M, Rammage L, Emma AJ. The irritable larynx syndrome. J Voice 1999;13:447–55.

72. Vertigan PE, Bone SL, Gibson PG. Laryngeal sensory dysfunction in laryngeal hypersensitivity syndrome. Respirol 2013;13:948–56.

73. Hilton E, Marsden P, Thurston A, et al. Clinical features of the urge-to-cough in patients with chronic cough. Respir Med 2015;109(6):701–7.

74. Won HK, Kang SY, Kang Y, et al. Cough-related laryngeal sensations and triggers in adults with chronic cough: symptom profile and impact. Allergy Asthma Immunol Res 2019;11(5):622–31.

75. Gibson PG, Vertigan AE. Management of chronic refractory cough. BMJ 2015;351:h5590.

76. Chung KF. Approach to chronic cough: the neuropathic basis for cough hypersensitivity syndrome. J Thoracic Dis 2014;6(Suppl 7): S699–707.

77. Song W-J, Morice AH. Cough hypersensitivity syndrome: a few more steps forward. Allergy Asthma Immunol Res 2017;9(5):394–402.

78. Widdicombe J, Fontana G. Cough: what's in a name? Eur Respir J 2006;28(1):10–5.

79. Payne RJ, Kost KM, Frenkiel S, et al. Laryngeal inflammation assessed using the reflux finding score in obstructive sleep apnea. Otolaryngol Head Neck Surg 2006;134(5):836–42.

80. Koufman JA. The otolaryngologic manifestations of gastroesophageal reflux disease (GERD): a clinical investigation of 225 patients using ambulatory 24-hour pH monitoring and an experimental investigation of the role of acid and pepsin in the development of laryngeal injury. Laryngoscope 1991; 101(4 pt 2 suppl 53):1–78.

81. Belafsky PC, Postma GN, Koufman JA. Validity and reliability of the reflux symptom index (RSI). J Voice 2002;16:274–7.

82. Belafsky P, Postma G, Koufman J. The validity and reliability of the reflux finding score (RFS). Laryngoscope 2001;111:1313–7.

83. Ford CN. Evaluation and management of laryngopharyngeal reflux. JAMA 2005;294(12):1534–40.

84. Novakovic D, MacKay S. Adult obstructive sleep apnoea and the larynx. Curr Opin Otolaryngol Head Neck Surg 2015;23(6):464–9.

85. He J, Wang C, Li W. Laryngopharyngeal reflux in obstructive sleep apnea-hypopnea syndrome: an updated meta-analysis. Nat Sci Sleep 2022;14: 2189–201.

86. Nguyen A, Jobin V, Payne R, et al. Laryngeal and velopharyngeal sensory impairment in obstructive sleep apnea. Sleep 2005;28:585–93.

87. Lee B, Woo P. Chronic cough as a sign of laryngeal sensory neuropathy: diagnosis and treatment. Ann Otol Rhinol Laryngol 2005;114(4):253–7.

88. Murry T, Branski RC, Yu K, et al. Laryngeal sensory deficits in patients with chronic cough and paradoxical vocal fold movement disorder. The Laryngoscope 2010;120(8):1576–81.

89. Greene SM, Simpson CB. Evidence for sensory neuropathy and pharmacologic management. Otolaryngol Clinics North Am 2010;43(1):67–72.

90. Benninger MS, Campagnolo A. Chronic laryngopharyngeal vagal neuropathy. Brazilian J Otorhinolaryngol 2018;84(4):401–3.

91. Cukier-Blaj S, Bewley A, Aviv JE, et al. Paradoxical vocal fold motion: a sensory-motor laryngeal disorder. Laryngoscope 2008;118(2):367–70.

92. Hanning CD. Laryngeal and velopharyngeal sensory impairment in obstructive sleep apnea. Sleep 2005;28(10):1335.

93. Kimoff RJ, Sforza E, Champagne V, et al. Upper airway sensation in snoring and obstructive sleep apnea. Am J Respir Crit Care 2001; 164(2):250–5.

94. Svanborg E, Ulander M, Brostrom A, et al. Palatal sensory function worsens in untreated snorers but not in CPAP-treated patients with sleep apnea, indicating vibration-induced nervous lesions. Chest 2020;157(5):1296–303.

95. Roy N, Merrill RM, Pierce J, et al. Evidence of possible irritable larynx syndrome in obstructive sleep apnea: an epidemiologic approach. J Voice 2021;35(6):932.e29–38.

96. Lin YS, Shen Y-J, Ou P-H, et al. HIF-1α-mediated, NADPH oxidase-derived ROS contributes to laryngeal airway hyperreactivity induced by intermittent hypoxia in rats. Front Physiol 2020;11:575260.

97. Poliacek I, Simera M, Veternik M, et al. The course of lung inflation alters the central pattern of tracheobronchial cough in cat – the evidence for volume feedback during cough. Respir Physiol Neruobiol 2016;229:43–50.

98. Tatar M, Hanacek J, Widdicombe J. The expiration reflex from the trachea and bronchi. Eur Respir J 2008;31:385–90.

99. Sullivan CE, Murphy E, Kozar LF, et al. Waking and ventilatory responses to laryngeal stimulation in sleeping dogs. J Appl Physiol Respir Environ Exerc Physiol 1978;45(5):681–9.

100. Sullivan CE, Kozar LF, Murphy E, et al. Arousal, ventilatory, and airway responses to bronchopulmonary stimulation in sleeping dogs. J Appl Physiol Respir Environ Exerc Physiol 1979;47(1): 17–25.

101. Hamilton RD, Winning AJ, Horner RL, et al. The effect of lung inflation on breathing in man during wakefulness and sleep. Respir Physiol 1988; 73(2):145–54.

102. George S, Suresh S. Vocal cord dysfunction: analysis of 27 cases and updated review of pathophysiology & management. Int Arch Otorhinolaryngol 2019;23(2):125–30.

103. Sant'Ambrogio FB, Mathew OP, Clark WD, et al. Laryngeal influences on breathing pattern and posterior cricoarytenoid muscle activity. J Appl Physiol (1985) 1985;58(4):1298–304.

104. Ferini-Strambi L. Neuropathic pain and sleep: a review. Pain Ther 2017;6(suppl 1):S19–23.

105. Ge TJ, Vetter J, Lai HH. Sleep disturbance and fatigue are associated with more severe urinary incontinence and overactive bladder. Urology 2017; 109:67–73.

106. Brignall K, Jayaraman B, Birring SS. Quality of life and psychosocial aspects of cough. Lung 2008; 186:S55–8.

107. Wright ML, Slovarp L, Reynolds J, et al. Prevalence of anxiety as a variable in treatment

outcomes for individuals with chronic refractory cough. Am J Speech Lang Pathol 2024;33(1): 476–84.

108. Coronado EG, Pantaleon-Martinez AM, Velazquez-Moctezuma J, et al. The bidirectional relationship between sleep and immunity against infections. J Immunol Res 2015;2015:678164.

109. Joo H, Moon J-Y, An TJ, et al. Revised Korean cough guidelines, 2020: Recommendations and summary statements. Tuberc Respir Dis 2021;84:263–73.

110. Rouadi PW, Idriss SA, Bousquet J, et al. WAO-ARIA consensus on chronic cough – Part II: phenotypes and mechanisms of abnormal cough presentation – Updates in COVID-19. World Allergy Organ J 2021;14(12):100618.

Does Obstructive Sleep Apnea Lead to Progression of Chronic Obstructive Pulmonary Disease

Walter T. McNicholas, MD[a,b],*

KEYWORDS

- Sleep disorders • Obstructive sleep apnea • Chronic obstructive pulmonary disease
- Overlap syndrome • Cardiovascular comorbidity • Outcomes

KEY POINTS

- The high prevalence of 10% for both OSA and COPD indicate a high likelihood of coexistence by chance alone, but bi-directional relationships have a significant impact on the overlap of the two disorders.
- Factors such as obesity and right heart failure increase the likelihood of OSA in patients with COPD, whereas lung hyperinflation diminishes the likeihood.
- OSA may aggravate COPD by promoting airway inflammation and cigarette smoking in patients with COPD may aggravate upper airway inflammation.
- Patients with OSA-COPD overlap are at higher risk of cardiovascular comorbidity than those with either disorder alone, which is likely contributed to by the greater degree of nocturnal oxygen desaturation reported in overlap patients.
- CPAP therapy in patients with the overlap syndrome is associated with improved survival compared to those not treated, and similar to the survival of patients with COPD alone, which emphasises the clinical benefit of identifying coexisting OSA in patients with COPD.

INTRODUCTION

Chronic obstructive pulmonary disease (COPD) and obstructive sleep apnea (OSA) are both highly prevalent disorders, so the likelihood of chance overlap is high. However, there is evidence of bidirectional interactions between the 2 disorders that influence both the likelihood of occurrence and progression of each one.[1,2] While effective therapy of OSA has been demonstrated to improve outcomes in patients with COPD, this may not be true for untreated OSA. This aspect is highly relevant, as the general population prevalence of OSA is very high, being estimated as close to 1 billion adults worldwide,[3] and most of these patients are undiagnosed. While most of these patients have isolated sleep-disordered breathing (SDB) rather than the clinical syndrome associated with relevant clinical features,[4] this high prevalence is relevant to COPD, as there is evidence that the coexistence of OSA and COPD is associated with more profound nocturnal oxygen desaturation (NOD) than COPD alone.[5,6] The present article reviews the impact of untreated OSA on the progression of COPD, which in many cases will reflect the impact of unrecognized OSA in COPD patients.

Funding: This work is supported by the European Union's Horizon 2020 research and innovation programme under grant agreement no. 965417.
[a] Department of Respiratory and Sleep Medicine, St. Vincent's Hospital Group, Dublin, Ireland; [b] School of Medicine and the Conway Research Institute, University College, Dublin, Ireland
* Department of Respiratory and Sleep Medicine, St. Vincent's Hospital Group, St. Vincent's Private Hospital, Suite 5, Herbert Avenue, Merrion Road, Dublin 4, Ireland.
E-mail address: walter.mcnicholas@ucd.ie

sleep.theclinics.com

EPIDEMIOLOGY AND BIDIRECTIONAL RELATIONSHIPS BETWEEN CHRONIC OBSTRUCTIVE PULMONARY DISEASE AND OBSTRUCTIVE SLEEP APNEA IN THE OVERLAP SYNDROME

The global prevalence of COPD according to the Global Initiative for Chronic Obstructive Lung Disease criteria of forced expiratory volume during the first second/forced vital capacity ratio less than 0.7 has been estimated in a recent systematic review at 10% of the adult general population.[7] The prevalence is highest in the population over 65 years, in the Western Pacific region and lowest in the Americas. Globally, male sex, smoking, low body mass index (BMI), biomass exposure, and occupational exposure to dust or smoke are all major risk factors for COPD.

The global prevalence of OSA has been estimated at least as high as for COPD, although OSA prevalence is influenced by inconsistent definitions of the disorder. The traditional threshold for significant OSA defined as an apnea-hypopnea index (AHI) greater than 5 has been estimated to affect close to 1 billion of the adult population.[3] A higher threshold of AHI greater than 15, which is a level recognized by the American Academy of Sleep Medicine as a level of SDB that is clinically significant in the absence of relevant symptoms,[8] has been estimated at 425 million in the 30-year to 69-year age range. Even higher prevalence figures were reported in the Lausanne cohort study, where AHI greater than 15 was found in almost 50% of adult males.[9] However, this report found that symptomatic OSA occurred in less than 30% of those subjects with AHI greater than 15 and significant excess comorbidity was only found in the subcohort with AHI greater than 20.

While these reported high prevalence figures indicate that COPD and OSA are likely to occur together by chance association alone, several factors relating to each disorder will influence the likelihood of overlap.[10] For example, low BMI is a risk factor for COPD but is generally protective against OSA. Cigarette smoking is a strong risk factor for COPD and may also promote OSA by upper airway inflammation.[11] COPD is associated with poor sleep, especially stage rapid eye movement (REM) sleep[12] and therefore may be somewhat protective against OSA, which is typically more pronounced in REM.[13] COPD is not a uniform disorder but represents a spectrum of phenotypic variants ranging from the thin hyperinflated subtype (predominant emphysema "pink puffer" variant) to the heavier subtype associated with right heart failure (blue boater "bronchitis" variant). The lung hyperinflation and increased caudal traction associated with the predominant emphysema variant is protective against OSA, which is supported by a more negative critical closing pressure of the upper airway during sleep.[14] On the other hand, the high BMI and fluid retention associated with the predominant bronchitis variant promotes OSA by increased neck thickness and associated upper airway narrowing. Furthermore, rostral fluid shift in the recumbent position during sleep in patients with right heart failure due to COPD increases upper airway narrowing like that described in patients with congestive heart failure.[15] Also, skeletal myopathy, which occurs in many patients with advanced COPD,[16] may affect the upper airway dilating muscles, thus further predisposing to OSA.

Studies evaluating the prevalence of the overlap syndrome have produced differing results and most reports have evaluated the prevalence of OSA in patients with COPD. Estimates range from 1% to 3.6% for the prevalence of overlap syndrome in the general population, although much higher when prevalence is assessed in a dedicated OSA or COPD population, with the prevalence of COPD in OSA populations ranging from 7.6% to 55.7% and the prevalence of OSA in COPD populations ranging from 2.9% to 65.9%.[17] A report from the Sleep Heart Health Study cohort indicated no increase in SDB among patients with mild COPD,[18] but oxygen desaturations during sleep were greater in patients with the overlap compared to patients with either disorder alone. Also, the study population in this report was relatively old, where OSA appears to be less prevalent.[19] Bednarek and coworkers also reported no increased prevalence of OSA in subjects with COPD from a middle-aged general population of males and females, but reported greater sleeping oxygen desaturations in subjects with both COPD and OSA compared to COPD alone.[20] Studies including patients with moderate/severe COPD report a higher prevalence of the overlap and a recent report of peripheral artery tonometry in such patients report a prevalence of 47% for the overlap of COPD and OSA.[21] Other reports have also indicated a higher prevalence of OSA in patients with moderate or severe COPD.[22,23] These differing reports may reflect the different populations being studied and it is notable that the reports do not consider the differing COPD phenotypes. In this context, a report from the Genetic Epidemiology of COPD study found that the chronic bronchitis phenotype has a higher prevalence of OSA even after correcting for differences in BMI and lung function.[24] A higher BMI and positive smoking history positively correlate with the presence of OSA in patients with COPD.[22]

The possibility of OSA as a predisposing factor for COPD has been less extensively studied than the reverse association, and like studies of COPD, reports have produced differing results. One report indicated a higher prevalence of COPD and asthma in a cohort of patients with OSA as compared to a matched control population, which was especially so among female subjects.[25] However, another report based on a community study of 853 older men found a lower prevalence of COPD in those with SDB as compared to men without SDB.[19] OSA has been reported to exacerbate lower airway inflammation in COPD patients[26] and a study in mice found that chronic intermittent hypoxia induces inflammation and oxidative stress resulting in lung damage.[27] Thus, further research is needed on the relationships between COPD and OSA, especially regarding the influence of different COPD phenotypes on the prevalence of OSA and the outcomes of the overlap syndrome. Factors impacting the relationships between the 2 disorders are summarized in **Fig. 1**.

SLEEP-RELATED CONSEQUENCES OF THE OVERLAP SYNDROME

Sleep has effects on respiration that include adverse effects on neural control of breathing, reduced muscle function affecting especially the accessory muscles of respiration, and changes in lung mechanics that affect ventilation-perfusion relationships.[28] All these changes represent normal physiologic adaptations that result in no significant adverse consequences in normal subjects but may produce clinically significant decrements in gas exchange in patients with COPD. Changes in the control of breathing include reduced cortical inputs and chemoreceptor sensitivity. Accessory muscles most affected are the intercostal muscles, which are especially important in patients with COPD

where diaphragmatic flattening associated with hyperinflation may reduce the efficiency of this muscle. The intercostal muscles, being skeletal muscles, demonstrate diminished activity during sleep, especially during REM.[29] Furthermore, skeletal myopathy may occur in advanced COPD,[16] which further compounds the adverse impact on the accessory muscles during sleep. Changes in lung mechanics include increased airflow resistance and impaired ventilation-to-perfusion relationships. The overall effects of these adaptations in patients with COPD are to increase the likelihood of significant hypoxia and hypercapnia, which may have serious consequences that include an increased likelihood of death during sleep, especially during acute exacerbations.[30] NOD parallels awake hypoxemia and the increased likelihood of NOD in patients with COPD is a result of them being on or close to the steep portion of the oxyhemoglobin dissociation curve.

OSA is also associated with significant intermittent hypoxia during sleep in association with apnea and hypopnea, but arterial oxygen saturation (SaO2) usually reverts to the normal range in between these events[13] unless there are other comorbid factors such as major obesity.[31] The overall impact on gas exchange in patients with the overlap is to produce more profound oxygen desaturation during episodes of apnea or hypopnea and a greater likelihood of sustained desaturation in periods between these episodes, which increases the likelihood of complications such as pulmonary hypertension. However, coexisting OSA may compensate for sleep-related reduction in neural respiratory drive among patients with COPD in that it has been reported that hypoventilation during non-REM sleep in COPD alone is due to reduction of neural respiratory drive, but in overlap syndrome is due to increased upper airway resistance.[32]

Factors influencing likelihood of OSA in COPD

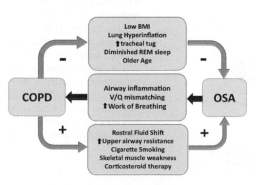

Fig. 1. Chronic obstructive pulmonary disease (COPD)–related factors that may promote or protect against the development of obstructive sleep apnea (OSA), and conversely, OSA-related factors that may promote the progression of COPD. (O'Neill, Emily; Ryan, Silke; McNicholas, Walter T.. Chronic obstructive pulmonary disease and obstructive sleep apnoea overlap: co-existence, comorbidity, or causality?. Current Opinion in Pulmonary Medicine 28(6):p 543-551, November 2022. https://doi.org/10.1097/MCP.0000000000000922.)

SYSTEMIC EFFECTS OF THE OVERLAP SYNDROME

COPD and OSA are each associated with an increased risk of cardiovascular comorbidity and there is strong evidence of overlapping cell and molecular mechanisms that contribute to this risk.[33] These mechanisms include systemic inflammation, oxidative stress, and sympathetic activation (**Fig. 2**). The intermittent hypoxia associated with OSA is especially likely to activate proinflammatory pathways such as that mediated by nuclear factor kappa-b [34] with downstream increase in tumor necrosis factor a (TNF-α) and interleukin-8.[35] This inflammatory pathway is believed to play an important role in the development and progression of atherosclerosis. Additional markers of inflammation such as C-reactive protein (CRP) have been reported to be elevated in patients with OSA, although comorbid obesity appears to play a significant role in this aspect.[36] COPD has also been reported to be associated with increased markers of inflammation including TNF-α and CRP.[37] Thus, it would be expected that patients with the overlap syndrome would have more pronounced evidence of systemic inflammation, although there have been few reports of this outcome. Patients with the overlap syndrome have greater arterial stiffness compared to those with COPD or OSA alone without greater nocturnal hypoxemia or inflammation, which may represent an additional factor in contributing to cardiovascular comorbidity.[38] Patients with the overlap syndrome have been reported to show autonomic changes associated with higher sympathetic and lower parasympathetic nervous system activity, as measured by heart rate changes, when compared with COPD or OSA alone.[39]

IMPACT OF THE OVERLAP ON CARDIOVASCULAR COMORBIDITY

Patients with COPD and OSA are at increased risk of cardiovascular comorbidity and there is emerging evidence that patients with the overlap syndrome are especially at risk. A meta-analysis of data from 11 studies including more than 45 million patients with COPD found higher prevalence of cardiovascular comorbidities in COPD patients compared to control subjects with an odds ratio (OR) of 1.9[40]. Regarding OSA, a meta-analysis of 17 prospective cohort studies reported an increased prevalence of total cardiovascular disease (OR 2.48) and an OR of 2.02 for stroke.[41] Cardiovascular disorders most closely associated with OSA are systemic hypertension and atrial fibrillation (AF),[42] and AF has been has been reported to have a higher incidence in patients with OSA-COPD overlap when compared to patients with OSA alone.[43] These considerations indicate that cardiovascular disease should be more prevalent in the overlap syndrome than either disorder alone, although the evidence in this respect is limited by the relatively small number of reported studies. However, a recent systematic review and meta-analysis of cardiovascular outcomes in COPD-OSA overlap patients confirmed a higher prevalence of cardiovascular diseases, especially ischemic heart disease, and systemic and pulmonary hypertension in overlap patients when compared to each disorder alone[44]

Pulmonary hypertension is especially prevalent in patients with the overlap syndrome when compared to either disorder alone.[5] This higher prevalence is likely a consequence of the greater degree of hypoxemia in patients with the overlap syndrome, especially during sleep.[6] Overlap

Inflammatory mechanisms in COPD and OSAS: implications for cardiovascular disease.

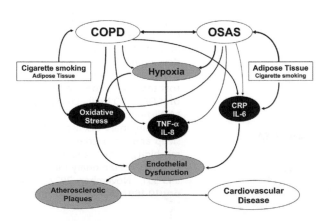

Fig. 2. Overlapping molecular mechanisms of systemic inflammation in chronic obstructive pulmonary disease (COPD) and obstructive sleep apnea syndrome (OSA). COPD and OSA are each associated with elevated levels of C-reactive protein (CRP) and interleukin (IL)-6, in addition to tumor necrosis factor (TNF)-a and IL-8, in addition to oxidative stress. Hypoxia is an important factor in increased TNF-a production in OSA, which is especially relevant in the overlap syndrome. Each inflammatory pathway has been associated with atherogenesis and subsequent cardiovascular disease. (McNicholas. AJRCCM 2009.)

patients also have a higher right ventricular mass index, likely because of pulmonary hypertension.[45] An expert consensus document has recommended polysomnography (PSG) to rule out OSA for all patients with pulmonary hypertension based on the consideration that therapy of OSA may benefit pulmonary hemodynamics.[46] A recent report based on data from the European Sleep Apnea Database cohort involving 5600 patients with OSA, found that a diagnosis of COPD increased the odds of heart failure (OR 1.75; 95% confidence interval [CI] 1.15–2.67) and systemic hypertension (OR 1.36; 95% CI 1.07–1.73). CT90 (cumulative time spent below SaO2 of 90%) was associated with increased risk of systemic hypertension, diabetes mellitus, and heart failure, whereas oxygen desaturation index was only related to hypertension and diabetes.[47] These data support another recent report involving a 5% national sample of Medicare beneficiaries that included 159,084 patients with COPD.[48] Cardiovascular diseases including coronary artery disease, congestive heart failure, and hypertension in addition to diabetes were more common in overlap patients compared to those with COPD alone. Another recent report of COPD patients in China indicated that patients with comorbid OSA had a higher prevalence of systemic hypertension and diabetes compared to patients with COPD alone, in addition to worse quality of life and more sleepiness.[49] Unsurprisingly, higher BMI and daytime sleepiness were significant risk factors for OSA. The higher prevalence of cardiovascular disease in the overlap syndrome is indirectly supported by the recent report indicating that hypoxic burden in OSA strongly predicts cardiovascular mortality.[50]

OUTCOMES OF THE OVERLAP SYNDROME

Patients with the overlap syndrome report worse quality of life compared to those with COPD alone using the Saint George Respiratory Questionnaire[51] and report higher scores of anxiety and depression on the Hospital Anxiety and Depression Scale.[49] Higher rates of cardiovascular events and all-cause mortality have been reported in patients with OSA-COPD overlap. A study of 10,149 patients clinically assessed for OSA reported that 30% had an AHI greater than 30, 25% demonstrated more than 10 minutes with a SaO2 less than 90%, and 12% had coexisting COPD.[52] Patients were followed for an average of 9.4 years. The investgators reported more nocturnal hypoxemia in overlap patients than either disorder alone together with a higher rate of cardiovascular morbidity and all-cause mortality. Cardiovascular

morbidity was more frequent in the group with COPD alone compared to those with severe OSA alone, and those with COPD alone had a greater hazard of composite adverse outcomes. The most important predictor of adverse cardiovascular outcomes was the cumulative time individuals with COPD spent with nocturnal hypoxemia. In contrast, another report of 6173 subjects from the Sleep Heart Health Study having home PSG assessed the influence of SDB and lung function on all-cause mortality.[53] Although lung function was negatively correlated with risk for all-cause mortality, the incremental contribution of lung function to mortality diminished with increasing severity of SDB. In a report from the 2005 to 2008 US National Health and Nutrition survey, OSA-COPD overlap patients had an adjusted hazard ratio (HR) for all-cause mortality of 2.4 and those with COPD alone had HR of 1.5 compared with those without either condition.[54] Interestingly, despite the higher mortality in overlap patients, OSA did not significantly increase mortality in patients with COPD in this survey.

Further insight into the impact of untreated OSA on disease progression in patients with COPD can be gained from studies of continuous positive airway pressure (CPAP) therapy in patients with the overlap syndrome by comparing patients who complied with therapy to patients who did not comply. Although such studies are observational in design and thus compromised by a lack of randomization to treatment, they offer insight into the natural progression of COPD in those patients who do not comply with CPAP therapy. A prospective study of 441 patients with the overlap syndrome treated with long-term CPAP reported that those patients who complied with CPAP had survival rates similar to a control group of 210 patients with COPD alone but overlap patients who did not comply with CPAP had higher mortality and a higher rate of severe COPD exacerbations resulting in hospitalization.[55] These findings were confirmed in another retrospective study of long-term CPAP therapy in 227 patients with the overlap syndrome.[56] Patients who did not comply with CPAP had a substantially lower survival rate than patients who complied, even compared to those who showed 2 to 4 hours nightly compliance. A recent retrospective observational study assessed the impact of positive airway pressure (PAP) therapy adherence on outcomes in 6810 Patients with OSA and COPD, of whom 2328 were nonadherent to PAP.[57] Compared with the year before commencing PAP, there were highly significant reductions in the number of emergency department visits, hospitalizations, and severe exacerbations during 2 years of CPAP therapy in adherent versus nonadherent patients. Furthermore, improvements in health status were paralleled by a reduction in associated health care costs. While these studies must be viewed with caution, as patients who do not comply with CPAP may also be noncompliant with other therapies, the consistent nature of the findings supports an adverse impact of untreated OSA on COPD outcomes.

SUMMARY

The bidirectional relationships between COPD and OSA underline the importance of identifying each disorder when it is present in an individual patient, especially as there are important shared mechanisms predisposing to cardiovascular comorbidity and the active treatment of coexisting OSA improves long-term outcomes in patients with COPD.

CLINICS CARE POINTS

- There are important bidirectional relationships between COPD and OSA that affect the pathophysiology of each disorder.
- The pink puffer phenotype of COPD protects against OSA by lung hyperinflation and low BMI, whereas the blue bloater phenotype predisposes to OSA by fluid retention.
- OSA may aggravate COPD by promoting airway inflammation.
- COPD-OSA overlap patients are at higher risk of cardiovascular comorbidity than either disorder alone due to factors such as greater NOD and sympathetic activation, which results in higher all-cause mortality.
- Active management of OSA with PAP improves COPD outcomes that include lower exacerbation rates compared to untreated patients.

DISCLOSURE

The author has nothing to disclose.

REFERENCES

1. Ioachimescu OC, McNicholas WT. Chronic obstructive pulmonary disease-obstructive sleep apnea overlap: more than a casual acquaintance. Am J Respir Crit Care Med 2022;206(2):139–41.
2. Gleeson M, McNicholas WT. Bidirectional relationships of comorbidity with obstructive sleep apnoea. Eur Respir Rev : an official journal of the European Respiratory Society 2022;31(164):210256.
3. Benjafield AV, Ayas NT, Eastwood PR, et al. Estimation of the global prevalence and burden of obstructive sleep apnoea: a literature-based analysis. Lancet Respir Med 2019;7(8):687–98.
4. McNicholas WT. Diagnosis of obstructive sleep apnea in adults. Proc Am Thorac Soc 2008;5(2):154–60.
5. Chaouat A, Weitzenblum E, Krieger J, et al. Association of chronic obstructive pulmonary disease and sleep apnea syndrome. Am J Respir Crit Care Med 1995;151(1):82–6.
6. McNicholas WT. Chronic obstructive pulmonary disease and obstructive sleep apnoea-the overlap syndrome. J Thorac Dis 2016;8(2):236–42.
7. Adeloye D, Song P, Zhu Y, et al, NIHR RESPIRE Global Respiratory Health Unit. Global, regional, and national prevalence of, and risk factors for, chronic obstructive pulmonary disease (COPD) in 2019: a systematic review and modelling analysis. Lancet Respir Med 2022;10(5):447–58.
8. Epstein LJ, Kristo D, Strollo PJ Jr, et al. Clinical guideline for the evaluation, management and long-term care of obstructive sleep apnea in adults. J Clin Sleep Med 2009;5(3):263–76.
9. Heinzer R, Vat S, Marques-Vidal P, et al. Prevalence of sleep-disordered breathing in the general population: the HypnoLaus study. Lancet Respir Med 2015;3(4):310–8.
10. McNicholas WT. COPD-OSA overlap syndrome: evolving evidence regarding epidemiology, clinical consequences, and management. Chest 2017;152(6):1318–26.
11. Renner B, Mueller CA, Shephard A. Environmental and non-infectious factors in the aetiology of pharyngitis (sore throat). Inflamm Res 2012;61(10):1041–52.
12. McSharry DG, Ryan S, Calverley P, et al. Sleep quality in chronic obstructive pulmonary disease. Respirology 2012;17(7):1119–24.
13. Deegan PC, McNicholas WT. Pathophysiology of obstructive sleep apnoea. Eur Respir J 1995;8(7):1161–78.
14. Biselli P, Grossman PR, Kirkness JP, et al. The effect of increased lung volume in chronic obstructive pulmonary disease on upper airway obstruction during sleep. J Appl Physiol 2015;119(3):266–71.
15. White LH, Bradley TD. Role of nocturnal rostral fluid shift in the pathogenesis of obstructive and central sleep apnoea. J Physiol 2013;591(5):1179–93.
16. Agusti A. Systemic effects of chronic obstructive pulmonary disease: what we know and what we don't know (but should). Proc Am Thorac Soc 2007;4(7):522–5.
17. Shawon MSR, Perret JL, Senaratna CV, et al. Current evidence on prevalence and clinical outcomes of co-morbid obstructive sleep apnea and chronic obstructive pulmonary disease: a systematic review. Sleep Med Rev 2017;32:58–68.

18. Sanders MH, Newman AB, Haggerty CL, et al. Sleep and sleep-disordered breathing in adults with predominantly mild obstructive airway disease. Am J Respir Crit Care Med 2003;167(1): 7–14.

19. Zhao YY, Blackwell T, Ensrud KE, et al. Sleep apnea and obstructive airway disease in older men: outcomes of sleep disorders in older men study. Sleep 2016;39(7):1343–51.

20. Bednarek M, Plywaczewski R, Jonczak L, et al. There is no relationship between chronic obstructive pulmonary disease and obstructive sleep apnea syndrome: a population study. Respiration 2005; 72(2):142–9.

21. Hansson D, Andersson A, Vanfleteren L, et al. Clinical impact of routine sleep assessment by peripheral arterial tonometry in patients with COPD. ERJ open research 2023;9(2).

22. Steveling EH, Clarenbach CF, Miedinger D, et al. Predictors of the overlap syndrome and its association with comorbidities in patients with chronic obstructive pulmonary disease. Respiration 2014; 88(6):451–7.

23. Soler X, Gaio E, Powell FL, et al. High prevalence of obstructive sleep apnea in patients with moderate to severe chronic obstructive pulmonary disease. Ann Am Thorac Soc 2015;12(8):1219–25.

24. Kim V, Han MK, Vance GB, et al. The chronic bronchitic phenotype of COPD: an analysis of the COPDGene Study. Chest 2011;140(3):626–33.

25. Greenberg-Dotan S, Reuveni H, Tal A, et al. Increased prevalence of obstructive lung disease in patients with obstructive sleep apnea. Sleep Breath 2014;18(1):69–75.

26. Wang Y, Hu K, Liu K, et al. Obstructive sleep apnea exacerbates airway inflammation in patients with chronic obstructive pulmonary disease. Sleep Med 2015;16(9):1123–30.

27. Tuleta I, Stockigt F, Juergens UR, et al. Intermittent hypoxia contributes to the lung damage by increased oxidative stress, inflammation, and disbalance in protease/antiprotease System. Lung 2016; 194(6):1015–20.

28. McNicholas WT. Impact of sleep in COPD. Chest 2000;117(suppl):48S–53S.

29. McNicholas WT. Impact of sleep on respiratory muscle function. Monaldi archives for chest disease = Archivio Monaldi per le malattie del torace 2002; 57(5–6):277–80.

30. McNicholas WT, FitzGerald MX. Nocturnal death among patients with chronic bronchitis and emphysema. BMJ 1984;289:878.

31. Ryan S, Crinion SJ, McNicholas WT. Obesity and sleep-disordered breathing—when two 'bad guys' meet. QJM 2014;107(12):949–54.

32. He B-T, Lu G, Xiao S-C, et al. Coexistence of OSA may compensate for sleep related reduction in neural respiratory drive in patients with COPD. Thorax 2016. https://doi.org/10.1136/thoraxjnl-2016-208467. [Epub ahead of print].

33. McNicholas WT. Chronic obstructive pulmonary disease and obstructive sleep apnea: overlaps in pathophysiology, systemic inflammation, and cardiovascular disease. Am J Respir Crit Care Med 2009;180(8): 692–700.

34. Ryan S, Taylor CT, McNicholas WT. Selective activation of inflammatory pathways by intermittent hypoxia in obstructive sleep apnea syndrome. Circulation 2005;112(17):2660–7.

35. Ryan S, Taylor CT, McNicholas WT. Predictors of elevated nuclear factor-kappaB-dependent genes in obstructive sleep apnea syndrome. Am J Respir Crit Care Med 2006;174(7):824–30.

36. Ryan S, Nolan GM, Hannigan E, et al. Cardiovascular risk markers in obstructive sleep apnoea syndrome and correlation with obesity. Thorax 2007; 62(6):509–14.

37. Broekhuizen R, Wouters EF, Creutzberg EC, et al. Raised CRP levels mark metabolic and functional impairment in advanced COPD. Thorax 2006;61(1): 17–22.

38. Shiina K, Tomiyama H, Takata Y, et al. Overlap syndrome: additive effects of COPD on the cardiovascular damages in patients with OSA. Respir Med 2012;106(9):1335–41.

39. Taranto-Montemurro L, Messineo L, Perger E, et al. Cardiac sympathetic hyperactivity in patients with chronic obstructive pulmonary disease and obstructive sleep apnea. COPD 2016;13(6):706–11.

40. Yin H-l, Yin S-q, Lin Q-y, et al. Prevalence of comorbidities in chronic obstructive pulmonary disease patients: a meta-analysis. Medicine 2017;96(19): e6836.

41. Dong J-Y, Zhang Y-H, Qin L-Q. Obstructive sleep apnea and cardiovascular risk: meta-analysis of prospective cohort studies. Atherosclerosis 2013; 229(2):489–95.

42. McNicholas WT. Obstructive sleep apnoea and comorbidity - an overview of the association and impact of continuous positive airway pressure therapy. Expet Rev Respir Med 2019;13(3):251–61.

43. Ganga HV, Nair SU, Puppala VK, et al. Risk of new-onset atrial fibrillation in elderly patients with the overlap syndrome: a retrospective cohort study. Journal of Geriatric Cardiology 2013;10(2):129–34.

44. Shah AJ, Quek E, Alqahtani JS, et al. Cardiovascular outcomes in patients with COPD-OSA overlap syndrome: a systematic review and meta-analysis. Sleep Med Rev 2022;63:101627.

45. Sharma B, Neilan TG, Kwong RY, et al. Evaluation of right ventricular remodeling using cardiac magnetic resonance imaging in co-existent chronic obstructive pulmonary disease and obstructive sleep apnea. COPD 2013;10(1):4–10.

46. McLaughlin VV, Archer SL, Badesch DB, et al. ACCF/AHA 2009 expert consensus document on pulmonary hypertension a report of the American college of cardiology foundation task force on expert consensus documents and the American heart association developed in collaboration with the American college of chest physicians; American thoracic society, inc.; and the pulmonary hypertension association. J Am Coll Cardiol 2009;53(17): 1573–619.

47. van Zeller M, Basoglu OK, Verbraecken J, et al. Sleep and cardiometabolic comorbidities in the obstructive sleep apnoea-COPD overlap syndrome: data from the European Sleep Apnoea Database. ERJ open research 2023;9(3).

48. Starr P, Agarwal A, Singh G, et al. Obstructive sleep apnea with chronic obstructive pulmonary disease among medicare beneficiaries. Ann Am Thorac Soc 2019;16(1):153–6.

49. Zhang P, Chen B, Lou H, et al. Predictors and outcomes of obstructive sleep apnea in patients with chronic obstructive pulmonary disease in China. BMC Pulm Med 2022;22(1):16.

50. Azarbarzin A, Sands SA, Stone KL, et al. The hypoxic burden of sleep apnoea predicts cardiovascular disease-related mortality: the osteoporotic fractures in men study and the sleep heart health study. Eur Heart J 2019;40(14):1149–57.

51. Mermigkis C, Kopanakis A, Foldvary-Schaefer N, et al. Health-related quality of life in patients with obstructive sleep apnoea and chronic obstructive pulmonary disease (overlap syndrome). Int J Clin Pract 2007;61(2):207–11.

52. Kendzerska T, Leung RS, Aaron SD, et al. Cardiovascular outcomes and all-cause mortality in patients with obstructive sleep apnea and chronic obstructive pulmonary disease (overlap syndrome). Ann Am Thorac Soc 2019;16(1):71–81.

53. Putcha N, Crainiceanu C, Norato G, et al. Influence of lung function and sleep-disordered breathing on all-cause mortality. a community-based study. Am J Respir Crit Care Med 2016;194(8):1007–14.

54. Du W, Liu J, Zhou J, et al. Obstructive sleep apnea, COPD, the overlap syndrome, and mortality: results from the 2005-2008 National Health and Nutrition Examination Survey. Int J Chron Obstruct Pulmon Dis 2018;13:665–74.

55. Marin JM, Soriano JB, Carrizo SJ, et al. Outcomes in patients with chronic obstructive pulmonary disease and obstructive sleep apnea: the overlap syndrome. Am J Respir Crit Care Med 2010;182(3):325–31.

56. Stanchina ML, Welicky LM, Donat W, et al. Impact of CPAP use and age on mortality in patients with combined COPD and obstructive sleep apnea: the overlap syndrome. J Clin Sleep Med : JCSM 2013;9(8): 767–72.

57. Sterling KL, Pépin JL, Linde-Zwirble W, et al. Impact of positive airway pressure therapy adherence on outcomes in patients with obstructive sleep apnea and chronic obstructive pulmonary disease. Am J Respir Crit Care Med 2022;206(2):197–205.

Contribution of Obstructive Sleep Apnea to Asthmatic Airway Inflammation and Impact of Its Treatment on the Course of Asthma

Octavian C. Ioachimescu, MD, PhD, MBA[a,b,*]

KEYWORDS

- Asthma • Sleep apnea • Obstructive sleep apnea • Alternative overlap syndrome • Inflammation
- Positive airway pressure

KEY POINTS

- Asthma and obstructive sleep apnea (OSA) are very common respiratory disorders in the general population, and together constitute the so-called alternative overlap syndrome.
- Beyond their high prevalence, shared risk factors, and genetic linkages, bidirectional relationships exist between asthma and OSA.
- The accumulated evidence shows that OSA may contribute to asthma exacerbations, daytime and nighttime asthma symptoms, and poor quality of life.
- Continuous positive airway pressure therapy has been shown to improve outcomes of the comorbid asthma, especially in severe OSA and in those with poorly controlled asthma.

INTRODUCTION

Asthma and obstructive sleep apnea (OSA) are amongst the most common respiratory disorders in the general population, especially in the Western world. Approximately 10% of asthma patients have severe disease. Among individuals diagnosed with asthma, comorbid OSA is found in ~26%,[1] while moderate-to-severe OSA was found in 88% and 58% of cases of severe and moderate asthma, respectively.[2] The accumulated evidence shows that OSA may contribute to asthma exacerbations,[3] daytime and nighttime asthma symptoms,[4,5] and poor quality of life.[6] Beyond their high prevalence, shared risk factors, and genetic linkages, bidirectional relationships between asthma and OSA exist, each disorder affecting the other's presence and severity.[7–12] (**Fig. 1**) While coexistence of asthma and OSA in an individual may not represent a distinct disorder with a clear, unifying pathophysiology, it represents a syndrome, that is, a collection of common clinical manifestations. In order to avoid terminological confusion, this association has been coined as *alternative overlap syndrome* [vs the 'traditional' overlap syndrome, that is, chronic obstructive pulmonary disease-OSA association].[7]

We review in this article some of the salient links between constituents of the alternative overlap

[a] Clinical and Translational Science Institute of Southeast Wisconsin, Medical College of Wisconsin, Milwaukee, WI, USA; [b] Department of Medicine, Division of Pulmonary, Critical Care and Sleep Medicine, Medical College of Wisconsin, Milwaukee, WI, USA
* Clinical and Translational Science Institute of Southeast Wisconsin, Medical College of Wisconsin, Milwaukee, WI.
E-mail address: oioac@yahoo.com

Sleep Med Clin 19 (2024) 261–274
https://doi.org/10.1016/j.jsmc.2024.02.006
1556-407X/24/Published by Elsevier Inc.

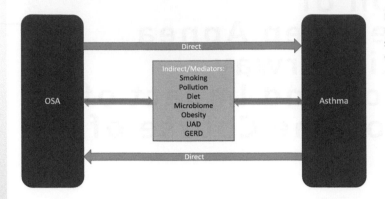

Fig. 1. Schematic representation of the relationships between obstructive sleep apnea and asthma, exerted via direct and indirect effects.

syndrome, with an emphasis on the effects of OSA or its treatment on inflammation in asthma. Noteworthy, cross-sectional and even longitudinal epidemiologic evaluations of OSA cohorts developing or with worsening asthma during follow-up cannot establish causal relationships, directionality, or the mediating influence of other factors. We will present, however, the data as we have it and allow biological plausibility to fill some of the existing gaps.

Pheno-Endotypic Interactions

Asthma symptoms are often worse at night, likely due to reduced lung volumes, decreased inspiratory muscle activity, eosinophil migration into the airways, reduced cortisol levels during the first part of the night, enhanced airway cellular inflammatory responsiveness, the presence of OSA, and so forth.

Asthma-OSA alternative overlap syndrome seems to be associated with worse morbidity and mortality compared with either disease alone.[9,13] In a cohort study of 4980 military veterans, we found a 10-year all-cause mortality of 63.5% for asthma-OSA overlap, 54.2% for asthma alone, and 60.4% for isolated OSA.[9] In OSA patients not on positive airway pressure (PAP) therapy, the risk of death was 1.3 (1.1–1.7) times higher than in those on PAP therapy.[9] Furthermore, in PAP-nonadherent OSA patients, the risk of death was 1.8 (1.1–2.8) times higher versus those who were PAP-adherent (≥70% nights and >4 hours/night).[9]

Multiple cross-sectional epidemiologic studies found that OSA is associated with worse asthma severity, increased frequency of exacerbation, and poor quality of life.[6,14–18] These associations have also been examined in several longitudinal studies. In the 10 to 11 years of follow-up among participants in the World Trade Center Health Registry, there was a trend for higher OSA prevalence associated with worse asthma control.[19] The

presence of OSA conferred 1.4 times higher risk of poorly controlled asthma and 1.5 increased risk of very poorly controlled asthma, even when adjusting for covariates such as body mass index (BMI).[19] In a prospective study on 146 participants with asthma and 157 matched controls, OSA was associated with higher risk of severe asthma exacerbation (realtive risk [RR] 14.2, 95% confidence interval [CI] 4.6–44.0) versus no OSA.[20] Contrary to these studies, in a 5-year follow-up of 177 subjects with difficult-to-control asthma, OSA was not associated with an increased risk of frequent, severe exacerbation.[21]

Genetic Factors

While our understanding of the genetics involving OSA is still limited, recent GWAS investigations[8] revealed several distinct genetic loci associated with the OSA risk. In addition, some of OSA comorbidities such as asthma share a common genetic background with OSA (r_g = 0.50, $P = 1.53 \times 10^{-8}$), even after adjustment for BMI ($r_g = 0.33, P = 2.6 \times 10^{-3}$). Other recent investigations evaluated the genetic connection between OSA and asthma through the use of bioinformatic capabilities.[22] The investigators found 5 hub crosstalk genes and several signaling pathways involved in the pathogenesis of OSA and asthma. By analyzing the differentially expressed genes of OSA and asthma, nucleotide-binding oligomerization domain (NOD)-like receptor (NLR) signaling pathway was found to be 1 key pathway in the development of the 2 diseases, even more significant than many other well-known pathways, including the tumor necrosis factor (TNF) signaling pathway, nuclear factor kappa-light-chain-enhancer of activated B cells (NF-κB) signaling pathway, and interleukin (IL)-17 signaling pathway. NLRs represent a member of intracellular innate immune sensors, capable of detecting microbial and injury-associated molecular patterns, and are widely regarded as having a central role in tissue homeostasis and innate immunity against microorganisms.[23] Interestingly, the synergy of NOD1 and NOD2 signaling pathways with the actions of toll-like receptors in the priming of T-helper-cell (Th)2 and Th17 immune responses, directly implicate NOD1 and NOD2 and their signaling pathways in several mechanisms and cell patterns related to asthma development and exacerbation.

Air Pollution and Smoking

A growing body of literature suggests that air pollution is a risk factor in the development or worsening of OSA.[24,25] Pollution can lead to increased inflammation in the upper airway, induce neuroinflammation, and disrupt neurotransmitter levels—all mechanisms involved in the etiopathogenesis of OSA. A recent article evaluated 204 studies on exposure to chemical pollutants versus sleep health and disorders.[25] Particulate matter (PM) and nitrogen dioxide (NO_2) were linked to poor sleep quality; tobacco smoke exposure in pediatric populations was associated with OSA; dioxins, polybrominated diphenyl ethers, and polychlorinated biphenyls were tied to sleep disruption and insomnia, and exposure to lead, mercury, and pesticides were also associated with insomnia.[25] Solvents such as toluene were associated with disrupted sleep timing and OSA. Gulf war illness exposures showed associations with poor sleep quality, insomnia, OSA, and altered sleep architecture.[25] Another article examined the association between air pollution and OSA in the general population, and potential effect modifications by seasonality, temperature, and humidity.[24] The investigators found a relationship between air pollution and OSA, even when the pollution levels were below the recommended air quality guidelines, and seasonal pollution variability remained an important modifier. Indoor air quality, while important, is often not assessed, and high levels of indoor pollution are likely even in areas with low outdoor pollution.[24] Zhang and colleagues[26] conducted time series analyses on individual-level, longitudinal, at-home sleep monitoring data from smart devices among 51,842 Chinese telephone users, in relationship to fine PM, NO_2, carbon monoxide, and sulfur dioxide levels. Each quartile increment in the moving average concentration of air pollutants (during sleep and in the previous 2 days) was associated with a 1.1% to 4.3% increase in the risk of OSA exacerbation, an increase in the apnea-hypopnea index (AHI) of 0.05 to 0.17 events/h, and a decrease in peripheral oxygen saturation by 0.003% to 0.014%. This large-scale, nationwide, longitudinal study provided compelling evidence that short-term exposure to air pollution may worsen OSA.[26]

The Wisconsin Sleep Cohort study also reported that compared with never smokers, current smokers had a significantly greater risk of snoring (odds ratio [OR] 2.3) and of moderate/severe OSA (OR 4.4). Heavy smokers ($\geq$40 cigarettes/day) had the greatest risk of mild OSA (OR 6.7) and of moderate/severe OSA (OR 40.5). After adjustment for confounders, former smoking was not related to snoring or OSA anymore.[27] A more recent study done in the general population of France reconfirmed that OSA is more frequent among current smokers.[28]

The pathophysiological connections remain incompletely elucidated. Some investigators suggested that an increase in inflammation of the upper airways, as confirmed by biopsy of uvular mucosa lamina propria, could lead to a decrease in the overall diameter of the airways.[29] In another possible mechanism, active smoking and nicotine exposure seem to reduce N3 duration,[30,31] which is a 'protective' sleep stage for the development of OSA. Others suggest that the nicotine withdrawal may lead to an increase in sleep-disordered breathing through a decrease in the tone of the upper airways.[27,32–34]

Sleep Fragmentation

Various investigators postulated that the impaired sleep architecture itself may be important in the OSA-asthma interactions.[35] Sleep fragmentation and frequent arousals, which are common features in OSA, may cause an increase in airway resistance and blunting of the arousal response to bronchoconstriction.[35] Furthermore, early studies of OSA demonstrated that patients with asthma were breathing more irregularly (with hypopnea, apnea, and hyperpnea) in rapid eye movement (REM) sleep than those without asthma.[36] This may be related to the increased cholinergic outflow that occurs during REM sleep, which in turn modulates the caliber and reactivity of the lower airways.[36] In a recent study, a low arousal threshold (as determined by a validated clinical score,[37] yet using a home sleep apnea test device) was present in 71% of patients with alternative overlap syndrome versus 31% of patients with OSA alone (P=.002), significant even after adjustment for BMI or OSA severity.[38] This was in contrast with previous investigations, which showed that a low arousal threshold was more frequently seen in nonobese asthma patients.[39]

Chronic Intermittent Hypoxia

In OSA, respiratory events lead to hypoxia and reoxygenation, with the generation of reactive oxygen species and oxidative stress, ultimately leading to tissue damage and upper airway inflammation. The oxidative stress cascade involves downstream inflammation, sympathetic tone surcharges, endothelial dysfunction, and broncho-constriction.[11] Another possible trigger for reflex bronchoconstriction is via carotid body stimulation by the hypoxic stimulus accompanying obstructive apneas.[40] Oxidative stress may also play an essential role in the development of chronic systemic inflammation in OSA.[41–43] Broytman and colleagues[44] showed that intermittent hypoxia superimposed on allergic lower airway inflammation in rats alters the airway inflammation toward monocyte or macrophage-predominant phenotype and induces matrix remodeling that leads to small airway basement membrane thinning and large airway fibrosis, with airflow obstruction and emphysema-like areas in the lung periphery. In subsequent investigations, the investigators found that intermittent hypoxia did not influence the house dust mite (HDM)–induced alterations in lung function, but worsened the airway hyperreactivity (AHR) to methacholine (to the largest degree in HDM-challenged rats and predominantly in the distal airways), exerted detrimental effects on the elastic properties of the respiratory system, and upregulated some allergic responses to HDM.[45] In another study, on male brown Norway rats exposed to 14-day intermittent hypoxia or room air for 6 hours a day, the investigators found that methacholine significantly induced an augmented bronchoconstriction in hypoxia-exposed rats versus room air controls.[46] Moreover, hypoxic exposure led to heightened lung inflammation, as reflected by increased neutrophilic infiltration, higher concentrations of IL-6 and prostaglandin E2 in bronchoalveolar lavage fluid, and lung lipid peroxidation. Hypoxic-induced AHR and lung inflammation were completely abolished by daily intraperitoneal injection of N-acetylcysteine (an antioxidant) or ibuprofen (a cyclooxygenase inhibitor), but not by apocynin (an inhibitor of NADPH oxidase) or vehicle.[46]

Inflammation

Repetitive, complete, or partial collapse of the upper airway during sleep ultimately leads to vibratory mechanical stress, trauma, and subsequent inflammation, including subepithelial edema and inflammatory cell infiltration of nasal passages, uvula, soft palate, and pharyngeal walls.[47–53] In addition, inflammation in OSA is also the result of the severe chronic intermittent hypoxia (CIH) experienced in this disorder.[54–57] In a recent study on 89 patients with OSA, 28 snorers, and 26 healthy controls, pharyngeal lavage and plasma samples were collected at baseline and after a 1-year of follow-up. Inflammatory cells were evaluated by flow cytometry; IL-6, IL-8, and TNF-α were evaluated by immunoassays.[53] In pharyngeal lavage, CD4+ T-cells, IL-6, and IL-8 were higher in OSA patients than in snorers or healthy controls, and the AHI correlated significantly with CD4+, IL-6, and IL-8. Further, pharyngeal lavage inflammatory biomarkers decreased significantly, but not in plasma after 1 year of therapy with continuous positive airway pressure (CPAP) or surgery.[53]

Initially, it was found that CD4+ T helper lymphocytes played an important role in the inflammatory cascades of asthma. Subsequently, specific T-helper subsets (Th1, Th2) were characterized. The Th2 cells were critical in promoting eosinophilic airway inflammation and the generation of Th2 cytokines like IL-4, 5, and 13.[58] Consequently, an initial categorization nomenclature of Th2-high and Th2-low asthma was used, with an eosinophilic profile dominating the former, while a pauci-granulocytic, neutrophilic, or mixed profile characterized the latter. More recently, the discovery of innate lymphoid cells type and their ability to produce large amounts of type 2 (T2) immune-response cytokines improved our understanding of the inflammatory pathways of asthma beyond Th subtypes.[59] This led to the modification of the endotypic categorization of asthma into T2-high and T2-low/non-T2 groups. The use of additional biomarkers, such as total and specific immuno-globulin (Ig) E, skin prick testing, and fractional exhaled nitric oxide , has allowed for further stratification of endotypes and phenotypes within the broader T2-high versus T2-low schema. This classification has been used to develop targeted therapies, directed at specific cytokines or molecules implicated in these endotypes, which revolutionized asthma management, particularly the difficult-to-treat or severe asthma.[60,61]

OSA and CIH may also induce central nervous system inflammation and impair cognitive function.[56,62–65] Further, hypoxia-induced inflammation alters respiratory chemoreflexes and motor plasticity. This may contribute to the underlying pathophysiology, as OSA-induced inflammation may compromise spontaneous respiratory compensation, exacerbating the primary respiratory disorder.[36]

A close relationship between local (eg, airway) and systemic inflammation constitutes the spillover hypothesis, which suggests that the overflow of inflammatory cytokines, chemoattractant factors, and/or inflammatory cells from a local source into blood stream is responsible for the observed systemic inflammation.[66] In OSA, this is characterized by elevation of serum proinflammatory cytokines and chemokines such as TNF-α, C-reactive protein, 8-isoprostane, IL-6, and so forth.[47,67-71] Recently, Nadeem and colleagues[72] concluded that those with OSA, on average, had higher levels of systemic inflammatory markers than healthy controls. Systemic inflammation may also contribute to weakening of the respiratory muscles[73] and destabilizing the loop gain and respiratory control, thus impairing the protective airway patency mechanisms.[36]

Endothelial Dysfunction

Repetitive changes in blood flow associated with apneas can lead to vascular wall changes and endothelial dysfunction in the upper airway vasculature. Endothelial dysfunction can further contribute to inflammation and may be responsible for the cardiovascular consequences often seen in OSA. Conversely, while most attention on the pathogenesis of asthma has focused on the role of airway epithelial inflammation and smooth muscle hypertrophy,[74] asthma is also associated with vascular abnormalities that include increased number of capillaries in the bronchial walls, a process associated with vasodilation, capillary leak, and edema, contributing to airway constriction and microvascular remodeling.[75,76] Some investigators assessed plasma levels of endothelial microparticles, the membrane vesicles that are shed by endothelial cells during activation or apoptosis, in nonsmoker patients with asthma, and suggested a novel endotype of highly allergic asthma, with elevated IgE and eosinophil levels, which may have particularly high burden of endothelial activation and/or dysfunction.[77]

Airway Angiogenesis

Asthma is also associated with enhanced airway wall angiogenesis and microvascular remodeling.[75] These airway vascular abnormalities are associated with increased blood flow, microvascular permeability, and edema, contributing to the influx of inflammatory cells and airway narrowing. The increase in airway wall vascularity likely reflects a local increase in angiogenesis, an active process involving endothelial cell activation, proliferation, and apoptosis.[76] Some proposed that vascular endothelial growth factor (VEGF) might play a role in the pathogenesis of both asthma and OSA.[11] VEGF is a multifaceted, highly conserved cytokine, with a plethora of biological effects, including angiogenesis, carcinogenesis, and inflammation.[78] VEGF is a hypoxia-sensitive glycoprotein, and OSA and asthma can promote its expression.[40] VEGF may contribute to bronchial

inflammation, AHR, and vascular remodeling in those patients.[40] Although the relationship between the elevated VEGF levels in OSA and asthma is conceivable, no conclusive data are currently available.

Leptin

Leptin is a protein produced by adipose tissue, which circulates systemically and acts on the hypothalamus to induce satiety and increase metabolism.[79] Leptin was found elevated in OSA patients, without associated satiety, that is, the so-called leptin resistance phenomenon.[35] Furthermore, the evidence of local leptin production in the respiratory compartment supports the concept that leptin plays an important role in respiration, lung development, and in the pathogenesis of various respiratory disorders.[80] Coupled with the increased levels of serum leptin observed in OSA, the proinflammatory effects of leptin suggest that this hormone might also be relevant to asthma exacerbations in OSA.[80] This was supported by previous investigations, which showed that leptin might contribute to airway hyperresponsiveness.[81]

Fluid Shifts

Cao and colleagues[82,83] showed that generation of deep, negative intrathoracic pressures against occluded upper airway during OSAs increase intrathoracic fluid return and narrow small airways in individuals with asthma. The investigators simulated the effects of OSA by generating negative pleural pressures during Mueller maneuver (MM) to assess its effect on thoracic fluid volume (TFV) and on small airways. In both groups, TFV increased more with MM than during normal breathing. In the healthy group, no significant reactance changes were seen with either MM or normal breathing. In asthma patients, MM induced significantly greater narrowing of small airways than normal breathing, and these changes were also greater than those in healthy controls. The oscillometric changes induced by MM suggested small airway narrowing only in participants with asthma. This suggested that, while rostral fluid shift into the neck predisposes to OSA, fluid shift into the thorax induced by OSA comorbid with asthma may worsen the latter at night, by narrowing small airways and increasing airflow resistance.[82,83]

Chrono-Biologic Effects

Hypoxia increases the activity of HIF-1α, which in turn modulates expression of circadian clock genes. The balance between HIF-1α and CLOCK pathways can be altered in hypoxic states, including CIH of OSA.[84,85] Moreover, sleep and circadian rhythms become impaired with aging, which is very relevant for OSA pathogenesis in adults. Among changes seen with aging, HIF-1α induces a deficit in mitochondrial biogenesis, with impaired energy-dependent cellular processes, including tissue repair pathways.[86] Mitochondrial dysfunction can lead to the accumulation of reactive oxygen species, which can damage deoxyribonucleic acid (DNA) and disrupt circadian clock functions. The classical biological stressors that modulate mitochondrial protein acetylation include alterations in caloric levels and redox signaling, and the major enzyme orchestrating deacetylation is the mitochondrial-enriched sirtuin SIRT3. The SIRT3 modulates mitochondrial homeostasis and its target proteins include mediators of energy metabolism and mitochondrial redox stress adaptive program proteins.[87] Perturbation of such protein leads to inflammasome activation and to the chronic inflammation associated with aging known as inflammaging.[87] Inflammation, in turn, can activate the NF-κB transcription factor, which can repress the transcription of the clock genes; this process becomes a cycle, since the circadian clock regulates the expression of genes involved in DNA repair and in the oxidative stress response. In summary, emerging evidence suggests that sleep disorders, immunosenescence, inflammaging, and the effects of CIH are closely related and further studies are needed.

Obesity

Obesity is an established risk factor for both OSA and asthma. Approximately 60% of moderate-to-severe OSA cases are attributed to overweight or obesity.[88] Using data from a large cohort study, Peppard and colleagues[89] estimated that approximately 10% of weight gain increases AHI by 32%, while a 10% weight loss decreases AHI by 26%. Similarly, weight gain has been shown to increase the risk of asthma in adults.[90] Using data from National Health and Nutrition Examination Surgery, people gaining greater than 29 kg from young to middle adulthood had a 1.5 higher risk of asthma (95% CI 1.2–2.0) compared with those with stable weight (weight change $\leq$2.5 kg).[90] Weight loss interventions using diet and/or exercise, as well as bariatric surgery, have been shown to improve asthma control.[91–93] A meta-analysis of 6 randomized controlled trials (RCTs) of successful weight loss showed improved asthma-related quality of life, asthma control, and lung function (forced expiratory volume in 1 second [FEV$_1$], forced vital capacity [FVC], and total lung capacity).[94] Abdominal obesity and supine position during sleep lead

to a reduced functional residual capacity, which can diminish the longitudinal tracheal tug, increasing the propensity of the upper airway to collapse, hence a higher chance of developing or aggravating OSA.

Obesity appears to have a causal role in asthma too, as prospective studies show that obesity precedes asthma onset,[95–97] and weight gain is associated with the development of asthma in susceptible individuals.[96,98] Asthma risk is increased by 50% in overweight and obese individuals.[99] There are 2 predominant phenotypes of obese asthma, with significantly different inflammatory profiles[100] One of the phenotypes is represented by early-onset allergic asthma, which typically develops in childhood and is characterized by type 2 inflammation; obesity is not always present, but when it is, it aggravates asthma symptoms; this phenotype does not completely resolve with weight loss.[100] Late-onset nonatopic asthma is another phenotype, in which the disease onset is during adulthood, typically in older obese women, with non-T2 inflammation refractory to corticosteroids and more likely to resolve with weight loss.[100]

In obese asthma patients, weight loss is highly recommended. In uncontrolled studies, bariatric surgery improved asthma outcomes, including symptoms, medication use, and exacerbation rates.[101–103] In a 3-arm trial that randomized overweight or obese adults with asthma to either dietary intervention, exercise intervention, or both, it was found that 5% to 10% weight loss resulted in improved asthma control in 58% and better quality of life in 83% of participants, irrespective of the intervention.[92] In 1 outlier study, Forno and colleagues[104] demonstrated improvement in asthma control after bariatric surgery only in those who had metabolic syndrome. The overwhelming evidence, however, shows that weight loss improves asthma outcomes.[105]

Physical exercise and better diet are also good prescriptions for obese asthma patients, even without significant weight loss. Energy-dense, high-fat, and low-fiber diets are typically obesogenic[106] and proinflammatory.[107] Clinical intervention studies show that fatty acids induce airway inflammation,[108] while soluble fiber meals reduce airway inflammation and improve asthma control,[109,110] and high fruit and vegetable intake reduces exacerbation risk.[111,112] In addition to weight control, physical exercise has a broad range of benefits, including reduction in the all-cause mortality, cardiovascular disease, type 2 diabetes, depression, and cancer. Physical activity consistently decreases asthma exacerbation rates and health care utilization and improves asthma quality of life among all asthma subjects.[113,114] Freitas and colleagues[91] have shown that, independent of weight loss, asthma control can be improved in obese asthma patients via an exercise intervention, where a corresponding improvement in aerobic capacity is achieved.

Gastroesophageal Reflux Disorder

Several investigators found evidence of gastroesophageal reflux disorder (GERD) in 58% to 62% of patients with OSA.[35] One theory states that the significant drop in negative intrathoracic pressures caused by upper airway obstruction (similar to MM) can predispose to retrograde movement of gastric content.[115] An alternative theory states that arousals following respiratory events are associated with swallowing of saliva and upper airway secretions, which leads to a relaxation of the lower esophageal sphincter and distal esophageal gastric refluxate. Conversely, nocturnal GERD may lead to a higher arousal index, reduced sleep quantity and quality, plus laryngeal edema, all leading potentially to increased upper airway collapsibility. Conflicting data exist for these theories.[116] CPAP decreases GERD symptoms, implying that this treatment may be efficacious for both diseases.[117]

Epidemiologic data suggest that GERD occurs in 30% to 80% of asthma patients.[118] GERD may induce asthma directly by microaspiration, with respiratory mucosal injury by gastric (acid and pepsin) or duodenal (bile acids and trypsin) contents, and indirectly, via vagally mediated mechanisms to reflex bronchospasm.[35,119] Hence, it is thought that OSA-induced acid reflux may play a role in triggering asthma symptoms.[119] Esophageal manometry and a 24-hour esophageal pH testing demonstrate frequent GERD in the absence of overt symptoms in stable asthma patients,[120] although majority of subjects reported cough due to laryngopharyngeal reflux independent of other reflux symptoms.[121] Nevertheless, the association between these 3 conditions remains complex.[35]

Previous studies demonstrate variable associations of GERD with asthma severity and exacerbations.[105] In a cross-sectional study on 152 subjects, GERD was found a significant risk factor (OR 4.9, CI 1.4–17.8) for recurrent exacerbations after covariate adjustment.[17] Furthermore, GERD has been associated with exacerbation frequency in large asthma cohort studies.[122,123] Using data from the Severe Asthma Research Project, Denlinger and colleagues[123] found an increased rate of asthma exacerbations in those with GERD (RR 1.6, CI 1.3–2.0).

Upper Airway Disease

Chronic nasal obstruction is caused by anatomic factors (eg, septal deviation, nasal valve incompetence, craniofacial abnormalities) or by inflammatory disorders (eg, allergic or nonallergic rhinitis, chronic rhinosinusitis with or without polyps). A recent study found that ~ 35% of OSA patients have nasal obstruction ≥3 nights/week before PAP initiation, and that this subgroup reported more daytime sleepiness.[124] OSA patients also compute higher baseline scores for measures of sinonasal disease versus healthy controls.[125] Nasal passages account for greater than 50% of the total airway resistance.[126] Recumbent posture during sleep increases further nasal venous engorgement, leading to higher resistance and decreased airflow, a phenomenon augmented in patients with baseline congestion.[127] Several studies have found no association between nasal resistance and OSA, while others showed correlations between nasal resistance or volume and AHI or oxygen desaturation index, while Virkkula and colleagues[128] found this effect to be greater in nonobese subjects. Overall, the correlation between objective nasal resistance and subjective reports of nasal obstruction is poor.[129] The fact that upper airway obstruction is often a multilevel, dynamic collapse might explain why single-level nasal surgery is often unsuccessful.[130]

Microbiome

The microbiome is a complex ecosystem of bacteria, viruses, fungi, and such microorganisms, which coexists with the host and dynamically interacts with its cells and immune and metabolic processes.[131] Currently, most microbiome investigations focus on bacteria.[132,133] The effect of gut microbiome on the function of the respiratory system is complex.[131,133] Furthermore, common risk factors for lung disease (diet, pollution, smoking), or their physiologic correlates (hypoxemia, sleep fragmentation) may also alter the gut microbiome.

Intestinal microbiome itself may play a role in the development of atopic asthma.[134] According to the hygiene hypothesis, a secular reduction in infections in the Western world was accompanied by a rise in allergic and autoimmune diseases.[135] Indeed, germ-free mice exhibit predominantly a type 2 inflammatory phenotype[136] and have less CD4+ T cells in the lamina propria, with a higher Th2/Th1 ratio.[137]

Diet strongly influences the composition of the gut bacteriome.[138] It is known that due to fragmented sleep and leptin resistance, patients with OSA tend to consume high-calorie, carbohydrate-rich, and lipid-rich diets.[139] Sleep fragmentation and restriction, hallmarks of OSA, may also disrupt gut microbiome via an increase in appetite.[140]

Few studies have investigated intestinal microbiome in OSA.[141,142] Ko and colleagues[143] studied 93 adult patients with OSA and 20 controls, and found significant microbiome differences only at genus level, with decreased abundances of a few short-chain fatty acid (SCFA)–producing bacteria, which could lead to epithelial barrier disruption. The investigators also showed a significant relationship between *Prevotella* enterotype and OSA.[144] In a study on 60 OSA patients and 12 controls, abundances of several genera were lower in OSA, and SCFA-producing bacteria were in an inverse relationship with the presence of hypertension.[145] Bikov and colleagues[146] reported in OSA participants lower abundances of *Actinobacteria* phylum, bacteria which produce the sleep-promoting gamma-aminobutyric acid; therefore, low *Actinobacteria* could contribute to increased arousals in OSA. They also noted higher abundances of *Proteobacteria* phylum, which have been correlated with IL-6 levels.[147] Finally, Wang and colleagues[148] concluded that OSA was associated with increased ratios of *Firmicutes/Bacteroides* and decreased *Clostridium* XIVa.

Obstructive Sleep Apnea Treatment Effects

CPAP therapy, which acts a pneumatic split for the upper airway, has been shown to improve outcomes of the comorbid asthma, especially in severe OSA or in those with poorly controlled asthma.[149] In a survey of 1586 subjects on CPAP therapy for OSA, asthma was reported in 13% of cases.[150] Self-reported asthma severity and the use of rescue medication decreased with CPAP.[150] In a study of 20 adults with asthma and OSA, 6-week CPAP therapy improved AHI and quality of life, but not AHR.[151] In another study, on 100 people with asthma, 54%, 33%, and 13% had severe, moderate, or mild OSA, respectively.[152] After 3 months of CPAP, asthma control was good in 70% participants (vs 41% at baseline) and the Asthma Control Test (ACT) score improved.[152] In a prospective study of 99 adults with alternative overlap syndrome, CPAP improved Asthma Control Questionnaire score at 6 months, decreased percentage of uncontrolled asthma from 41% to 17%, reduced asthma exacerbation rate to 17% (from a baseline of 35% in the preceding 6 months), and increased asthma-specific quality of life.[153] In 37 subjects with asthma and OSA randomized to 3-month CPAP versus control, no differences in ACT score were seen between the 2 groups, but CPAP group had improved daytime sleepiness and better quality

of life scores.[154] While current evidence on the association between OSA, asthma, and PAP therapy relies heavily on data from observational studies, RCTs are urgently needed to understand the impact of PAP therapy and optimal PAP usage to achieve better asthma control. The use of alternative therapies for OSA, such as hypoglossal nerve stimulators, mandibular advancement devices, or surgery, versus asthma outcomes are also needed.

Several studies have shown that OSA may worsen pulmonary function in asthmatics, while its reversibility with CPAP is unclear. Body weight could partially explain a decline in pulmonary function in patients with OSA. A recent meta-analysis showed that %predicted FEV_1 (%FEV_1) was lower in adult asthma patients complicated with OSA, but the trend did not reach statistical significance.[155] In a case-control study of 30 asthma patients versus 12 age-matched, gender-matched, and BMI-matched controls, alternative overlap syndrome participants had higher BMI and lower %FEV_1 versus those with asthma alone.[156] In this study, higher BMI, GERD, and %FEV_1 were independent predictors of OSA. In a retrospective study of 466 subjects, there was a dose-dependent association between the decrease in FEV_1 and the increase in AHI.[157] The annual decline in FEV_1 was greater in those with severe OSA versus those with mild/moderate OSA or normal group; by contrast, BMI was not associated with an annual decline in FEV_1.[157] Good adherence to CPAP therapy also mitigated the FEV_1 decline in asthma patients with severe OSA. As such, mean decline in FEV_1 after CPAP use was 41 mL, significantly lower than before CPAP initiation, that is, 69 mL.[157] In a cohort of 4329 subjects followed for 10 years, FEV_1 and FVC declined more rapidly in subjects with high OSA risk versus those with low OSA risk.[158] These declines were associated with increased BMI between visits and OSA symptoms.[158] When the analysis was adjusted for weight changes, only those with asthma had a significant association between OSA symptom score and decline in lung function, suggesting that OSA may impact asthma outcomes independently of weight changes.[158]

While CPAP therapy has been shown to improve asthma symptoms and response to corticosteroid therapy,[159] little is known about the potential mechanisms underlying these observations. A recent study suggested that this may be mediated via a reduction in proinflammatory cytokines associated with asthma, thus improving responsiveness to corticosteroid therapy.[160] CPAP therapy reduced systemic inflammation in both patients with isolated OSA and in those with asthma plus OSA. IL-4 was higher at baseline in the OSA with asthma group versus OSA group. Its levels were significantly reduced in the OSA with asthma group following CPAP treatment.[160]

There is some conflicting evidence regarding whether PAP therapy attenuates AHR. Six-week CPAP therapy improved AHI, but not airway responsiveness, as measured by a provocation test in 20 adults with asthma and OSA.[151] A prospective study of 99 asthmatic adults with OSA reported a significantly reduced percentage of subjects with positive bronchodilator response after 6 months of CPAP therapy.[153] In 57 people with OSA and 13 controls, exhaled nitric oxide remained higher in OSA subjects versus controls, even after using CPAP therapy.[71] AHR to methacholine did not differ between OSA and controls at baseline, but increased after CPAP use.[71] In 16 asthmatic adults, CPAP use was associated with an enhanced bronchodilator response to albuterol and reduced AHR to methacholine.[161] Another study performed in stable asthma participants with normal spirometry showed reduced AHR to methacholine after CPAP use of only 7 days.[162]

Very limited evidence exists on the effects of alternative therapies for OSA on asthma. In a survey of subjects with asthma and OSA on oral appliances, 1-month of oral appliance therapy improved AHI and asthma control.[88] The lack of objective measurements of adherence and comparison with CPAP requires further investigation.

In summary, the clinical characteristics and the pathophysiological mechanisms underlying alternative overlap syndrome, that is, the association between asthma and OSA, are beginning to become clearer. We have reviewed here the main effects that OSA may exert on the inflammation seen in asthma, and how PAP therapy may ameliorate some of these abnormalities. At this point, we need to invest in good translational investigations from clinic to the laboratory, and back to the clinic or bedside, to elucidate the complex causal interactions in alternative overlap syndrome.

REFERENCES

1. Teodorescu M, Broytman O, Curran-Everett D, et al. Obstructive sleep apnea risk, asthma burden, and lower airway inflammation in adults in the severe asthma Research program (SARP) II. J Allergy Clin Immunol Pract 2015;3(4):566–575 e1.
2. Julien JY, Martin JG, Ernst P, et al. Prevalence of obstructive sleep apnea-hypopnea in severe versus moderate asthma. J Allergy Clin Immunol 2009;124(2):371–6.
3. Li X, Cao X, Guo M, et al. Trends and risk factors of mortality and disability adjusted life years for chronic respiratory diseases from 1990 to 2017: systematic analysis for the Global Burden of Disease Study 2017. BMJ 2020;368:m234.
4. Teodorescu M, Polomis DA, Teodorescu MC, et al. Association of obstructive sleep apnea risk or diagnosis with daytime asthma in adults. J Asthma 2012;49(6):620–8.
5. Teodorescu M, Polomis DA, Gangnon RE, et al. Sleep duration, asthma and obesity. J Asthma 2013;50(9):945–53.
6. Kim MY, Jo EJ, Kang SY, et al. Obstructive sleep apnea is associated with reduced quality of life in adult patients with asthma. Ann Allergy Asthma Immunol 2013;110(4):253–7, 257 e1.
7. Ioachimescu OC, Teodorescu M. Integrating the overlap of obstructive lung disease and obstructive sleep apnoea: OLDOSA syndrome. Respirology 2013;18(3):421–31.
8. Strausz S, Ruotsalainen S, Ollila HM, et al. Genetic analysis of obstructive sleep apnoea discovers a strong association with cardiometabolic health. Eur Respir J 2021;57(5):2003091.
9. Ioachimescu OC, Janocko NJ, Ciavatta MM, et al. Obstructive lung disease and obstructive sleep apnea (OLDOSA) cohort study: 10-year assessment. J Clin Sleep Med 2020;16(2):267–77.
10. Khatri SB, Ioachimescu OC. The intersection of obstructive lung disease and sleep apnea. Cleve Clin J Med 2016;83(2):127–40.
11. Puthalapattu S, Ioachimescu OC. Asthma and obstructive sleep apnea: clinical and pathogenic interactions. J Investig Med 2014;62(4):665–75.
12. Teodorescu M, Barnet JH, Hagen EW, et al. Association between asthma and risk of developing obstructive sleep apnea. JAMA 2015;313(2):156–64.
13. Bouloukaki I, Fanaridis M, Testelmans D, et al. Overlaps between obstructive sleep apnoea and other respiratory diseases, including COPD, asthma and interstitial lung disease. Breathe 2022;18(3):220073.
14. Ozden Mat D, Firat S, Aksu K, et al. Obstructive sleep apnea is a determinant of asthma control independent of smoking, reflux, and rhinitis. Allergy Asthma Proc 2021;42(1):e25–9.
15. Teodorescu M, Polomis DA, Hall SV, et al. Association of obstructive sleep apnea risk with asthma control in adult. Chest 2010;138(3):543–50.
16. Teodorescu M, Polomis DA, Gangnon RE, et al. Asthma control and its relationship with obstructive sleep apnea (OSA) in older adults. Sleep Disord 2013;2013:251567.
17. ten Brinke A, Sterk PJ, Masclee AA, et al. Risk factors of frequent exacerbations in difficult-to-treat asthma. Eur Respir J 2005;26(5):812–8.

18. Tay TR, Radhakrishna N, Hore-Lacy F, et al. Comorbidities in difficult asthma are independent risk factors for frequent exacerbations, poor control and diminished quality of life. Respirology 2016;21(8): 1384–90.

19. Jordan HT, Stellman SD, Reibman J, et al. Factors associated with poor control of 9/11-related asthma 10-11 years after the 2001 World Trade Center terrorist attacks. J Asthma 2015;52(6):630–7.

20. Wang Y, Liu K, Hu K, et al. Impact of obstructive sleep apnea on severe asthma exacerbations. Sleep Med 2016;26:1–5.

21. Yii ACA, Tan JHY, Lapperre TS, et al. Long-term future risk of severe exacerbations: distinct 5-year trajectories of problematic asthma. Allergy 2017; 72(9):1398–405.

22. Que Y, Meng H, Ding Y, et al. Investigation of the shared gene signatures and molecular mechanisms between obstructive sleep apnea syndrome and asthma. Gene 2023;896:148029.

23. Alvarez-Simon D, Ait Yahia S, de Nadai P, et al. NOD-like receptors in asthma. Front Immunol 2022;13:928886.

24. Clark DPQ, Son DB, Bowatte G, et al. The association between traffic-related air pollution and obstructive sleep apnea: a systematic review. Sleep Med Rev 2020;54:101360.

25. Wallace DA, Gallagher JP, Peterson SR, et al. Is exposure to chemical pollutants associated with sleep outcomes? A systematic review. Sleep Med Rev 2023;70:101805.

26. Zhang Q, Wang H, Zhu X, et al. Air pollution may increase the sleep apnea severity: a nationwide analysis of smart device-based monitoring. Innovation 2023;4(6):100528.

27. Wetter DW, Young TB, Bidwell TR, et al. Smoking as a risk factor for sleep-disordered breathing. Arch Intern Med 1994;154(19):2219–24.

28. Balagny P, Vidal-Petiot E, Renuy A, et al. Prevalence, treatment and determinants of obstructive sleep apnoea and its symptoms in a population-based French cohort. ERJ Open Res 2023;9(3). https://doi.org/10.1183/23120541.00053-2023.

29. Kim KS, Kim JH, Park SY, et al. Smoking induces oropharyngeal narrowing and increases the severity of obstructive sleep apnea syndrome. J Clin Sleep Med 2012;8(4):367–74.

30. Zhang L, Samet J, Caffo B, et al. Cigarette smoking and nocturnal sleep architecture. Am J Epidemiol 2006;164(6):529–37.

31. Mauries S, Bertrand L, Frija-Masson J, et al. Effects of smoking on sleep architecture and ventilatory parameters including apneas: results of the Tab-OSA study. Sleep Med X 2023;6:100085.

32. Benowitz NL, Kuyt F, Jacob P 3rd. Circadian blood nicotine concentrations during cigarette smoking. Clin Pharmacol Ther 1982;32(6):758–64.

33. Gothe B, Strohl KP, Levin S, et al. Nicotine: a different approach to treatment of obstructive sleep apnea. Chest 1985;87(1):11–7.

34. Wetter DW, Fiore MC, Baker TB, et al. Tobacco withdrawal and nicotine replacement influence objective measures of sleep. J Consult Clin Psycho 1995;63(4):658–67.

35. Antonaglia C. Obstructive sleep apnea syndrome (OSAS) and asthma: a simple association: a new syndrome or a cluster? J Biomed Res Environ Sci 2022;3:944–52.

36. Huxtable AG, Vinit S, Windelborn JA, et al. Systemic inflammation impairs respiratory chemoreflexes and plasticity. Respir Physiol Neurobiol 2011;178(3):482–9.

37. Edwards BA, Eckert DJ, McSharry DG, et al. Clinical predictors of the respiratory arousal threshold in patients with obstructive sleep apnea. Am J Respir Crit Care Med 2014;190(11):1293–300,

38. Antonaglia C, Passuti G, Giudici F, et al. Low arousal threshold: a common pathophysiological trait in patients with obstructive sleep apnea syndrome and asthma. Sleep Breath 2023;27(3): 933–41.

39. Gray EL, McKenzie DK, Eckert DJ. Obstructive sleep apnea without obesity is common and difficult to treat: evidence for a distinct pathophysiological phenotype. J Clin Sleep Med 2017;13(1): 81–8.

40. Alkhalil M, Schulman E, Getsy J. Obstructive sleep apnea syndrome and asthma: what are the links? J Clin Sleep Med 2009;5(1):71–8.

41. Ryan S, McNicholas WT. Intermittent hypoxia and activation of inflammatory molecular pathways in OSAS. Arch Physiol Biochem 2008;114(4):261–6.

42. Greenberg H, Ye X, Wilson D, et al. Chronic intermittent hypoxia activates nuclear factor-kappaB in cardiovascular tissues in vivo. Biochem Biophys Res Commun 2006;343(2):591–6.

43. Jelic S, Le Jemtel TH. Inflammation, oxidative stress, and the vascular endothelium in obstructive sleep apnea. Trends Cardiovasc Med 2008;18(7): 253–60.

44. Broytman O, Braun RK, Morgan BJ, et al. Effects of chronic intermittent hypoxia on allergen-induced airway inflammation in rats. Am J Respir Cell Mol Biol 2015;52(2):162–70.

45. Teodorescu M, Song R, Brinkman JA, et al. Chronic intermittent hypoxia increases airway hyperresponsiveness during house dust mites exposures in rats. Respir Res 2023;24(1):189.

46. Low T, Lin TY, Lin JY, et al. Airway hyperresponsiveness induced by intermittent hypoxia in rats. Respir Physiol Neurobiol 2022;295:103787.

47. Hatipoglu U, Rubinstein I. Inflammation and obstructive sleep apnea syndrome: how many ways do I look at thee? Chest 2004;126(1):1–2.

48. Paulsen FP, Steven P, Tsokos M, et al. Upper airway epithelial structural changes in obstructive sleep-disordered breathing. Am J Respir Crit Care Med 2002;166(4):501–9.

49. Zakkar M, Sekosan M, Wenig B, et al. Decrease in immunoreactive neutral endopeptidase in uvula epithelium of patients with obstructive sleep apnea. Ann Otol Rhinol Laryngol 1997;106(6):474–7.

50. Llorente Arenas EM, Vicente Gonzalez EA, Marin Trigo JM, et al. [Histologic changes in soft palate in patients with obstructive sleep apnea]. An Otorrinolaringol Ibero-Am 2001;28(5):467–76. Cambios histologicos en el paladar blando en pacientes con apnea obstructiva del sueno.

51. Boyd JH, Petrof BJ, Hamid Q, et al. Upper airway muscle inflammation and denervation changes in obstructive sleep apnea. Am J Respir Crit Care Med 2004;170(5):541–6.

52. Puig F, Rico F, Almendros I, et al. Vibration enhances interleukin-8 release in a cell model of snoring-induced airway inflammation. Sleep 2005; 28(10):1312–6.

53. Vicente E, Marin JM, Carrizo SJ, et al. Upper airway and systemic inflammation in obstructive sleep apnoea. Eur Respir J 2016;48(4):1108–17.

54. Wills-Karp M. Immunologic basis of antigen-induced airway hyperresponsiveness. Annu Rev Immunol 1999;17:255–81.

55. Decramer M, Rennard S, Troosters T, et al. COPD as a lung disease with systemic consequences–clinical impact, mechanisms, and potential for early intervention. COPD 2008;5(4):235–56.

56. Gozal D. Sleep, sleep disorders and inflammation in children. Sleep Med 2009;10(Suppl 1):S12–6.

57. McDonald VM, Simpson JL, Higgins I, et al. Multidimensional assessment of older people with asthma and COPD: clinical management and health status. Age Ageing 2011;40(1):42–9.

58. Venkayya R, Lam M, Willkom M, et al. The Th2 lymphocyte products IL-4 and IL-13 rapidly induce airway hyperresponsiveness through direct effects on resident airway cells. Am J Respir Cell Mol Biol 2002;26(2):202–8.

59. Spits H, Di Santo JP. The expanding family of innate lymphoid cells: regulators and effectors of immunity and tissue remodeling. Nat Immunol 2011;12(1):21–7.

60. Fitzpatrick AM, Chipps BE, Holguin F, et al. T2-"Low" asthma: overview and management strategies. J Allergy Clin Immunol Pract 2020;8(2):452–63.

61. Kuruvilla ME, Lee FE, Lee GB. Understanding asthma phenotypes, endotypes, and mechanisms of disease. Clin Rev Allergy Immunol 2019;56(2): 219–33.

62. McNicholas WT. Obstructive sleep apnea and inflammation. Prog Cardiovasc Dis 2009;51(5): 392–9.

63. Ryan S, Taylor CT, McNicholas WT. Systemic inflammation: a key factor in the pathogenesis of cardiovascular complications in obstructive sleep apnoea syndrome? Thorax 2009;64(7):631–6.

64. Inancli HM, Enoz M. Obstructive sleep apnea syndrome and upper airway inflammation. Recent Pat Inflamm Allergy Drug Discov 2010;4(1):54–7.

65. Kimoff RJ, Hamid Q, Divangahi M, et al. Increased upper airway cytokines and oxidative stress in severe obstructive sleep apnoea. Eur Respir J 2011;38(1):89–97.

66. Teichert T, Vossoughi M, Vierkotter A, et al. Investigating the spill-over hypothesis: analysis of the association between local inflammatory markers in sputum and systemic inflammatory mediators in plasma. Environ Res 2014;134:24–32.

67. Chua AP, Aboussouan LS, Minai OA, et al. Long-term continuous positive airway pressure therapy normalizes high exhaled nitric oxide levels in obstructive sleep apnea. J Clin Sleep Med 2013; 9(6):529–35.

68. Carpagnano GE, Kharitonov SA, Resta O, et al. 8-Isoprostane, a marker of oxidative stress, is increased in exhaled breath condensate of patients with obstructive sleep apnea after night and is reduced by continuous positive airway pressure therapy. Chest 2003;124(4):1386–92.

69. Goldbart AD, Krishna J, Li RC, et al. Inflammatory mediators in exhaled breath condensate of children with obstructive sleep apnea syndrome. Chest 2006;130(1):143–8.

70. Li AM, Hung E, Tsang T, et al. Induced sputum inflammatory measures correlate with disease severity in children with obstructive sleep apnoea. Thorax 2007;62(1):75–9.

71. Devouassoux G, Levy P, Rossini E, et al. Sleep apnea is associated with bronchial inflammation and continuous positive airway pressure-induced airway hyperresponsiveness. J Allergy Clin Immunol 2007;119(3):597–603.

72. Nadeem R, Molnar J, Madbouly EM, et al. Serum inflammatory markers in obstructive sleep apnea: a meta-analysis. J Clin Sleep Med 2013;9(10): 1003–12.

73. Reid MB, Lannergren J, Westerblad H. Respiratory and limb muscle weakness induced by tumor necrosis factor-alpha: involvement of muscle myofilaments. Am J Respir Crit Care Med 2002;166(4): 479–84.

74. Holgate ST, Wenzel S, Postma DS, et al. Asthma. Nat Rev Dis Primers 2015;1(1):15025.

75. Harkness LM, Ashton AW, Burgess JK. Asthma is not only an airway disease, but also a vascular disease. Pharmacol Ther 2015;148:17–33.

76. Watson EC, Grant ZL, Coultas L. Endothelial cell apoptosis in angiogenesis and vessel regression. Cell Mol Life Sci 2017;74(24):4387–403.

77. Strulovici-Barel Y, Kaner RJ, Crystal RG. High apoptotic endothelial microparticle levels measured in asthma with elevated IgE and eosinophils. Respir Res 2023;24(1):180.

78. Ferrara N, Gerber HP, LeCouter J. The biology of VEGF and its receptors. Nat Med 2003;9(6):669–76.

79. Jacono FJ, Mayer CA, Hsieh YH, et al. Lung and brainstem cytokine levels are associated with breathing pattern changes in a rodent model of acute lung injury. Respir Physiol Neurobiol 2011;178(3):429–38.

80. Taille C, Rouvel-Tallec A, Stoica M, et al. Obstructive sleep apnoea modulates airway inflammation and remodelling in severe asthma. PLoS One 2016;11(3):e0150042.

81. Sideleva O, Suratt BT, Black KE, et al. Obesity and asthma: an inflammatory disease of adipose tissue not the airway. Am J Respir Crit Care Med 2012;186(7):598–605.

82. Cao X, Bradley TD, Bhatawadekar SA, et al. Effect of simulated obstructive apnea on thoracic fluid volume and airway narrowing in asthma. Am J Respir Crit Care Med 2021;203(7):908–10.

83. Cao X, de Oliveira Francisco C, Bradley TD, et al. Association of obstructive apnea with thoracic fluid shift and small airways narrowing in asthma during sleep. Nat Sci Sleep 2022;14:891–9.

84. Hunyor I, Cook KM. Models of intermittent hypoxia and obstructive sleep apnea: molecular pathways and their contribution to cancer. Am J Physiol Regul Integr Comp Physiol 2018;315(4):R669–87.

85. Yang MY, Lin PW, Lin HC, et al. Alternations of circadian clock genes expression and oscillation in obstructive sleep apnea. J Clin Med 2019;8(10):1634.

86. Yuan Y, Cruzat VF, Newsholme P, et al. Regulation of SIRT1 in aging: roles in mitochondrial function and biogenesis. Mech Ageing Dev 2016;155:10–21.

87. Sack MN. The role of SIRT3 in mitochondrial homeostasis and cardiac adaptation to hypertrophy and aging. J Mol Cell Cardiol 2012;52(3):520–5.

88. Young T, Peppard PE, Taheri S. Excess weight and sleep-disordered breathing. J Appl Physiol 2005;99(4):1592–9.

89. Peppard PE, Young T, Palta M, et al. Longitudinal study of moderate weight change and sleep-disordered breathing. JAMA 2000;284(23):3015–21.

90. Wang T, Zhou Y, Kong N, et al. Weight gain from early to middle adulthood increases the risk of incident asthma later in life in the United States: a retrospective cohort study. Respir Res 2021;22(1):139.

91. Freitas PD, Ferreira PG, Silva AG, et al. The role of exercise in a weight-loss program on clinical control in obese adults with asthma. A randomized controlled trial. Am J Respir Crit Care Med 2017;195(1):32–42.

92. Scott HA, Gibson PG, Garg ML, et al. Dietary restriction and exercise improve airway inflammation and clinical outcomes in overweight and obese asthma: a randomized trial. Clin Exp Allergy 2013;43(1):36–49.

93. van Huisstede A, Rudolphus A, Castro Cabezas M, et al. Effect of bariatric surgery on asthma control, lung function and bronchial and systemic inflammation in morbidly obese subjects with asthma. Thorax 2015;70(7):659–67.

94. Okoniewski W, Lu KD, Forno E. Weight loss for children and adults with obesity and asthma. A systematic review of randomized controlled trials. Ann Am Thorac Socy 2019;16(5):613–25.

95. Shaheen SO, Sterne JA, Montgomery SM, et al. Birth weight, body mass index and asthma in young adults. Thorax 1999;54(5):396–402.

96. Camargo CA Jr, Weiss ST, Zhang S, et al. Prospective study of body mass index, weight change, and risk of adult-onset asthma in women. Arch Intern Med 1999;159(21):2582–8.

97. Guerra S, Sherrill DL, Bobadilla A, et al. The relation of body mass index to asthma, chronic bronchitis, and emphysema. Chest 2002;122(4):1256–63.

98. Beckett WS, Jacobs DR Jr, Yu X, et al. Asthma is associated with weight gain in females but not males, independent of physical activity. Am J Respir Crit Care Med 2001;164(11):2045–50.

99. Beuther DA, Sutherland ER. Overweight, obesity, and incident asthma: a meta-analysis of prospective epidemiologic studies. Am J Respir Crit Care Med 2007;175(7):661–6.

100. Bates JHT, Poynter ME, Frodella CM, et al. Pathophysiology to phenotype in the asthma of obesity. Ann Am Thorac Soc 2017;14(Supplement_5):S395–8.

101. Dixon JB, Chapman L, O'Brien P. Marked improvement in asthma after Lap-Band surgery for morbid obesity. Obes Surg 1999;9(4):385–9.

102. Dhabuwala A, Cannan RJ, Stubbs RS. Improvement in co-morbidities following weight loss from gastric bypass surgery. Obes Surg 2000;10(5):428–35.

103. Macgregor AM, Greenberg RA. Effect of surgically induced weight loss on asthma in the morbidly obese. Obes Surg 1993;3(1):15–21.

104. Forno E, Zhang P, Nouraie M, et al. The impact of bariatric surgery on asthma control differs among obese individuals with reported prior or current asthma, with or without metabolic syndrome. PLoS One 2019;14(4):e0214730.

105. Althoff MD, Ghincea A, Wood LG, et al. Asthma and three colinear comorbidities: obesity, OSA, and GERD. J Allergy Clin Immunol Pract 2021;9(11):3877–84.

106. Jessri M, Wolfinger RD, Lou WY, et al. Identification of dietary patterns associated with obesity in a nationally representative survey of Canadian adults: application of a priori, hybrid, and simplified dietary pattern techniques. Am J Clin Nutr 2017; 105(3):669–84.

107. Wood LG. Diet, obesity, and asthma. Ann Am Thorac Soc 2017;14(Supplement_5):S332–8.

108. Wood LG, Garg ML, Gibson PG. A high-fat challenge increases airway inflammation and impairs bronchodilator recovery in asthma. J Allergy Clin Immunol 2011;127(5):1133–40.

109. Halnes I, Baines KJ, Berthon BS, et al. Soluble fibre meal challenge reduces airway inflammation and expression of GPR43 and GPR41 in asthma. Nutrients 2017;9(1):57.

110. McLoughlin R, Berthon BS, Rogers GB, et al. Soluble fibre supplementation with and without a probiotic in adults with asthma: a 7-day randomised, double blind, three way cross-over trial. EBioMedicine 2019;46:473–85.

111. Wood LG, Garg ML, Powell H, et al. Lycopene-rich treatments modify noneosinophilic airway inflammation in asthma: proof of concept. Free Radic Res 2008;42(1):94–102.

112. Wood LG, Garg ML, Smart JM, et al. Manipulating antioxidant intake in asthma: a randomized controlled trial. Am J Clin Nutr 2012;96(3):534–43.

113. Nyenhuis SM, Dixon AE, Ma J. Impact of lifestyle interventions targeting healthy diet, physical activity, and weight loss on asthma in adults: what is the evidence? J Allergy Clin Immunol Pract 2018;6(3): 751–63.

114. Panagiotou M, Koulouris NG, Rovina N. Physical activity: a missing link in asthma care. J Clin Med 2020;9(3):706.

115. Fahy JV. Type 2 inflammation in asthma–present in most, absent in many. Nat Rev Immunol 2015; 15(1):57–65.

116. Lim KG, Morgenthaler TI, Katzka DA. Sleep and nocturnal gastroesophageal reflux: an update. Chest 2018;154(4):963–71.

117. Tawk M, Goodrich S, Kinasewitz G, et al. The effect of 1 week of continuous positive airway pressure treatment in obstructive sleep apnea patients with concomitant gastroesophageal reflux. Chest 2006;130(4):1003–8.

118. Sandur V, Murugesh M, Banait V, et al. Prevalence of gastro-esophageal reflux disease in patients with difficult to control asthma and effect of proton pump inhibitor therapy on asthma symptoms, reflux symptoms, pulmonary function and requirement for asthma medications. J Postgrad Med 2014;60(3):282–6.

119. Murugesan N, Saxena D, Dileep A, et al. Update on the role of FeNO in asthma management. Diagnostics 2023;13(8):1428.

120. Harding SM, Guzzo MR, Richter JE. The prevalence of gastroesophageal reflux in asthma patients without reflux symptoms. Am J Respir Crit Care Med 2000;162(1):34–9.

121. Harding SM, Guzzo MR, Richter JE. 24-h esophageal pH testing in asthmatics: respiratory symptom correlation with esophageal acid events. Chest 1999;115(3):654–9.

122. Denlinger LC, Phillips BR, Ramratnam S, et al. Inflammatory and comorbid features of patients with severe asthma and frequent exacerbations. Am J Respir Crit Care Med 2017;195(3):302–13.

123. Blakey JD, Price DB, Pizzichini E, et al. Identifying risk of future asthma attacks using UK medical record data: a respiratory effectiveness group initiative. J Allergy Clin Immunol Pract 2017;5(4): 1015–1024 e8.

124. Varendh M, Andersson M, Bjornsdottir E, et al. Nocturnal nasal obstruction is frequent and reduces sleep quality in patients with obstructive sleep apnea. J Sleep Res 2018;27(4):e12631.

125. Moxness MHS, Bugten V, Thorstensen WM, et al. Sinonasal characteristics in patients with obstructive sleep apnea compared to healthy controls. Int J Otolaryngol 2017;2017:1935284.

126. Ferris BG Jr, Mead J, Opie LH. Partitioning of respiratory flow resistance in man. J Appl Physiol 1964;19:653–8.

127. Calvo-Henriquez C, Chiesa-Estomba C, Lechien JR, et al. The recumbent position affects nasal resistance: a systematic review and meta-analysis. Laryngoscope 2022;132(1):6–16.

128. Virkkula P, Maasilta P, Hytonen M, et al. Nasal obstruction and sleep-disordered breathing: the effect of supine body position on nasal measurements in snorers. Acta Otolaryngol 2003;123(5): 648–54.

129. Stewart MG, Smith TL. Objective versus subjective outcomes assessment in rhinology. Am J Rhinol 2005;19(5):529–35.

130. Schoustra E, van Maanen P, den Haan C, et al. The role of isolated nasal surgery in obstructive sleep apnea therapy-A systematic review. Brain Sci 2022;12(11):1446.

131. Cho I, Blaser MJ. The human microbiome: at the interface of health and disease. Nat Rev Genet 2012;13(4):260–70.

132. Enaud R, Prevel R, Ciarlo E, et al. The gut-lung Axis in health and respiratory diseases: a place for inter-organ and inter-kingdom crosstalks. Front Cell Infect Microbiol 2020;10:9.

133. Bingula R, Filaire M, Radosevic-Robin N, et al. Desired turbulence? Gut-lung Axis, immunity, and lung cancer. J Oncol 2017;2017:5035371.

134. Frati F, Salvatori C, Incorvaia C, et al. The role of the microbiome in asthma: the Gut(-)Lung Axis. Int J Mol Sci 2018;20(1):123.

135. Okada H, Kuhn C, Feillet H, et al. The 'hygiene hypothesis' for autoimmune and allergic diseases: an update. Clin Exp Immunol 2010;160(1):1–9.

136. Herbst T, Sichelstiel A, Schar C, et al. Dysregulation of allergic airway inflammation in the absence of microbial colonization. Am J Respir Crit Care Med 2011;184(2):198–205.

137. Huang YJ, Boushey HA. The microbiome in asthma. J Allergy Clin Immunol 2015;135(1):25–30.

138. Singh RK, Chang HW, Yan D, et al. Influence of diet on the gut microbiome and implications for human health. J Transl Med 2017;15(1):73.

139. Gileles-Hillel A, Kheirandish-Gozal L, Gozal D. Biological plausibility linking sleep apnoea and metabolic dysfunction. Nat Rev Endocrinol 2016;12(5):290–8.

140. Poroyko VA, Carreras A, Khalyfa A, et al. Chronic sleep disruption alters gut microbiota, induces systemic and adipose tissue inflammation and insulin resistance in mice. Sci Rep 2016;6:35405.

141. Collado MC, Katila MK, Vuorela NM, et al. Dysbiosis in snoring children: an interlink to comorbidities? J Pediatr Gastroenterol Nutr 2019;68(2):272–7.

142. Valentini F, Evangelisti M, Arpinelli M, et al. Gut microbiota composition in children with obstructive sleep apnoea syndrome: a pilot study. Sleep Med 2020;76:140–7.

143. Ko CY, Liu QQ, Su HZ, et al. Gut microbiota in obstructive sleep apnea-hypopnea syndrome: disease-related dysbiosis and metabolic comorbidities. Clin Sci (Lond) 2019;133(7):905–17.

144. Ko CY, Fan JM, Hu AK, et al. Disruption of sleep architecture in Prevotella enterotype of patients with obstructive sleep apnea-hypopnea syndrome. Brain Behav 2019;9(5):e01287.

145. Ko CY, Su HZ, Zhang L, et al. Disturbances of the gut microbiota, sleep architecture, and mTOR signaling pathway in patients with severe obstructive sleep apnea-associated hypertension. Int J Hypertens 2021;2021:9877053.

146. Yunes RA, Poluektova EU, Dyachkova MS, et al. GABA production and structure of gadB/gadC genes in Lactobacillus and Bifidobacterium strains from human microbiota. Anaerobe 2016;42:197–204.

147. Smith RP, Easson C, Lyle SM, et al. Gut microbiome diversity is associated with sleep physiology in humans. PLoS One 2019;14(10):e0222394.

148. Wang F, Liu Q, Wu H, et al. The dysbiosis gut microbiota induces the alternation of metabolism and imbalance of Th17/Treg in OSA patients. Arch Microbiol 2022;204(4):217.

149. Davies SE, Bishopp A, Wharton S, et al. Does Continuous Positive Airway Pressure (CPAP) treatment of obstructive sleep apnoea (OSA) improve asthma-related clinical outcomes in patients with co-existing conditions?- A systematic review. Respir Med 2018;143:18–30.

150. Kauppi P, Bachour P, Maasilta P, et al. Long-term CPAP treatment improves asthma control in patients with asthma and obstructive sleep apnoea. Sleep Breath 2016;20(4):1217–24.

151. Lafond C, Series F, Lemiere C. Impact of CPAP on asthmatic patients with obstructive sleep apnoea. Eur Respir J 2007;29(2):307–11.

152. Cisneros C, Iturricastillo G, Martinez-Besteiro E, et al. Obstructive sleep apnea: the key for a better asthma control? Sleep Med 2023;101:135–7.

153. Serrano-Pariente J, Plaza V, Soriano JB, et al. Asthma outcomes improve with continuous positive airway pressure for obstructive sleep apnea. Allergy 2017;72(5):802–12.

154. Ng SSS, Chan TO, To KW, et al. Continuous positive airway pressure for obstructive sleep apnoea does not improve asthma control. Respirology 2018;23(11):1055–62.

155. Wang D, Zhou Y, Chen R, et al. The relationship between obstructive sleep apnea and asthma severity and vice versa: a systematic review and meta-analysis. Eur J Med Res 2023;28(1):139.

156. Zidan M, Daabis R, Gharraf H. Overlap of obstructive sleep apnea and bronchial asthma: effect on asthma control. Egypt J Chest Dis Tuberc 2015;64:425–30.

157. Wang TY, Lo YL, Lin SM, et al. Obstructive sleep apnoea accelerates FEV(1) decline in asthmatic patients. BMC Pulm Med 2017;17(1):55.

158. Emilsson OI, Sundbom F, Ljunggren M, et al. Association between lung function decline and obstructive sleep apnoea: the ALEC study. Sleep Breath 2021;25(2):587–96.

159. Yim S, Fredberg JJ, Malhotra A. Continuous positive airway pressure for asthma: not a big stretch? Eur Respir J 2007;29(2):226–8.

160. Mahboub B, Kharaba Z, Ramakrishnan RK, et al. Continuous positive airway pressure therapy suppresses inflammatory cytokines and improves glucocorticoid responsiveness in patients with obstructive sleep apnea and asthma: a case-control study. Ann Thorac Med 2022;17(3):166–72.

161. Lin HC, Wang CH, Yang CT, et al. Effect of nasal continuous positive airway pressure on methacholine-induced bronchoconstriction. Respir Med 1995;89(2):121–8.

162. Busk M, Busk N, Puntenney P, et al. Use of continuous positive airway pressure reduces airway reactivity in adults with asthma. Eur Respir J 2013;41(2):317–22.

Obstructive Sleep Apnea Effects on Chronic Airway Disease Exacerbations—Missed Opportunities for Improving Outcomes in Chronic Obstructive Pulmonary Disease and Asthma

Marta Marin-Oto, MD[a], Jose M. Marin, MD[b],*

KEYWORDS

- Sleep • Obstructive sleep apnea • Chronic obstructive pulmonary disease • Overlap syndrome
- Chronic obstructive pulmonary disease exacerbation • Asthma • Asthma exacerbation

KEY POINTS

- Obstructive sleep apnea (OSA), asthma, and chronic obstructive pulmonary disease (COPD) are the most prevalent respiratory disorders.
- COPD and asthma exacerbations are fundamental health outcomes in the prognosis of both entities.
- OSA is an independent risk factor to explain the increased prevalence and severity of exacerbations in COPD and asthma.
- In cases of OSA/COPD or OSA/asthma syndrome, continuous positive airway pressure treatment can reduce COPD and asthma exacerbations. This treatment should be indicated in accordance with the available OSA management guidelines.

KEY/ESSENTIAL HEADINGS: OBSTRUCTIVE SLEEP APNEA AND CHRONIC AIRWAY DISEASE EXACERBATIONS

Introduction

Chronic obstructive pulmonary disease (COPD), bronchial asthma, and obstructive sleep apnea (OSA) constitute the 3 most prevalent chronic respiratory diseases worldwide. Using the Global Initiative for Chronic Obstructive Lung Disease (GOLD) definition of COPD (forced expiratory volume during the first second (FEV_1)/forced vital capacity (FVC) < 0.7), the current prevalence of COPD is estimated between 9% and 12%.[1] In a recent modeling study, it is projected that COPD prevalence will increase by 23% from now to 2050 especially among women and in low-to-middle–income countries.[2] Asthma prevalence data reported around the world are highly variable, probably because the diagnosis of asthma largely falls on an exclusively clinical definition without the need for confirmation with a specific complementary test. In the United States,

[a] Respiratory Department, University of Zaragoza School of Medicine, Hospital Clínico Universitario, San Juan Bosco 15, Zaragoza 50009, Spain; [b] Department of Medicine, University of Zaragoza School of Medicine, Hospital Universitario Miguel Servet, Domingo Miral, s/n, Zaragoza 50009, Spain
* Corresponding author.
E-mail address: jmmarint@unizar.es

Sleep Med Clin 19 (2024) 275–282
https://doi.org/10.1016/j.jsmc.2024.02.007
1556-407X/24/

using Behavioral Risk Factor Surveillance System data, it was estimated that in 2020, 9% of adults had been diagnosed with asthma.[3] In the case of OSA, the prevalence depends on the cutoff of the apnea-hypopnea index (AHI) that is considered for its diagnosis. Considering AHI cutoffs greater than 5, OSA figures could currently be around 50% of the adult population in the United States.[4] It is evident that the high prevalence of these 3 entities separately implies the frequent coincidence of COPD/OSA and asthma/OSA in the same patient. However, no population-based epidemiologic studies have been carried out to accurately estimate the prevalence of these overlap syndromes in the general population. In any case, it is noteworthy that more than 80% of patients with COPD or OSA are not diagnosed and therefore adequately treated.[1,4] This has important consequences for health outcomes of patients suffering from these overlap syndromes.

COPD and asthma exacerbations, especially if they require hospitalization, are associated with considerable morbidity and mortality and are the main components of the health care costs due to these diseases worldwide.[1,5] In this article, the authors review the role of the coexistence of OSA as an aggravating factor to develop exacerbations in patients with asthma or COPD, and how the treatment of OSA can efficiently modify health outcomes of these respiratory diseases.

Definitions

At present, we suspect COPD when a patient presents with respiratory symptoms and a history of risk for COPD (eg, exposure to tobacco smoke or other toxic inhalants). In these cases, spirometry confirms the diagnosis if the post-bronchodilator ratio FEV_1/FVC is less than 0.7.[1] On the other hand, according to the Global Initiative for Asthma (GINA), the diagnosis of asthma is defined as the history of respiratory symptoms that vary in intensity and over time together with variable expiratory airflow limitation.[5] There is no global agreement on how to define OSA, but we mostly understand that a patient suffers from OSA when he/she shows more than 5 apneas or hypopneas per hour of sleep (AHI) in a sleep study.[5] We define the coincidence of OSA in patients with COPD or asthma as COPD/OSA and asthma/OSA overlap syndromes, respectively.[1,5] Both, COPD and asthma are chronic inflammatory bronchopulmonary diseases. In asthma, inflammation is mostly limited to the airways and airway obstruction is characteristically variable in most patients. In COPD, pulmonary inflammation is also associated with airway remodeling, peribronchial fibrosis, destruction of alveolar airspace (emphysema), and

vascular changes with a wide variation among patients.[6] The final consequences of these changes lead to a persistent airflow limitation and impaired functional capacity. A differential aspect between asthma and COPD is the evidence that the latter is associated with frequent comorbidities that will develop at younger ages compared to subjects without COPD.[7]

As defined by the GOLD initiative, an acute exacerbation of COPD (AECOPD) is a clinical event characterized by increased dyspnea and/or cough and sputum that worsens in less than 14 days which may be accompanied by tachypnea and/or tachycardia and is often associated with increased local and systemic inflammation caused by infection, pollution, or other insult to the airways.[1] Asthma exacerbations are episodes characterized by a progressive increase in respiratory symptoms such as dyspnea, cough, wheezing, or chest tightness and a progressive decrease in lung function; they represent a change from the patient's usual status that is sufficient to require a change in treatment.[5]

LINK BETWEEN OBSTRUCTIVE SLEEP APNEA AND CHRONIC OBSTRUCTIVE PULMONARY DISEASE

In patients with COPD, some frequent comorbid conditions are also OSA risk factors (**Fig. 1**). One-third of patients with COPD are active smokers and another 50% are ex-smokers. Patients who are active smokers have more upper airway inflammation and collapsibility than nonsmokers.[8] In a cross-sectional study, cigarette smoking history was associated with early onset of OSA and AHI increased as mean pack-years increased.[9] Therefore, tobacco is a determinant of the pathogenesis

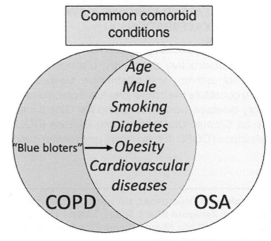

Fig. 1. Risk factors and comorbidities shared by patients with chronic obstructive pulmonary disease (COPD) and obstructive sleep apnea (OSA).

of both entities, COPD and OSA. Quitting tobacco smoking results in a deceleration in disease progression and reduces the risk of exacerbations in smokers with COPD.[10]

Unlike in OSA, obesity is not a risk factor for developing COPD. However, a specific phenotype of a COPD patient, bloated, bronchitic, overweight, and sleepy, has been defined for decades. This is the typical "blue bloater" patient who characteristically shows a tendency toward hypoxemia and carbon dioxide retention and who, we now know, most of the time suffers from OSA.[11] In contrast, there is an inverse relationship between AHI and the percentage of emphysema, which is preferably found in thin COPD patients.[12] As the disease progresses, many COPD patients develop fluid retention as a consequence of the administration of systemic corticosteroids or the development of right heart failure. At night, fluid retention contributes to rostral redistribution into the neck, peripharyngeal fluid accumulation, and upper airway narrowing, thereby facilitating OSA.[13] Some therapies for COPD such as systemic steroids may produce accumulation of fat in the parapharyngeal tissues and myopathies of the pharyngeal muscles, which increased upper airway collapsibility.[14] Today, a clear understanding of the pathophysiological links between OSA and COPD remains elusive. However, in patients with COPD-OSA overlap, clinical outcomes are poorer than in either disease alone.

LINK BETWEEN OBSTRUCTIVE SLEEP APNEA AND ASTHMA

OSA increases asthma burden and is associated with poor asthma control.[5] Independent of obesity and other confounders, it appears that OSA aggravates asthma through non-eosinophilic inflammatory pathways.[15] GINA recognized the importance of OSA as a comorbid condition for an appropriate management of this disease, and they recommended performing a sleep study to investigate the coexistence of OSA in patients with severe asthma, difficult-to-control asthma, and asthma associated with obesity.[5]

Obesity is the most common risk factor for OSA, but it is also a risk factor for asthma with a "dose-response" effect of increasing body mass index (BMI), which at the same time can increase the risk of incident asthma, especially in women.[16] OSA is very common in patients with chronic rhinosinusitis and nasopharyngeal polyps because they lead to increasing intrathoracic and pharyngeal negative pressure, which promotes upper airway collapse.[17] Many patients with non-atopic asthma and most patients with atopic asthma suffer from nasal problems including chronic rhinosinusitis and nasal polyps.

Therefore, it is possible that asthmatics with this type of chronic nasal pathology simultaneously present with OSA, and it is advisable to rule out the coexistence of OSA through a sleep study in patients with a rapid evolution of their asthma. Another risk for OSA among some asthmatics is the need for frequent bursts or continuous use of oral steroids. This treatment can augment the tendency to obesity in addition to producing accumulation of fat in the parapharyngeal tissues and myopathies of the pharyngeal muscles, as in COPD.[18]

RISK FACTORS FOR CHRONIC OBSTRUCTIVE PULMONARY DISEASE EXACERBATIONS

One of the main objectives of COPD management is to avoid AECOPDs. This is because exacerbations accelerate the lung function decline, worsen patients' quality of life, and increase mortality.[19] In general, as patients with COPD progress in their natural history, they present an increase in AECOPDs. However, there is a great interindividual variability in the frequency and severity of exacerbations. There are well-established risk factors for AECOPDs such as being an active smoker,[20] being exposed to a polluted environment,[21] or having a history of previous exacerbations[22] (**Fig. 2**). Risk factors for AECOPDs related to the characteristics of the disease itself include greater functional impairment,[23] emphysema on chest computed tomography,[24] and the coexistence of pulmonary hypertension.[25] COPD patients who have a chronic bronchitic phenotype[26] or coexistent bronchiectasis[27] also are at increased risk of AECOPDs. Among the many blood biomarkers studies carried out in recent years, it has been shown that a higher level of eosinophils is associated with a greater risk of exacerbations and are predictors of a better therapeutic response to inhaled corticosteroids.[28–30]

As stated earlier, patients with COPD suffer more comorbidities and at a younger age than subjects in the population without COPD.[7] Among more than 72 comorbidities significantly present in patients with COPD compared to subjects without COPD, there is a group of 12 entities ("comorbidome") that are associated with a greater risk of exacerbations and death.[31] An exhaustive review of each comorbid condition is not the purpose of this article.

OBSTRUCTIVE SLEEP APNEA AS A RISK FACTOR FOR CHRONIC OBSTRUCTIVE PULMONARY DISEASE EXACERBATIONS
Obesity

Underweight and overweight are important predictors of poor outcomes in COPD. In the Genetic

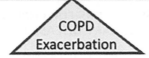

Aggravating factors:	Protective factors:
• Previous exacerbations • Active smoking • Air pollution • More severe COPD • Bronchitic phenotype • Emphysema • Higher eosinophils • Comorbidities (OSA)	• Smoking cessation • Vaccination • Pharmacotherapy • Oxygen therapy • Education • Physical activity • Good management of comorbidities (OSA)

COPD Exacerbation

Fig. 2. Aggravating and protective factors for chronic obstructive pulmonary disease (COPD) exacerbation. OSA, obstructive sleep apnea.

Epidemiology of COPD (COPDGene) study, a large multicenter cohort of subjects with GOLD stages 2 through 4 COPD, increasing severity of obesity was associated independently with greater odds of AECOPDs.[32] In 1 retrospective study, Goto and colleagues showed that COPD patients undergoing bariatric surgery had a reduced risk of hospitalization for AECOPDs.[33] However, at baseline, sleep study was not performed in these studies so OSA cannot be ruled out and therefore the specific role of obesity with/without OSA on incident AECOPD could not be assessed. The intermediate mechanisms that explain the increase of AECOPD with obesity and its reduction with bariatric surgery have not been established. It is known that obesity and associated metabolic dysfunction increase the levels of circulating inflammatory biomarkers such as white blood cell count, C-reactive protein, and fibrinogen levels which are characteristically elevated in patients with frequent COPD exacerbations.[34] On the other hand, obesity reduces the lung's defense capacity against viruses and bacteria.[35,36] Therefore, it is possible that weight loss reduces exacerbations in patients with obesity (with/without associated OSA) by restoring immune function against respiratory infections (**Fig. 3**). In any case, the relationship between obesity and AECOPDs is far from being elucidated given that some randomized control trials (RCTs) have shown that overweight or obese patients do not have an increased risk of AECOPD as compared to normal weight COPD patients.[37] But again, no sleep studies were done in those RCTs to identify the coexistence of OSA in obese participants.

Obstructive Sleep Apnea

Few studies have evaluated if COPD patients with OSA (overlap syndrome), with or without associated obesity, have more risk of exacerbations than COPD without OSA. In our observational cohort which includes subjects referred for evaluation of suspected OSA, spirometry in addition to sleep study was performed at baseline and patients were treated accordingly based on current OSA and COPD guidelines.[38] Three groups were pre-specified: OSA with continuous positive airway pressure (CPAP), OSA without CPAP, and COPD alone. All 3 groups had similar markers of COPD severity. After a mean of 9.6-year follow-

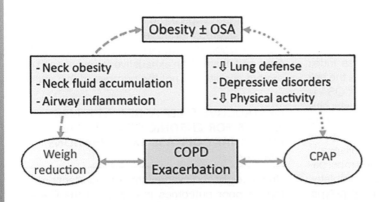

Fig. 3. Intermediate mechanism in obesity and obstructive sleep apnea (OSA) as a risk factor for chronic obstructive pulmonary disease (COPD) exacerbations. CPAP, continuous positive airway pressure.

up, at least 1 hospitalization because of COPD exacerbation occurred in 39.5% patients with COPD alone and in 61.4% patients with COPD/OSA overlap untreated with positive airway pressure (PAP) (adjusted relative risk, 1.70 [95% confidence interval (CI), 1.21–2.38]). These patients also had a greater risk of hospital readmission. In line with these results, a recent retrospective study showed that among patients hospitalized for COPD exacerbation, those with OSA had higher readmission and mortality rates than those without OSA.[39] Finally, among COPD patients included in the Long-Term Oxygen Treatment Trial, those at intermediate to high risk of OSA (modified STOP-BANG [snoring history, tiredness during the day, observed apnea, high blood pressure, BMI>35 kg/m2 (or 30 kg/m2), age>50 years, neck circumference>40 cm, and gender (male)] score ≥ 3) relative to low risk (score<3) had increased frequency of COPD exacerbations (adjusted incidence rate ratio: 1.78, 95% CI, 1.10–2.89).[40] This evidence, however, is considered insufficient by the GOLD to recommend performing sleep studies in all patients with COPD who are admitted for an exacerbation. However, this initiative advocates for the assessment of OSA-specific sleep symptoms among patients with severe COPD.[1]

Observational and population studies also suggest that the increased risk for AECOPDs in patients with overlap syndrome may be mitigated with PAP.[38,40–43] For example, in our mentioned prospective clinical-based study, patients with overlap syndrome treated with CPAP had no increased risk for severe exacerbations compared with patients with COPD only.[38] In addition, overlap patients treated with CPAP had a reduction of mortality. A lower risk of AECOPDs was also obtained in retrospective studies of COPD/OSA overlap patients engaged in Health Plans and Medicare that were treated or not treated with CPAP.[40,42] In these studies, the impact on mortality was not assessed. These real-life studies in any case indicate "association" and not "causation" of the effect of CPAP on the reduction of exacerbations in patients with overlap syndrome. Given the impact of AECOPDs on health care cost and on the progression of the disease, it is fully justified to confirm these findings through a randomized trial. Also, because bilevel positive airway pressure therapy is widely used for severe AECOPDs and for stable hypercapnic COPD patients, this form of PAP therapy should be evaluated in OSA/COPD overlap syndrome.

OSA is associated with a number of factors that may favor AECOPDs in patients with overlap syndrome. Characteristically, in patients with OSA, diabetes and metabolic syndrome are more prevalent, and it is known that these comorbidities favor the development of AECOPDs.[44] In OSA, depressive disorders are frequent and related with the OSA severity.[45] Similarly, anxiety or depression in COPD patients is also a risk factor for AECOPDs.[46] Daytime sleepiness and fatigue are not frequent in COPD alone but in those with overlap syndrome, these daytime symptoms can decrease physical activity and worsen health outcomes.[47] What is very relevant when recognizing the presence of these intermediate mechanisms that aggravate the risk of AECOPDs is that many of them are reversed by weight reduction and/or with CPAP treatment in cases of overlap syndrome. This is what happens with the improvement of diabetes[48] and anxiety/depression[49] with CPAP therapy in OSA patients, but it remains to be clarified whether this beneficial effect of CPAP also occurs in patients with overlap syndrome.

OBSTRUCTIVE SLEEP APNEA AS A RISK FACTOR FOR ASTHMA EXACERBATIONS

The main trigger for asthma exacerbations are external agents such as microorganisms, pollens, or pollutants. However, these episodes are more frequent in patients with uncontrolled asthma symptoms or with poor adherence to appropriate therapy and/or significant comorbidities.[5] Among the comorbidities that increase the risk of exacerbations, the GINA consensus points to obesity, chronic rhinosinusitis, and gastroesophageal reflux.[5] Interestingly, these comorbidities are also very common in subjects with OSA and therefore, in patients with OSA/asthma overlap, they may act as potentiating mechanisms of asthmatic exacerbations.

In a large observational series of patients with asthma, logistic regression analysis on comorbid factors shows that psychological dysfunction (odd ratio [OR] 10.8), recurrent respiratory tract infections (OR 6.9), gastroesophageal reflux (OR 4.9), severe nasal sinus disease (OR 3.7), and OSA (OR 3.4) were significantly associated with frequent exacerbations.[50] These results are not surprising since it is known that snoring and OSA trigger nocturnal asthma attacks in patients with OSA/asthma.[51] In the World Trade Center Health Registry, among patients with asthma there was a higher OSA prevalence with worse asthma control adjusting for BMI.[52] Among Chinese patients with asthma, OSA was associated with higher risk of severe asthma exacerbations compare to non-OSA asthmatics (relative risk 14.23).[53] The intermediate mechanisms by which OSA may worsen the health outcomes of people with asthma are unknown. The authors previously demonstrated that OSA is associated with upper airway inflammation as evidenced by an increase in inflammatory biomarkers obtained from pharyngeal lavage.[54] This fact is in agreement with a high fraction of exhaled nitric oxide level obtained in untreated OSA patients.[55] Of interest is that these airway inflammatory markers were reduced with CPAP treatment in both studies.

CPAP therapy in patients with OSA/asthma overlap syndrome appears to improve quality of life, especially in severe OSA and poorly controlled asthma.[56] However, evidence is mainly derived from observational studies of short duration. In fact, a meta-analysis found CPAP improved daytime or nighttime asthma symptoms but did not show an improvement in asthma control or asthma exacerbations.[57] Currently, the effect of CPAP on the health outcomes in patients with asthma and OSA has not been elucidated and randomized trials are necessary to definitively evaluate this effect. Till there is further understanding of this relationship between OSA and asthma, in patients with OSA/asthma overlap syndrome, the management of both entities separately (asthma and OSA) should be carried out in accordance with the clinical management guidelines for each of the entities.

SUMMARY

In patients with COPD and asthma, exacerbations determine the natural history of both diseases. Patients with both respiratory diseases who suffer from OSA as a comorbidity (overlap syndromes) have a higher risk of exacerbations and hospitalization. In cases of OSA/COPD and OSA/asthma in which CPAP treatment is indicated, adequate adherence to therapy appears to reduce exacerbations and their severity, especially in OSA/COPD overlap. However, there is a lack of randomized trials that definitively demonstrate this evidence.

CLINICS CARE POINTS

- Both, in patients with COPD and with asthma, exacerbations are frequent, worsen the quality of life, accelerate functional deterioration, and increase morbidity and mortality.

- Among the main risk factors for developing more frequent and more severe exacerbations, the coexistence of certain comorbidities such as OSA is well established in COPD and its importance in asthma is less evident.

- OSA is a modifiable risk factor through effective treatment using CPAP or other specific therapies (eg, weight reduction) and therefore a sleep study should be considered in cases of COPD or asthma with severe exacerbations.

- There is no robust evidence based on randomized trials of the long-term effect of CPAP on the potential reduction of COPD or asthma exacerbations. Until then, the management of the coexistence of OSA in patients with OSA/COPD or OSA/asthma overlap syndromes should be carried out according to the OSA clinical management guidelines.

DISCLOSURE

Both authors report no conflicts of interest.

REFERENCES

1. Global Initiative for Chronic Obstructive Lung Disease (GOLD). Global strategy for the diagnosis, management, and prevention of chronic obstructive pulmonary disease. Available at: https://goldcopd.org/digital-gold-report/. [Accessed 22 December 2023].
2. Boers E, Barrett M, Su JG, et al. Global burden of chronic obstructive pulmonary disease through 2050. JAMA Netw Open 2023;6(12):e2346598.
3. Qin X, Pate CA, Zahran HS. Adult asthma prevalence and trend analysis by urban-rural status across sociodemographic characteristics-United States, 2012-20. J Allergy Clin Immunol Glob 2023;2(2):100085.
4. Benjafield AV, Ayas NT, Eastwood PR, et al. Estimation of the global prevalence and burden of obstructive sleep apnoea: a literature-based analysis. Lancet Respir Med 2019;7(8):687–98.
5. Global initiative for asthma. Global strategy for asthma management and prevention. 2023. Available at: www.ginasthma.org. [Accessed 22 December 2023].
6. Agustí A, Hogg JC. Update on the pathogenesis of chronic obstructive pulmonary disease. N Engl J Med 2019;381(13):1248–56.
7. Divo MJ, Celli BR, Poblador-Plou B, et al. Chronic obstructive pulmonary disease (COPD) as a disease of early aging: evidence from the EpiChron cohort. PLoS One 2018;13(2):e0193143.
8. Kim KS, Kim JH, Park SY, et al. Smoking induces oropharyngeal narrowing and increases the severity of obstructive sleep apnea syndrome. J Clin Sleep Med 2012;8(4):367–74.
9. Varol Y, Anar C, Tuzel OE, et al. The impact of active and former smoking on the severity of obstructive sleep apnea. Sleep Breath 2015;19(4):1279–84.
10. Scanlon PD, Connett JE, Waller LA, et al, Lung Health Study Research Group. Smoking cessation and lung function in mild-to-moderate chronic obstructive pulmonary disease. The Lung Health Study. Am J Respir Crit Care Med 2000;161(2 Pt 1):381–90.

11. Flenley DC. Sleep in chronic obstructive lung disease. Clin Chest Med 1985;6(4):651–61.

12. Krachman SL, Tiwari R, Vega ME, et al. Effect of emphysema severity on the apnea-hypopnea index in smokers with obstructive sleep apnea. Ann Am Thorac Soc 2016;13(7):1129–35.

13. Yumino D, Redolfi S, Ruttanaumpawan P, et al. Nocturnal rostral fluid shift: a unifying concept for the pathogenesis of obstructive and central sleep apnea in men with heart failure. Circulation 2010; 121(14):1598–605.

14. McNicholas WT. Chronic obstructive pulmonary disease and obstructive sleep apnea: overlaps in pathophysiology, systemic inflammation, and cardiovascular disease. Am J Respir Crit Care Med 2009;180(8):692–700.

15. Teodorescu M, Broytman O, Curran-Everett D, et al. Obstructive sleep apnea risk, asthma burden, and lower airway inflammation in adults in the Severe Asthma Research Program (SARP) II. J Allergy Clin Immunol Pract 2015;3(4):566–75.

16. Beuther DA, Sutherland ER. Overweight, obesity, and incident asthma: a meta-analysis of prospective epidemiologic studies. Am J Respir Crit Care Med 2007;175(7):661–6.

17. Young T, Finn L, Kim H. Nasal obstruction as a risk factor for sleep disordered breathing. J Allergy Clin Immunol 1997;99(2):S757–62.

18. Yigla M, Tov N, Solomonov A, et al. Difficult-to-control asthma and obstructive sleep apnea. J Asthma 2003;40(8):865–71.

19. Seemungal TA, Donaldson GC, Paul EA, et al. Effect of exacerbation on quality of life in patients with chronic obstructive pulmonary disease. Am J Respir Crit Care Med 1998;157(5 Pt 1):1418–22.

20. Sundh J, Johansson G, Larsson K, et al. The phenotype of concurrent chronic bronchitis and frequent exacerbations in patients with severe COPD attending Swedish secondary care units. Int J Chron Obstruct Pulmon Dis 2015;10(1):2327–34.

21. Li J, Sun S, Tang R, et al. Major air pollutants and risk of COPD exacerbations: a systematic review and meta-analysis. Int J Chron Obstruct Pulmon Dis 2016;11(1):3079–91.

22. Hurst JR, Vestbo J, Anzueto A, et al. Susceptibility to exacerbation in chronic obstructive pulmonary disease. N Engl J Med 2010;363(12):1128–38.

23. Marin JM, Carrizo SJ, Casanova C, et al. Prediction of risk of COPD exacerbations by the BODE index. Respir Med 2009;103(3):373–8.

24. Han MK, Kazerooni EA, Lynch DA, et al. Chronic obstructive pulmonary disease exacerbations in the COPDGene study: associated radiologic phenotypes. Radiology 2011;261(1):274–82.

25. Wells JM, Washko GR, Han MK, et al. Pulmonary arterial enlargement and acute exacerbations of COPD. N Engl J Med 2012;367(10):913–21.

26. Burgel PR, Nesme-Meyer P, Chanez P, et al. Cough and sputum production are associated with frequent exacerbations and hospitalizations in COPD subjects. Chest 2009;135(4):975–82.

27. Ni Y, Shi G, Yu Y, et al. Clinical characteristics of patients with chronic obstructive pulmonary disease with comorbid bronchiectasis: a systemic review and meta-analysis. Int J Chron Obstruct Pulmon Dis 2015;10(1):1465–75.

28. Bafadhel M, Peterson S, De Blas MA, et al. Predictors of exacerbation risk and response to budesonide in patients with chronic obstructive pulmonary disease: a post-hoc analysis of three randomised trials. Lancet Respir Med 2018;6(2):117–26.

29. Pascoe S, Locantore N, Dransfield MT, et al. Blood eosinophil counts, exacerbations, and response to the addition of inhaled fluticasone furoate to vilanterol in patients with chronic obstructive pulmonary disease: a secondary analysis of data from two parallel randomised controlled trials. Lancet Respir Med 2015;3(6):435–42.

30. Singh D, Agusti A, Martinez FJ, et al. Blood eosinophils and chronic obstructive pulmonary disease: a global initiative for chronic obstructive lung disease Science Committee 2022 review. Am J Respir Crit Care Med 2022;206(1):17–24.

31. Divo M, Cote C, de Torres JP, et al. Comorbidities and risk of mortality in patients with chronic obstructive pulmonary disease. Am J Respir Crit Care Med 2012;186(2):155–61.

32. Lambert AA, Putcha N, Drummond MB, et al. COPDGene Investigators. Obesity is associated with increased morbidity in moderate to severe COPD. Chest 2017;151(1):68–77.

33. Goto T, Tsugawa Y, Faridi MK, et al. Reduced risk of acute exacerbation of COPD after bariatric surgery: a self-controlled case series study. Chest 2018; 153(3):611–7.

34. Thomsen M, Ingebrigtsen TS, Marott JL, et al. Inflammatory biomarkers and exacerbations in chronic obstructive pulmonary disease. JAMA 2013;309(22): 2353–61.

35. Neidich SD, Green WD, Rebeles J, et al. Increased risk of influenza among vaccinated adults who are obese. Int J Obes 2017;41(9):1324–30.

36. Ubags ND, Burg E, Antkowiak M, et al. A comparative study of lung host defense in murine obesity models. insights into neutrophil function. Am J Respir Cell Mol Biol 2016;55(2):188–200.

37. Putcha N, Anzueto AR, Calverley PMA, et al. Mortality and exacerbation risk by body mass index in patients with COPD in TIOSPIR and UPLIFT. Ann Am Thorac Soc 2022;19(2):204–13.

38. Marin JM, Soriano JB, Carrizo SJ, et al. Outcomes in patients with chronic obstructive pulmonary disease and obstructive sleep apnea: the overlap syndrome. Am J Respir Crit Care Med 2010;182(3):325–31.

39. Naranjo M, Willes L, Prillaman BA, et al. Undiagnosed OSA may significantly affect outcomes in adults admitted for COPD in an inner-city hospital. Chest 2020;158(3):1198–207.

40. Donovan LM, Feemster LC, Udris EM, et al. Poor outcomes among patients with chronic obstructive pulmonary disease with higher risk for undiagnosed obstructive sleep apnea in the LOTT Cohort. J Clin Sleep Med 2019;15(1):71–7.

41. Ioachimescu OC, Janocko NJ, Ciavatta M-M, et al. Obstructive lung disease and obstructive sleep apnea (OLDOSA) cohort study: 10-year assessment. J Clin Sleep Med 2020;16(2):267–77.

42. Singh G, Agarwal A, Zhang W, et al. Impact of PAP therapy on hospitalization rates in Medicare beneficiaries with COPD and coexisting OSA. Sleep Breath 2019;23(2):193–200.

43. Sterling KL, Pépin JL, Linde-Zwirble W, et al. Impact of positive airway pressure therapy adherence on outcomes in patients with obstructive sleep apnea and chronic obstructive pulmonary disease. Am J Respir Crit Care Med 2022;206(2):197–205.

44. Castan-Abad MT, Montserrat-Capdevila J, Godoy P, et al. Diabetes as a risk factor for severe exacerbation and death in patients with COPD: a prospective cohort study. Eur. J. Public Health 2020;30(4):822–7.

45. Chen YH, Keller JK, Kang JH, et al. Obstructive sleep apnea and the subsequent risk of depressive disorder: a population-based follow-up study. J Clin Sleep Med 2013;9(5):417–23.

46. Yohannes AM, Mulerova H, Lavoie K, et al. The association of depressive symptoms with rates of acute exacerbations in patients with COPD: results from a 3-year longitudinal follow-up of the ECLIPSE Cohort. J Am Med Dir Assoc 2017;18(11):955–9.

47. Ramon MA, Ter Riet G, Carsin AE, et al, PAC-COPD Study Group. The dyspnoea-inactivity vicious circle in COPD: development and external validation of a conceptual model. Eur Respir J 2018;52(3): 1800079.

48. Martınez-Ceron E, Barquiel B, Bezos AM, et al. Effect of continuous positive airway pressure on glycemic control in patients with obstructive sleep apnea and type 2 diabetes. A randomized clinical trial. Am J Respir Crit Care Med 2016;194(4):476–85.

49. Jackson ML, Tolson J, Schembri R, et al. Does continuous positive airways pressure treatment improve clinical depression in obstructive sleep apnea? A randomized wait-list controlled study. Depress Anxiety 2021;38(5):498–507.

50. ten Brinke A, Sterk PJ, Masclee AA, et al. Risk factors of frequent exacerbations in difficult-to-treat asthma. Eur Respir J 2005;26(5):812–8.

51. Chan CS, Woolcock AJ, Sullivan CE. Nocturnal asthma: role of snoring and obstructive sleep apnea. Am Rev Respir Dis 1988;137(6):1502–4.

52. Jordan HT, Stellman SD, Reibman J, et al. Factors associated with poor control of 9/11-related asthma 10-11 years after the 2001 World Trade Center terrorist attacks. J Asthma 2015;52(6):630–7.

53. Wang Y, Liu K, Hu K, et al. Impact of obstructive sleep apnea on severe asthma exacerbations. Sleep Med 2016;26(10):1–5.

54. Vicente E, Marin JM, Carrizo SJ, et al. Upper airway and systemic inflammation in obstructive sleep apnoea. Eur Respir J 2016;48(4):1108–17.

55. Chua AP, Aboussouan LS, Minai OA, et al. Long-term continuous positive airway pressure therapy normalizes high exhaled nitric oxide levels in obstructive sleep apnea. J Clin Sleep Med 2013; 9(6):529–35.

56. Serrano-Pariente J, Plaza V, Soriano JB, et al. Asthma outcomes improve with continuous positive airway pressure for obstructive sleep apnea. Allergy 2017;72(8):802–12.

57. Davies SE, Bishopp A, Wharton S, et al. Does Continuous Positive Airway Pressure (CPAP) treatment of obstructive sleep apnoea (OSA) improve asthma-related clinical outcomes in patients with co-existing conditions?- A systematic review. Respir Med 2018;143(10):18–30.

Untreated Obstructive Sleep Apnea in Interstitial Lung Disease and Impact on Interstitial Lung Disease Outcomes

Andrea S. Melani, MD*, Sara Croce, MD, Maddalena Messina, MD,
Elena Bargagli, MD

KEYWORDS

- Obstructive sleep apnea (OSA) • Interstitial lung disease (ILD) • Sleep-related breathing disorders
- Respiratory disturbance index • Sleep Apnea Quality of Life Index • the Sleep Quality Scale
- the Functional Outcomes of Sleep Questionnaire • the Pittsburgh Sleep Quality Index

KEY POINTS

- Obstructive sleep apnea (OSA), a highly prevalent sleep-related breathing disorder, is very common in subjects with interstitial lung disease (ILD).
- OSA is underdiagnosed in subjects with ILD. The presence of OSA in subjects with ILD does not significantly change symptoms as compared to subjects with ILD without OSA. Subjects with ILD and OSA often suffer from a disproportionate hypoxemic burden during sleep.
- It has been supposed that OSA might predispose to ILD in early stages of the disease. Other studies have suggested that ILD might predispose or aggravate OSA.
- The overlap of OSA, sleep-related hypoxemia, and ILD may be associated with poor prognosis and ILD progression.

INTRODUCTION

According to the revised third edition of the International Classification of Sleep Disorders,[1] sleep-related breathing disorders (SBDs) are clinically relevant abnormalities of breathing that occur during sleep and may or may not be present while awake. SBDs include sleep apnea syndromes and other sleep-related hypoxemic disturbances. Obstructive sleep apnea (OSA) syndrome is the most common SBD.[1]

The coexistence of OSA and interstitial lung diseases (ILDs) has been known for many decades,[2,3] but recently it has been shown that this associations is common and clinically relevant.[4–27] OSA is now identified as an important comorbidity in idiopathic pulmonary fibrosis (IPF), the most common and severe variety of ILD.[28] The relationship between ILD and OSA is an interesting but not well-defined topic. It is not clear (1) whether OSA is more common in subjects with ILD than in general healthy population, (2) whether OSA predisposes to ILD, or/and (3) whether ILD predisposes to OSA. It is also not understood (4) whether the symptoms of subjects with OSA and ILD are similar to those of the associated diseases, or enhanced or reduced, (5) whether the coexistence of both diseases worsens ILD prognosis, and (6) what the best therapy is for each of the 2 diseases when they co-occur.

Respiratory Diseases Unit, Department of Medicine, Surgery and Neurosciences, University of Siena, Siena 53100, Italy
* Corresponding author.
E-mail address: a.melani@ao-siena.toscana.it

Sleep Med Clin 19 (2024) 283–294
https://doi.org/10.1016/j.jsmc.2024.02.008
1556-407X/24/

The aim of this narrative review is to analyze the frequency, the characteristics, the outcome, and the management of the co-occurrence of OSA and ILD.

OBSTRUCTIVE SLEEP APNEA: DEFINITION, DIAGNOSIS, EPIDEMIOLOGY, CLINICS, OUTCOMES, AND TREATMENT

OSA is characterized by repeated episodes of complete cessation (apnea) or significant decrease in airflow (hypopnea) due to the collapse of pharynx during sleep. The diagnosis of OSA[1] requires the presence of at least 5 episodes per hour of sleep associated with related symptoms, or at least 15 episodes independently of the presence of symptoms. Accordingly, monitoring during sleep is required for the diagnosis of OSA. In-laboratory polysomnography (PSG) is the gold standard to diagnose OSA and grade its severity.[29] PSG gives the respiratory disturbance index (RDI) that represents the number of respiratory effort-related arousals, apneas, and hypopneas per hour of sleep. Based on the RDI, OSA severity is traditionally categorized into mild (5–14.9), moderate (15–29.9), and severe (≥30).[30] PSG is time-consuming, expensive, and of limited availability, preventing widespread use. Portable type III monitoring systems (respiratory sleep polygraphy without neurologic parameters) offer the opportunity to increase diagnostic capacity for OSA. These devices give the apnea/hypopnea index (AHI; thereafter this term will indicate RDI and AHI except than otherwise specified) that represents the number of apneas and hypopneas per hour of estimated sleep.[29] Home type III systems are becoming ubiquitous for diagnosing OSA even if it is at the expense of reduced accuracy.[29,30] Type III monitoring devices usually underestimate disease severity as the sleep time is estimated and not objectively measured, and cortical arousals during sleep cannot be diagnosed.[31] The American Academy of Sleeping Medicine defines hypopnea as a change in airflow associated with a 3% oxygen desaturation or a cortical arousal but allows an alternative definition that requires a change in airflow associated with a 4% oxygen desaturation without the need for cortical arousals.[31] Type IV monitoring systems, such as nocturnal oximetry monitoring devices, are usually not recommended to diagnose OSA in the presence of concomitant chronic lung diseases[32,33] even if they are sometimes used to screen for OSA in subjects with ILD.[30]

OSA is a highly prevalent syndrome.[34] It has been estimated that, worldwide, almost 500 million adults aged 30 to 69 years have moderate-to-severe OSA.[34] However, the prevalence of OSA differs between studies depending on the diagnostic methodology used (including different devices and scoring criteria used[35]) and the characteristics of the studied population. In the seminal community-based Wisconsin Sleep Cohort study, among adults aged 30 to 70 years, based on an AHI value of 15 events/h or greater, approximately 13% of men and 6% of women had moderate-to-severe OSA[36]; using the definition of an AHI of 5 events/h or greater associated with hypersomnia (defined as Epworth Sleepiness Scale score >10), the prevalence of OSA was 14% in men and 5% in women.[36] In the more recent population based HypnoLaus Sleep Cohort Study, based on an AHI of 15 events/h or greater, 50% of men and 23% of women in the age group of 35 to 75 years showed moderate-to-severe OSA[37]; using the definition of an AHI of 5 events/h or greater associated with hypersomnia (defined as Epworth Sleepiness Scale score >10), the prevalence of OSA was 15% in male individuals and 7% in female individuals.[37]

Symptoms of OSA are not specific and common to other sleeping disturbances. The most common symptoms associate with OSA are unrefreshing sleep, daytime sleepiness, insomnia, awakening with gasping or choking sensation, loud snoring, witnessed apneas, and fatigue.[4–27] These symptoms are associated with sedentary life, poor exercise tolerance, and impaired quality of life. Several specific patient-reported tools, such as the Sleep Apnea Quality of Life Index, the Sleep Quality Scale, the Functional Outcomes of Sleep Questionnaire (FOSQ), and the Pittsburgh Sleep Quality Index, have been used to define the impact of OSA on quality of sleep and life. Excessive daytime sleepiness, possibly the most typical symptom of subjects with OSA, is often measured using the Epworth Sleepiness Scale. Other questionnaires, such as the STOP-BANG and the Berlin questionnaire, have been used as screening tools in groups of subjects at high risk of OSA, but their role to diagnose OSA is weak.[38]

OSA is associated with repeated phasic oxyhemoglobin desaturations, arousals, oxidative stress, excessive release of catecholamines, intrathoracic pressure swings, and low-grade chronic inflammation.[34] Severe untreated OSA has been associated with metabolic and cardiovascular accidents and reduced survival.[34] The gold standard for treating adults with clinically significant OSA is regular use of a positive airway pressure (PAP) during sleep. PAP treatment, compared to no therapy, improves excessive sleepiness, quality of life, and comorbid hypertension.[39,40]

INTERSTITIAL LUNG DISEASE: DEFINITION, DIAGNOSIS, EPIDEMIOLOGY, CLINICS, OUTCOMES, AND TREATMENT

ILDs represent a heterogeneous group of chronic diffuse pulmonary infiltrative disorders, mostly characterized by lung inflammation and fibrosis, classified according to etiologic, clinical, radiological, and histopathological findings.[28,41] Some ILDs are limited to the lungs, such as IPF, which accounts for about a quarter of ILD cases.[28] Other ILDs occur in a background of systemic diseases, such as sarcoidosis and connective tissue disease-related ILD.[41] The adjusted estimated prevalence of IPF ranges from 0.33 to 4.51 per 10,000 cases worldwide.[28] It is estimated that in Europe approximately 40,000 new cases of IPF and progressive pulmonary fibrosis are being diagnosed each year.[28,42] The clinical presentation of ILD is not specific and similar to other chronic lung diseases. Exertional dyspnea, fatigue, and dry cough are the most typical symptoms in subjects with ILD. Although the natural history of ILD other than IPF is variable, approximately one-third of subjects with non-IPF ILD show evolution with the loss of lung function and progression of disease.[28,41–44] IPF and progressive ILD have a detrimental effect on quality of life, with high rates of hospitalization. When left untreated, these diseases have a median survival of 3 to 5 years.[28,41–43]

Subjects with IPF also suffer from poor sleep quality and efficiency, increased arousals, and sleep fragmentation, independently of the presence of OSA.[5,6,45–48] Similar findings are also observed in mixed ILD populations.[18,21] Several parameters have been used to predict ILD progression and survival. They include the decline in forced vital capacity (FVC) and gas exchange (ie, diffusing capacity of the lung for carbon monoxide, DL_{co}), the distance walked in the 6 minute walk test and related exertional oxyhemoglobin desaturation, the extension of chest lesions on high-resolution computed tomography, the deterioration of quality of life by specific patient-reported tools, such as the Saint George Respiratory Questionnaire and the King's Brief ILD questionnaire, or composite tools, such as the Gender, Age and Physiology-ILD and the composite physiologic index.[29,41–44]

Over the last years, advances have been made in pharmacologic treatment of IPF and progressive ILD. Two antifibrotic drugs reduce the decline in lung function in subjects with IPF and may also reduce exacerbations, disease progression, hospitalization, and survival. Immunosuppressant agents have been used in subjects with progressive ILD. The combination of antifibrotics and immunosuppressants is reasonable in progressive ILD to slow the disease course.[44,49]

INTERACTION BETWEEN INTERSTITIAL LUNG DISEASE AND OBSTRUCTIVE SLEEP APNEA
Prevalence and Characteristics of Subjects with IPF or Mixed interstitial lung disease and obstructive sleep apnea

Twenty-four cross-sectional or prospective studies performed with type I to III polygraphies have evaluated the prevalence of OSA in subjects with ILD (**Table 1**).[4–27] Fifteen studies have included subjects with only IPF, other studies have included populations with mixed ILD. As ILD is a relatively uncommon condition, the sample sizes of these studies have been relatively small, ranging from 9[15] to 100[19] subjects. A few studies have included a small control group, comprised healthy persons,[16,18,19] asthmatics,[7] or patients with chronic obstructive pulmonary disease.[23] No substantial differences in severity and frequency of OSA between subjects with IPF and other ILD are observed, but firm conclusions cannot be drawn as approximately half of the populations in studies with mixed ILD had IPF. Overall, OSA seems to be common in subjects with IPF and ILD. Male sex, overweight, and older age, which are established risk factors for OSA,[34,36,37] also prevail in subjects with IPF.

Independently of the presence of OSA, subjects with ILD experience increased arousals, sleep fragmentation, reduced slow wave sleep, and sleep efficiency.[5,6,18,21,25,46,47] Most studies found no substantial differences in sleep architecture between subjects with ILD with OSA and without OSA.[5,6,18,21,25,46,47] Most studies did not report significant differences in sleep-related symptoms between subjects with ILD and OSA and those with only ILD.[5–26] Excessive daytime somnolence, possibly the most typical symptom of subjects with OSA, was reported by only 22% of subjects with IPF and OSA.[48] In addition subjects with moderate-to-severe OSA often suffered from daytime fatigue (75%), insomnia (67%), and nocturnal cough (56%), typically seen in subjects with ILD.[48] In a population of 34 consecutively enrolled subjects with IPF undergoing PSG, almost 3/4ths suffered from an SDB, but less of 10% reported excessive daytime sleepiness.[46] In another population of 49 subjects with mixed ILD, hypersomnia (reported as a score to the epworth sleepiness scale [ESS] >10) was observed in 18% of cases.[17] Another study in 50 subjects with mixed ILD reported excessive daytime sleepiness (ESS score ≥10) in 10% of cases.[10] Pillai and colleagues[7] reported lower

Table 1
Cross-sectional and prospective studies evaluating the prevalence and some characteristics of obstructive sleep apnea in populations with IPF and ILD

First Author	Year of Publication	Sample Size, No.	Study Subjects (%IPF)	Age, years	Male, %	BMI	FVC % Pred	DLco % Pred	AHI, % ≥5/≥15	AHI	ODI	CT90%
Aydogdu	2006	37	ILD(49)	54	43	NA	NA	66	65/30	NA[a]	NA	NA
Lancaster	2009	50	IPF	65	68	32	58–73	38–48	88/68	NA[a]	NA	NA
Mermigkis	2010	34	IPF	65	62	27	72.5	54	59/15	9	9.5	21
Pillai	2012	54	ILD(41)	69	54	30	64	43	65/37	24[b]	NA	NA
Pitsiou	2012	33	IPF	69	79	NA	NA	NA	24/6	7[b]	NA	NA
Kolilekas	2013	31	IPF	68	77	29	78	44	90/52	NA[a]	NA	17
Pihtili	2013	50	ILD(27)	54	28	26	85	72	68/30	11[a]	14[d]	6
Mermigkis	2015	92	IPF	70	68	NA	NA	NA	85/65	NA[a]	NA	NA
Reid	2015	27	IPF	71	70	29	NA	83	22/NA	17[b]	NA	18
Lee	2016	20	IPF	68	NA	29	82	51	45/NA	NA[b]	NA	19
Bosi	2017	35	IPF	68	77	23	72	46	71.5/31	11[a]	11[d]	7.5
Gille	2017	45	IPF	69	84	28	73	45	89/62	NA[a]	NA	3–27
Schertel	2017	9	IPF	67	89	NA	58	41	75/22	NA[b]	NA	NA
Ahmed	2018	20	IPF	48	30	32	NA	NA	50/NA	13[a]	NA	25
Cardoso	2018	49	ILD(24)	62	53	26	86	66	69/24	11[b]	11[c]	8.4
Mavroudi	2018	40	ILD(47)	62	70	29	84	NA	67/7	8[a]	8?	NA
Canora	2019	100	ILD(54)	68	NA	28	69	49	79/33	11[b]	3[d]	5
Sarac	2019	79	ILD(20)	55	52	29	81	66	67/54	22[a]	14[c]	11
Troy	2019	92	ILD(48)	66	55	31	77	54	65/33	7[a]	8[c]	2.5
Tudorarache	2019	23	IPF	68	57	28	71	44	83/63	NA[b]	NA	NA
Zhang	2019	77	ILD(74)	65	75	25	75	52	87/62	NA[a]	NA	NA
Papadogiannis	2021	45	IPF	72	67	30	82	60	84/64	25	24	30

Valecchi	2023	46	ILD (24)	60	65	30	83.5	57	64/33	17[b]	15[d]	25
Hagmeyer	2023	74	IPF	74	76	27	71	54	40/NA	13[a]	NA	NA
Bordas	2023	50	IPF	73	74	28	90	NA	NA/58	NA	NA	NA

Abbreviations: NA, not available; IPF, idiopathic pulmonary fibrosis; ILD, interstitial lung disease; BMI, body mass index; FVC, forced vital capacity, DLco, diffusion capacity for carbon monoxide; AHI, apnea-hypopnea index; ODI, oxyhemoglobin desaturation index; CT90, percentage of estimated total sleep time with an oxygen saturation level <90%; Data are reported as percentage or mean.

[a] PSG.
[b] type III monitoring device.
[c] ODI3.
[d] ODI4.

Courtesy of Melani A.S, Sara Croce, Maddalena Messina, and Elena Bargagli.

scores of hypersomnia in 49 subjects with ILD than in a control group of asthmatics. Subjects with ILD and OSA often showed impaired quality of life.[5,6,18,21–25,46–48]

Sleep-related hypoxemia is common and often severe in subjects with OSA and ILD.[2–27] Of note, sleep oximetry monitoring of some subjects with OSA does not show a saw-tooth appearance (the typical picture of OSA) but even prolonged desaturations.[50] These sustained oxyhemoglobin desaturations, which are common in subjects with chronic lung diseases,[51] are usually related to hypoventilation or ventilation/perfusion mismatching during sleep. Bye and colleagues[2] observed marked sleep oximetry desaturations in 69% of 13 subjects with ILD. Perez-Padilla and colleagues[4] found that 11 patients with ILD had cumulative percentage time with oxyhemoglobin saturation less than 90% in sleep (CT90, a parameter commonly used to define severity of sleeping hypoxemia) much lower than that of healthy controls (43% vs 0.2%). Clark and colleagues[52] performed an overnight oximetry in a population of 67 patients with ILD (60 of them with IPF) with mild impairment in lung function (mean FVC 80% and awakening resting arterial oxygen tension (Pao_2) 69 mm Hg), observing that 9 out of 48 patients (18%) had a CT90 greater than 30%. Some authors found that patients with IPF can show overnight oximetry desaturation independently of the presence of OSA. Mermigkis and colleagues[6] reported a CT90 of 12% in 14 patients with IPF without any evidence of OSA. Of note, sleep-related hypoxemia seems to be only weakly correlated with impaired quality of life.[46] Another large retrospective study in a mixed ILD population of 134 subjects[53] found that more than a third of subjects showed a CT90 of 20% or more and sleep oximetry desaturations can occur in the context of mild ILD and be disproportionate to the extent of the underlying lung disease; in fact, 78% of subjects with sleep-related hypoxemia did not have resting daytime hypoxemia.[53]

Coexistence of Untreated obstructive sleep apnea and interstitial lung disease: Outcomes

Some prospective studies suggest that elevated AHI and/or sleep-related hypoxemia are associated to poor prognosis in subjects with ILD.[9,13,21,27] We evaluated a population of 46 subjects with mixed ILD and found that the only sleep parameter independently related to a progressive course (defined as time to either death or a >10% fall in FVC below baseline) was an AHI greater than 30 (hazard ratio [HR], 7.53; 95% confidence interval [CI], 1.83–30.64; P = .005).[27] Another Italian study, evaluating the impact of

sleep breathing disturbances on prognosis of 35 subjects with IPF with a median follow-up of 12 months, found that sleep-related hypoxemia (defined as sleeping saturation level ≤88% for ≥5 minutes) was associated with disease progression, independently of the AHI.[13] Previously, one study in 31 patients with IPF (of whom 10 succumbed to disease and 21 were still alive at the end of monitoring) found that sleeping nadir oxygen saturation, but not AHI, was associated with survival.[9] Troy and colleagues[21] found that CT90 and not AHI was the only sleep parameter predictive of either overall survival or progression-free survival (defined as time to either death, transplantation, fall in FVC 10% or greater within 6 months, fall in DL_{co} 15% or greater within 6 months, and/or development of new or worsening PH on serial echocardiography; HR, 1.01; 95% CI, 1.00–1.02; P = .038). Recently another study using a type IV monitoring device found in 102 subjects with ILD that nocturnal hypoxemia evaluated as CT90 greater than 10% was associated with a more rapid decline in both quality of life as measured by the King's Brief Interstitial Lung Disease questionnaire (P = .005), increased risk of disease progression (HR, 7.8; 95% CI, 2.8–21.4; P < .001) and higher all-cause mortality at 1 year (HR, 8.21; 95% CI, 2.40–28.1; P < .001).[54] Larger retrospective studies seem to confirm these findings. Corte and colleagues[53] found an association between oxygen desaturation index (ODI) and survival (HR, 1.04; 95% CI, 1.00, 1.06; P = .009) in a group of 134 subjects with mixed ILD. Another single-center Korean study found that the CT90 was a risk factor for mortality (HR, 1.08; 95% CI, 1.02–1.14; P = .007) in a group of 167 patients with IPF (including 108 subjects with concomitant confirmed OSA with a type 4 portable device) followed for a mean period of 27 months.[55] A Canadian study seems to add some further evidence to the usefulness of OSA screening in subjects with IPF. Using an administrative database, the authors found that the group of 201 patients with IPF undergoing PSG (used as a surrogate of likelihood of having OSA with subsequent diagnosis and treatment) had significantly reduced rates of respiratory-related hospitalization (HR, 0.43; 95% CI, 0.24–0.75; P = .003) and all-cause mortality (HR, 0.49; 95% CI, 0.30–0.80; P = .004) compared to the matched controls.[56]

Results of PAP Treatment in Subjects with Mixed interstitial lung disease and obstructive sleep apnea

Mermigkis and colleagues[57] started PAP therapy in a group of 12 patients with IPF and moderate-to-severe OSA. They found a significant improvement in quality of life evaluated by the FOSQ at 1, 3, and 6 months after PAP initiation. Another multicenter study started PAP treatment in 60 newly diagnosed patients with IPF and moderate-to-severe OSA and found that after 1 year of treatment, only the group with good PAP adherence showed statistically significant improvement in all measured generic and specific quality of life and sleep quality questionnaires. The most striking improvements were in the FOSQ (P = .0002), and in the Fatigue Severity Scale (P = .0007), an instrument used to evaluate daytime fatigue. They also observed an improved survival (P = .01) at 24 months after PAP treatment.[48] In another study, effective PAP treatment in 45 patients with newly diagnosed IPF lead to a significant improvement in excessive daytime sleepiness, fatigue, sleep quality, and life expectancy at a 7 year follow-up period.[24] These results seem to show that long-term effective PAP treatment is feasible in subjects with OSA and ILD, even if the same group[48,57] recognize that PAP adherence may be difficult in subjects that often have complaints of nocturia, insomnia, and nocturnal cough due to claustrophobia, poor mask fit and excessive air leakage. A real-world data study showed that the use of PAP had limited impact on disease progression and survival.[58] This 20 year observational retrospective study involving subjects with mixed ILD (2.5% of whom had IPF) did not find improvements in all-cause mortality or progression-free survival either among patients with OSA versus those without or among those adherent with PAP versus those not using PAP. However, in the subset of subjects requiring supplemental oxygen in addition to PAP therapy, adherence to PAP therapy was associated with significantly better progression-free survival.[58] In-laboratory CPAP titration is recommended in patients with OSA and chronic lung diseases.[39,40] This practice is time-consuming and not always available. The role of automatic-PAP (APAP) titration has been investigated in 25 patients with fibrotic ILD and moderate-to-severe OSA or mild OSA with excessive daytime sleepiness and/or cardiovascular disease.[17] Four out of 25 patients refused APAP treatment, 2 patients died before starting treatment, and 2 others reported APAP intolerance due to claustrophobia and/or insomnia and were excluded after 1 week of unsuccessful attempts. In the remaining 17 patients, good APAP adherence was noted 1 month after APAP initiation,[17] showing that autotitration is feasible.

IS THERE A PATHOGENETIC LINK BETWEEN OBSTRUCTIVE SLEEP APNEA AND INTERSTITIAL LUNG DISEASE?

In the last few years, several studies have suggested that OSA may predispose to ILD and vice versa. As shown in **Fig. 1**, the relationship between OSA and ILD might also be bidirectional.

Can obstructive sleep apnea Predispose to interstitial lung disease?

Some studies seem to suggest that OSA might contribute to the development of ILD, even in the earlier phases. The cross-sectional Multi-Ethnic Study of Atherosclerosis (MESA) included 1690 adults (mean age 68 years, mean FVC of 97% predicted) without any selection criteria based on respiratory or sleep disturbances who performed thoracic computed tomographic (CT) imaging and in-home PSG. Almost a third of participants had an AHI of 15 or greater.[59] There was an association between AHI of 15 or greater and subclinical ILD (6.1% high-attenuation areas increment; 95% CI, 0.5–12; P = .03 and 2.3-fold increased odds of interstitial lung abnormalities; 95% CI, 1.3–4.1; P = .005) among participants with normal body weights.[59] OSA severity in a subsample of 99 subjects with normal body weight was associated with elevated serum biomarkers of alveolar injury and extracellular matrix remodeling.[59] More recently, using data from the MESA study, participants with an AHI value of 15 events/h or greater and in the highest hypoxic burden quartile had increases in high-attenuation areas on chest CT imaging of 11.3% (95% CI, 3.7%–19.4%) and 9.9% (95% CI, 1.4%–19.0%) per 10 years, respectively. Subjects with AHI of 15 events/h or greater also showed a more rapid decline in FVC compared to the other group.[60] Sleep-related sustained and/or intermittent hypoxemia might cause lung fibrosis. Several animal studies have shown that chronic, intermittent hypoxemia may predispose to pulmonary fibrosis through oxidative and inflammatory pathways.[61,62] Intermittent hypoxia–reoxygenation episodes sustain the overexpression of proinflammatory substances, such as matrix metalloproteinase-7, surfactant protein A, Krebs von der Lungen-6, which may induce or aggravate alveolar epithelial cell injury,[63] cytokines with fibrogenic potential,[14] and the hypoxia-inducible factor 1(HIF-1). HIF1, in turn, promotes angiogenesis and lung fibrosis.[64] Of note, the HIF-1 signaling pathway is inhibited with nintedanib, a tyrosine-kinase antagonist used to treat IPF, which blocks profibrotic processes in the extracellular matrix.[65] Intermittent hypoxia induces the release of endothelin-1 that acts as a

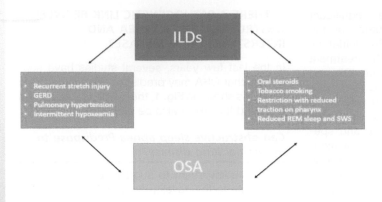

Fig. 1. The relationship between OSA and ILD. GERD, gastroesophageal reflux disease; REM, rapid eye movement; SWS, slow wave sleep. (*Courtesy* of Melani A.S, Sara Croce, Maddalena Messina and Elena Bargagli.)

vasoconstrictor on smooth muscle cells in pulmonary arteries leading to increased pulmonary blood pressures.[66] Pulmonary hypertension is not infrequent in subjects with moderate-to-severe untreated OSA. In the largest study to date, which included 220 consecutive subjects with OSA with AHI of 20 or greater using right heart catheterization (the gold standard to diagnose pulmonary hypertension), Chaouat and colleagues found a prevalence of pulmonary hypertension in 17% of cases.[67] These authors did not find a clear relationship between the severity of OSA and the development of pulmonary hypertension.[67] The prevalence of pulmonary hypertension complicating ILD, which is not insignificant at an early stage, increases up to 90% in patients with ILD listed for lung transplantation.[68] Pulmonary arterial hypertension is associated with reduced survival in subjects with ILD.[68] Hagmeyer and colleagues[26] subjected 74 subjects with IPF to PSG and cardiopulmonary exercise testing finding that pulmonary hypertension might be the pathophysiological link between breathing respiratory disturbances and ILD. Troy and colleagues[21] found a relationship between sleep-related hypoxemia (reported as CT90 ≥ 10%) and pulmonary hypertension at baseline echocardiography; moreover, CT90 also predicted new or worsening pulmonary hypertension. Another study in 33 prospectively investigated subjects with IPF found an inverse correlation between nocturnal oxyhemoglobin saturation levels and echocardiographically estimated systolic pulmonary arterial pressure ($P = .002$).[8] In a retrospective cohort study the group of subjects with ILD and pulmonary hypertension (defined as mean pulmonary artery pressure on right heart catheterization ≥20 mm Hg) showed lower CT90 (17% vs 6%, $P = .03$) and sleep efficiency (62% vs 72%, $P = .03$) compared to patients with ILD without pulmonary hypertension.[69] Of note, effective PAP treatment has been

associated with reduced levels of angiogenetic cytokines, such as the vascular endothelial growth factor, regulated by HIF-1.[70] Recurrent gastroesophageal reflux induced by intrathoracic pressure swings associated with OSA[71] might be another mechanism that can lead to the development or the progression of ILD. The link between lung fibrosis and gastroesophageal reflux is well established.[22] Gastroesophageal reflux is also linked to an increased risk of exacerbations in subjects with IPF.[72] A last mechanism by which OSA might be implicated in the pathogenesis of ILD is mechanical. OSA is characterized by repeated forced inspirations against a closed glottis. These tractions can lead to recurrent injuries in peripheral lung tissues predisposing to or aggravating lung fibrosis.[73] Wang and colleagues found that effective PAP therapy in subjects with OSA can reduce gastroesophageal reflux and mechanical trauma to the trachea during the apnea events.[74]

Can interstitial lung disease Predispose to obstructive sleep apnea?

ILD is associated with some pathophysiological mechanisms with the potential to sustain or aggravate OSA and sleep-related hypoxemia. Many subjects with chronic lung diseases, who were not severely hypoxemic at rest while awake, underwent greater degree of hypoxemia during an apnea than that of subjects with normal lung function, even for the same degree of upper airway collapse. This is also demonstrated in subjects with ILD.[50,51] A reduction in lung volumes, typical of advanced ILD, may translate into diminished caudal traction to the pharynx, which in turn predisposes to airway collapse.[75] Of note, among studies of subjects with ILD, there were conflicting findings on the value of lung function parameters in predicting the association with OSA: one study showing that the AHI was related to FVC%

predicted,[13] but others observed a weak[21] or no association[5,7,27] between AHI and FVC% predicted. Perhaps, the measurements of lung function in the supine position maintained during sleep might have a contribution to understand that relationship between ILD and OSA.[25]

Prolonged use of systemic corticosteroids is common in subjects with ILD[76] and may increase the risk of OSA.[77] Corticosteroid use causes fluid retention. Rostral fluid shift during sleep in the recumbent position may, in turn, predispose to upper airway obstruction by airway narrowing.[78] In addition, corticosteroids cause skeletal muscle atrophy and central neck fat redistribution that may also predispose to weight gain.[76]

Subjects with ILD have frequent nocturnal symptoms causing increased arousals and sleep fragmentation, reduced slow wave sleep and sleep efficiency.[5,6,18,21,25,46,47] These factors may cause ventilatory instability that, in turn, may predispose to OSA.[79,80]

SUMMARY

In a recent review, Karuga and colleagues[81] concluded that OSA is more common in subjects with IPF than in the general healthy population. As studies evaluating the rates of OSA in subjects with IPF do not include a control healthy group, authors obtained this result deriving the rates of OSA in healthy controls matched for age, gender, body mass index, and race. Our narrative review confirms that OSA is highly prevalent both in subjects with IPF-only and in mixed ILD populations, but it is difficult to draw other conclusions from available studies for several reasons. First, monitoring devices used in sleep studies were different. Studies evaluating the prevalence of OSA in ILD populations have used different type III or IV monitoring devices and different scoring criteria to categorize OSA. Second, studies in ILD populations had small sample size and participants showed different characteristics. Third, inclusion criteria differed with variations in enrolments from referral clinics, inclusion based on symptoms or findings during clinic visits, or patient recruitment through clinics versus open invitation. However, it is clear that at present subjects with ILD are underdiagnosed for OSA and sleep-related hypoxemia. The finding of many previous studies that subjects with ILD and OSA had relatively mild symptoms compared to those with only ILD without OSA may have contributed to inadequate screening for underlying OSA and sleep-related hypoxemia in these populations. In addition, there is no guideline recommendation for OSA screening in subjects with ILD.

Some studies support the view that the coexistence of OSA and ILD may worsen outcomes. However, it is not defined which sleeping parameters (ie, AHI, ODI, lower nadir oxygen saturation levels, or CT90) are mostly associated with ILD progression. Further studies on the topic should confirm these findings and recommend the monitoring devices required for diagnosis of OSA and sleep-related disturbances in subjects with ILD and the parameters with greater predictive significance.

Three prospective studies suggest that subjects with ILD and OSA able to sustain long-term effective PAP treatment show a meaningful improvement. However, PAP adherence may be challenging in subjects with ILD. Studies evaluating the role of PAP in populations with ILD and OSA have used the AHI for OSA severity categorization. It is increasingly recognized that the AHI alone does not capture several components of OSA, but other aspects, such as hypoxic burden and hypersomnia can influence the risk of poor outcomes, and treatment response.[80–82] Recommendations should define characteristics of subjects with ILD requiring PAP treatment and the degree of adherence for giving benefits. In consideration of the hypoxic burden, the role of nocturnal oxygen therapy, eventually in association with PAP treatment, needs further investigation. Further studies should also evaluate the role of alternative therapies for OSA in subjects with ILD, such as positional treatment, and mandibular devices on outcomes.

We conclude that OSA and related hypoxic burden are common in subjects with ILD and seem to play a role in outcomes.

ACKNOWLEDGMENTS

All named authors contributed equally to the final article, including study conception and design, review of the searched literature, and drafting of the article. All authors contributed to the revision and approved the final version.

DISCLOSURE

S. Croce, M. Messina, A.S. Melani, and E. Bargagli have nothing to disclose. Funding: No funding or sponsorship was received for this study or publication of this article. Authorship: All named authors meet the International Committee of Medical Journal Editors criteria for authorship for this article, take responsibility for the integrity of the work as a whole, and have given their approval for this version to be published.

REFERENCES

1. American Academy of Sleep Medicine. Revised International Classification of sleep disorders. 3rd edition. Darien, IL: American Academy of Sleep Medicine; 2023.
2. Bye P, Issa F, Berthon-Jones M, et al. Studies of oxygenation during sleep in patients with interstitial lung disease. Am Rev Respir Dis 1984;129:27–32.
3. Perez-Padilla R, West P, Lertzman M, et al. Breathing during sleep in patients with interstitial lung disease. Am Rev Respir Dis 1985;132:224–322.
4. Aydoğdu M, Ciftçi B, Firat Güven S, et al. Interstisyel akciğer hastalarinda polisomnografi ile uyku özelliklerinin değerlendirilmesi [Assessment of sleep with polysomnography in patients with interstitial lung disease]. Tuberk Toraks 2006;54(3):213–21.
5. Lancaster LH, Mason WR, Parnell JA, et al. Obstructive sleep apnea is common in idiopathic pulmonary fibrosis. Chest 2009;136(3):772–8.
6. Mermigkis C, Stagaki E, Tryfon S, et al. How common is sleep-disordered breathing in patients with idiopathic pulmonary fibrosis? Sleep Breath 2010; 14(4):387–90.
7. Pillai M, Olson AL, Huie TJ, et al. Obstructive sleep apnea does not promote esophageal reflux in fibrosing interstitial lung disease. Respir Med 2012; 106(7):1033–9.
8. Pitsiou G, Bagalas V, Boutou A, et al. Should we routinely screen patients with idiopathic pulmonary fibrosis for nocturnal hypoxemia? Sleep Breath 2013;17(2):447–8.
9. Kolilekas L, Manali E, Vlami KA, et al. Sleep oxygen desaturation predicts survival in idiopathic pulmonary fibrosis. J Clin Sleep Med 2013;9(6):593–601.
10. Pihtili A, Bingol Z, Kiyan E, et al. Obstructive sleep apnea is common in patients with interstitial lung disease. Sleep Breath 2013;17(4):1281–8.
11. Reid T, Vennelle M, McKinley M, et al. Sleep-disordered breathing and idiopathic pulmonary fibrosis–is there an association? Sleep Breath 2015;19(2):719–21.
12. Lee RN, Kelly E, Nolan G, et al. Disordered breathing during sleep and exercise in idiopathic pulmonary fibrosis. QJM 2016;109(2):142.
13. Bosi M, Milioli G, Fanfulla F, et al. OSA and prolonged oxygen desaturation during sleep are Strong Predictors of poor outcome in IPF. Lung 2017; 195(5):643–51.
14. Gille T, Didier M, Boubaya M, et al. Collaborators Obstructive sleep apnoea and related comorbidities in incident idiopathic pulmonary fibrosis. Eur Respir J 2017;49(6):1601934.
15. Schertel A, Funke-Chambour M, Geiser T, et al. Novel insights in cough and breathing patterns of patients with idiopathic pulmonary fibrosis performing repeated 24-hour-respiratory polygraphies. Respir Res 2017;18(1):190.
16. Ahmed M, Awadalla NJ. Burden of sleep-related breathing disorders, air trapping, and obesity in idiopathic pulmonary fibrosis patients. Egypt J Chest Dis Tuberc 2018;67:300–5.
17. Cardoso AV, Pereira N, Neves I, et al. Obstructive sleep apnoea in patients with fibrotic diffuse parenchymal lung disease-characterization and treatment compliance assessment. Can J Respir Ther 2018; 54(2):35–40.
18. Mavroudi M, Papakosta D, Kontakiotis T, et al. Sleep disorders and health-related quality of life in patients with interstitial lung disease. Sleep Breath 2018; 22(2):393–400.
19. Canora A, Nicoletta C, Ghinassi G, et al. First description of the hyperpnea-hypopnea periodic breathing in patients with interstitial lung disease-obstructive sleep apnea: treatment implications in a real-life setting. Int J Environ Res Public Health 2019;16(23):4712.
20. Sarac S, Kavas M, Sahin M, et al. Relation of Warrick score and polysomnographic parameters in patients with interstitial lung disease. Med Sci Monit 2019;25: 2087–95.
21. Troy LK, Young IH, Lau EMT, et al. Nocturnal hypoxaemia is associated with adverse outcomes in interstitial lung disease. Respirology 2019;24(10): 996–1004.
22. Tudorache V, Traila D, Marc M, et al. Impact of moderate to severe obstructive sleep apnea on the cognition in idiopathic pulmonary fibrosis. PLoS One 2019;14(2):e0211455.
23. Zhang XL, Dai HP, Zhang H, et al. Obstructive sleep apnea in patients with fibrotic interstitial lung disease and COPD. J Clin Sleep Med 2019;15(12): 1807–15.
24. Papadogiannis G, Bouloukaki I, Mermigkis C, et al. Patients with idiopathic pulmonary fibrosis with and without obstructive sleep apnea: differences in clinical characteristics, clinical outcomes, and the effect of PAP treatment. J Clin Sleep Med 2021;17(3): 533–44.
25. Bordas-Martinez J, Salord N, Vicens-Zygmunt V, et al. Characterization of sleep-disordered breathing in idiopathic pulmonary fibrosis. Arch Bronconeumol 2023;59:768–71.
26. Hagmeyer L, Herkenrath SD, Treml M, et al. Sleep-related breathing disorders in idiopathic pulmonary fibrosis are frequent and may be associated with pulmonary vascular involvement. Sleep Breath 2023;27(3):961–71.
27. Valecchi D, Bargagli E, Pieroni MG, et al. Prognostic significance of obstructive sleep apnea in a population of subjects with interstitial lung diseases. Pulm Ther 2023;9(2):223–36.
28. Raghu G, Remy-Jardin M, Richeldi L, et al. Idiopathic pulmonary fibrosis (an Update) and progressive pulmonary fibrosis in adults: an Official ATS/

ERS/JRS/ALAT clinical practice guideline. Am J Respir Crit Care Med 2022;205(9):e18–47.

29. Grassion L, Gonzalez-Bermejo J, Arnulf I, et al. Diagnosing sleep disordered breathing in patients with chronic pulmonary disease: which test for which patient? Breathe 2023;19(1):220199.

30. Kapur VK, Auckley DH, Chowdhuri S, et al. Clinical practice guideline for diagnostic testing for adult obstructive sleep apnea: an American Academy of Sleep Medcine clinical practice guideline. J Clin Sleep Med 2017;13(3):479–504.

31. Malhotra RK, Kirsch DB, Kristo DA, et al. American Academy of Sleep Medicine Board of Directors. Polysomnography for obstructive sleep apnea should include arousal-based scoring: an American Academy of Sleep Medicine position statement. J Clin Sleep Med 2018;14(7):1245–7.

32. Lajoie AC, Sériès F, Bernard S, et al. Reliability of home nocturnal oximetry in the diagnosis of overlap syndrome in COPD. Respiration 2020;99(2):132–9.

33. Abrahamyan L, Sahakyan Y, Chung S, et al. Diagnostic accuracy of level IV portable sleep monitors versus polysomnography for obstructive sleep apnea: a systematic review and meta-analysis. Sleep Breath 2018;22(3):593–611.

34. Benjafield AV, Ayas NT, Eastwood PR, et al. Estimation of the global prevalence and burden of obstructive sleep apnoea: a literature-based analysis. Lancet Respir Med 2019;7(8):687–98.

35. Ng Y, Joosten SA, Edwards BA, et al. Oxygen desaturation index differs significantly between types of sleep Software. J Clin Sleep Med 2017;13(4):599–605.

36. Peppard PE, Young T, Barnet JH, et al. Increased prevalence of sleep-disordered breathing in adults. Am J Epidemiol 2013;177(9):1006–14.

37. Heinzer R, Vat S, Marques-Vidal P, et al. Prevalence of sleep-disordered breathing in the general population: the HypnoLaus study. Lancet Respir Med 2015;3(4):310–8.

38. Chiu HY, Chen PY, Chuang LP, et al. Diagnostic accuracy of the Berlin questionnaire, STOP-BANG, STOP, and Epworth sleepiness scale in detecting obstructive sleep apnea: a bivariate meta-analysis. Sleep Med Rev 2017;36:57–70.

39. Patil SP, Ayappa IA, Caples SM, et al. Treatment of adult obstructive sleep apnea with positive airway pressure: an American Academy of sleep medicine clinical practice guideline. J Clin Sleep Med 2019;15(2):335–43.

40. Patil SP, Ayappa IA, Caples SM, et al. Treatment of adult obstructive sleep apnea with positive airway pressure: an American Academy of sleep medicine systematic review, meta-analysis, and GRADE assessment. J Clin Sleep Med 2019;15(2):301–34.

41. Joy GM, Arbiv OA, Wong CK, et al. Prevalence, imaging patterns and risk factors of interstitial lung disease in connective tissue disease: a systematic review and meta-analysis. Eur Respir Rev 2023; 32(167):220210.

42. Aronson KI, Danoff SK, Russell AM, et al. Patient-centered outcomes Research in interstitial lung disease: an Official American thoracic Society Research statement. Am J Respir Crit Care Med 2021;204(2):e3–23. Erratum in: Am J Respir Crit Care Med. 2021 Sep 1;204(5):616.

43. Nasser M, Larrieu S, Si-Mohamed S, et al. Progressive fibrosing interstitial lung disease: a clinical cohort (the PROGRESS_ study). Eur Respir J 2021; 57(2):2002718.

44. Kreuter M, Swigris J, Pittrow D, et al. The clinical course of idiopathic pulmonary fibrosis and its association to quality of life over time: longitudinal data from the INSIGHTS-IPF registry. Respir Res 2019; 20(1):59.

45. Krishnan V, McCormack MC, Mathai SC, et al. Sleep quality and health-related quality of life in idiopathic pulmonary fibrosis. Chest 2008;134(4):693–8.

46. Bosi M, Milioli G, Parrino L, et al. Quality of life in idiopathic pulmonary fibrosis: the impact of sleep disordered breathing. Respir Med 2019;147:51–7.

47. Mermigkis C, Stagaki E, Amfilochiou A, et al. Sleep quality and associated daytime consequences in patients with idiopathic pulmonary fibrosis. Med Princ Pract 2009;18(1):10–5.

48. Mermigkis C, Bouloukaki I, Antoniou K, et al. Obstructive sleep apnea should be treated in patients with idiopathic pulmonary fibrosis. Sleep Breath 2015;19(1):385–91.

49. Copeland CR, Lancaster LH. Management of progressive fibrosing interstitial lung diseases (PF-ILD). Front Med 2021;8:743977.

50. Yasuda Y, Nagano T, Izumi S, et al. Analysis of nocturnal desaturation waveforms using algorithms in patients with idiopathic pulmonary fibrosis. Sleep Breath 2022;26(3):1079–86.

51. Hira HS, Sharma RK. Study of oxygen saturation, breathing pattern and arrhythmias in patients of interstitial lung disease during sleep. Indian J Chest Dis Allied Sci 1997;39(3):157–62.

52. Clark M, Cooper B, Singh S, et al. A survey of nocturnal hypoxaemia and health related quality of life in patients with cryptogenic fibrosing alveolitis. Thorax 2001;56:482–6.

53. Corte TJ, Wort SJ, Talbot S, et al. Elevated nocturnal desaturation index predicts mortality in interstitial lung disease. Sarcoidosis Vasc Diffuse Lung Dis 2012;29:41–50.

54. Myall KJ, West AG, Martinovic JL, et al. Nocturnal hypoxemia associates with symptom progression and mortality in patients with progressive fibrotic interstitial lung disease. Chest 2023;164(5):1232–42.

55. Lee JH, Jang JH, Park JH, et al. Prevalence and clinical impacts of obstructive sleep apnea in patients

with idiopathic pulmonary fibrosis: a single-center, retrospective study. PLoS One 2023;18(9):e0291195.

56. Vozoris NT, Wilton AS, Austin PC, et al. Morbidity and mortality reduction associated with polysomnography testing in idiopathic pulmonary fibrosis: a population-based cohort study. BMC Pulm Med 2021;21(1):185.

57. Mermigkis C, Bouloukaki I, Antoniou KM, et al. CPAP therapy in patients with idiopathic pulmonary fibrosis and obstructive sleep apnea: does it offer a better quality of life and sleep? Sleep Breath 2013;17(4):1137–43.

58. Adegunsoye A, Neborak JM, Zhu D, et al. CPAP adherence, mortality, and progression-free survival in interstitial lung disease and OSA. Chest 2020;158(4):1701–12.

59. Kim JS, Podolanczuk AJ, Borker P, et al. Obstructive sleep apnea and subclinical interstitial lung disease in the multi-ethnic study of atherosclerosis (MESA). Ann Am Thorac Soc 2017;14(12):1786–95.

60. Kim JS, Azarbarzin A, Podolanczuk AJ, et al. Obstructive sleep apnea and longitudinal changes in interstitial lung imaging and lung function: the MESA study. Ann Am Thorac Soc 2023;20(5):728–37.

61. Tuleta I, Stöckigt F, Juergens UR, et al. Intermittent hypoxia contributes to the lung damage by increased oxidative stress, inflammation, and disbalance in protease/antiprotease system. Lung 2016;194:1015–20.

62. Braun RK, Broytman O, Braun FM, et al. Chronic intermittent hypoxia worsens bleomycin-induced lung fibrosis in rats. Respir Physiol Neurobiol 2018;256:97–108.

63. Yang L, Gilbertsen A, Xia H, et al. Hypoxia enhances IPF mesenchymal progenitor cell fibrogenicity via the lactate/GPR81/HIF1α pathway. JCI Insight 2023;8(4):e163820.

64. Konigsberg IR, Borie R, Walts AD, et al. Molecular signatures of idiopathic pulmonary fibrosis. Am J Respir Cell Mol Biol 2021;65(4):430–41.

65. Epstein Shochet G, Bardenstein-Wald B, McElroy M, et al. Hypoxia inducible factor 1A supports a Pro-fibrotic Phenotype Loop in idiopathic pulmonary fibrosis. Int J Mol Sci 2021;22(7):3331.

66. Trakada G, Nikolaou E, Pouli A, et al. Endothelin-1 levels in interstitial lung disease patients during sleep. Sleep Breath 2003;7(3):111–8.

67. Chaouat A, Weitzenblum E, Krieger J, et al. Pulmonary hemodynamics in the obstructive sleep apnea syndrome. Results in 220 consecutive patients. Chest 1996;109(2):380–6.

68. Kacprzak A, Tomkowski W, Szturmowicz M. Pulmonary hypertension in the course of interstitial lung diseases-A personalised approach is needed to identify a dominant cause and provide an effective therapy. Diagnostics 2023;13(14):2354.

69. Simonson JL, Pandya D, Khan S, et al. Sleep architecture in patients with interstitial lung disease with and without pulmonary hypertension. Sleep Breath 2022;26(4):1711–5.

70. Qi JC, Zhang L, Li H, et al. Impact of continuous positive airway pressure on vascular endothelial growth factor in patients with obstructive sleep apnea: a meta-analysis. Sleep Breath 2019;23(1):5–12.

71. Shepherd KL, James AL, Musk AW, et al. Gastro-oesophageal reflux symptoms are related to the presence and severity of obstructive sleep apnoea. J Sleep Res 2011;20(1 Pt 2):241–9.

72. Collard HR, Moore BB, Flaherty KR, et al. Idiopathic pulmonary fibrosis clinical Research Network Investigators. Acute exacerbations of idiopathic pulmonary fibrosis. Am J Respir Crit Care Med 2007;176(7):63643.

73. Leslie KO. Idiopathic pulmonary fibrosis may be a disease of recurrent, tractional injury to the periphery of the aging lung: a unifying hypothesis regarding etiology and pathogenesis. Arch Pathol Lab Med 2012;136(6):591–600.

74. Wang L, Han H, Wang G, et al. Relationship between reflux diseases and obstructive sleep apnea together with continuous positive airway pressure treatment efficiency analysis. Sleep Med 2020;75:151–5.

75. Won CH, Kryger M. Sleep in patients with restrictive lung disease. Clin Chest Med 2014;35(3):505–12.

76. Melani AS, Croce S, Cassai L, et al. Systemic corticosteroids for treating respiratory diseases: less is better, but... when and How is it possible in real life? Pulm Ther 2023;9(3):329–44.

77. Berger G, Hardak E, Shaham B, et al. Preliminary prospective explanatory observation on the impact of 3-month steroid therapy on the objective measures of sleep-disordered breathing. Sleep Breath 2012;16(2):549–53.

78. White LH, Bradley TD. Role of nocturnal rostral fluid shift in the pathogenesis of obstructive and central sleep apnoea. J Physiol 2013;591(Pt 5):1179–93.

79. Si L, Zhang J, Wang Y, et al. Obstructive sleep apnea and respiratory center regulation abnormality. Sleep Breath 2021;25(2):563–70.

80. McNicholas WT, Pevernagie D. Obstructive sleep apnea: transition from pathophysiology to an integrative disease model. J Sleep Res 2022;31(4):e13616.

81. Karuga FF, Kaczmarski P, Szmyd B, et al. The association between idiopathic pulmonary fibrosis and obstructive sleep apnea: a systematic review and meta-analysis. J Clin Med 2022;11(17):5008.

82. Pevernagie DA, Gnidovec-Strazisar B, Grote L, et al. On the rise and fall of the apnea-hypopnea index: a historical review and critical appraisal. J Sleep Res 2020;29(4):e13066.

Obstructive Sleep Apnea and Sarcoidosis Interactions

Chitra Lal, MD

KEYWORDS

• Apnea • Sarcoidosis • Overlap • Fatigue • Hypoventilation

KEY POINTS

• Overlap of obstructive sleep apnea (OSA) with sarcoidosis is very common.
• Several clinical manifestations such as fatigue, hypersomnolence, cognitive deficits and pulmonary hypertension are common to both disorders.
• Early recognition and treatment of OSA and obesity hypoventilation syndrome in sarcoidosis patients can improve clinical symptoms and overall quality of life.

INTRODUCTION

Obstructive sleep apnea (OSA) is a very common condition and involves repetitive, episodic collapse of the upper airway, resulting in periodic oxygen desaturation. The worldwide prevalence of OSA, as defined by an apnea-hypopneas index (AHI) of $\geq$ 5 events/h and $\geq$ 15 events/h, is 936 million (95% confidence interval [CI] 903–970) adults aged 30 to 69 years and 425 million (399–450) adults aged 30 to 69 years, respectively.[1] This worldwide prevalence continues to increase due to various factors, including the obesity epidemic and greater awareness of this disorder.

Sarcoidosis is a multisystem granulomatous disorder which has a higher prevalence of OSA than found in the general population. OSA prevalence rates (as defined by an AHI $\geq$ 5 events/h) of between 17% and 67% [2–4] have been reported in sarcoidosis cohorts. In comparison, the prevalence of OSA in the general population is 9% in women and 24% in men in the 30-year to 60-year age group[5]

Many manifestations of sarcoidosis and OSA such as fatigue, cognitive impairment (CI), and pulmonary hypertension (PH) overlap. Hence there is significant interest in this overlap syndrome between OSA and sarcoidosis and its consequences.

EPIDEMIOLOGY, PREVALENCE, AND PATHOGENESIS OF OBSTRUCTIVE SLEEP APNEA-SARCOID OVERLAP SYNDROME

Given the high prevalence of OSA in sarcoidosis, there has been great interest in the reasons for this association. The OSASA study (The Prevalence of OSA in Sarcoidosis and Its Impact On Sleepiness, Fatigue, and Sleep-Associated Quality Of Life: A Cross-Sectional Study with Matched Controls) evaluated the prevalence of OSA and possible risk factors for OSA in sarcoidosis. 71 adult patients with sarcoidosis and 71 adult matched controls according to sex, age, and body mass index (BMI) were included. Measures such as Epworth Sleepiness Scale (ESS), Fatigue Assessment Scale (FAS), and Functional Outcomes of Sleep Questionnaire as well as home sleep apnea testing were performed. The risk of OSA was measured using the NoSAS score which includes neck circumference, obesity/BMI, snoring, age, and sex. The OSASA study found a 2.5-fold higher risk of mild OSA in sarcoidosis patients as compared with matched controls.[6] Sex, BMI, neck circumference, and NoSAS score were found to be positively associated with OSA in patients with sarcoidosis. On the other hand, age, steroid use, Scadding stages, inflammatory markers,

Pulmonary, Critical Care and Sleep Medicine, Medical University of South Carolina, 96 Jonathan Lucas Street, CSB 816, Msc 630, Charleston, SC 29425, USA
E-mail address: lalch@musc.edu

Sleep Med Clin 19 (2024) 295–305
https://doi.org/10.1016/j.jsmc.2024.02.010
1556-407X/24/© 2024 Elsevier Inc. All rights reserved.

and pulmonary function values were not associated with OSA in sarcoidosis patients. Thus, NoSAS score can be used to screen for OSA in sarcoidosis patients.

There is sound scientific basis as to why OSA would be more common in sarcoidosis and several hypotheses have been proposed in this regard. Sarcoidosis of the upper respiratory tract (SURT) may affect upper airway patency and increase the risk of OSA.[7] Biopsy confirmed SURT is seen in 2% to 3% of patients with sarcoidosis.[8] Nasal stuffiness, blockage, crusting, and anosmia are common initial manifestations of SURT.[9,10] While nasal disease is the commonest form of SURT, all parts of the upper respiratory tract can be affected. Laryngeal involvement can result in airway obstruction.[11] Thus SURT can increase the risk of OSA by causing upper airway obstruction. Skin lesions were found to be commonly associated with SURT in 92% of patients in 1 study, comprising of plaques, subcutaneous nodules, lupus pernio, and erythema nodosum.[12] In fact, patients with lupus pernio are at a higher risk of OSA.[3] The association between lupus pernio and OSA likely relates to the fact that lupus pernio is closely associated with SURT.[12]

An association between interstitial lung disease and OSA has also been reported.[4] Indeed, the severity of OSA as measured by the AHI and degree of hypoxemia is higher in sarcoidosis patients with parenchymal lung involvement as compared to those without parenchymal lung involvement.[13] Several mechanisms have been reported for this association. The decreased caudal traction on the upper airways can result in increased upper airway collapsibility and, hence, an increased risk of OSA.[14] Ventilatory system instability could also be a contributory factor due to heightened chemo-responsiveness and increased respiratory events during sleep.[14] In addition, rapid eye movement (REM) sleep is an atonic state, and some of these changes can be heightened during REM sleep, resulting in increased severity of OSA and hypoxemia in REM sleep.

A propensity for hypoxemia due to underlying lung disease can also increase the number of scored respiratory events, as hypopneas are defined by oxygen desaturation. This can result in a higher AHI in lung disease patients with associated hypoxemia, without any change in upper airway mechanics.[15]

Corticosteroids are the mainstay of treatment in sarcoidosis patients and may cause weight gain and thereby increase OSA risk.[15]

Salient recent studies evaluating OSA in sarcoidosis are listed in **Table 1**.

SCREENING FOR OBSTRUCTIVE SLEEP APNEA IN SARCOIDOSIS PATIENTS

Traditional risk factors for OSA, such as obesity and enlarged neck circumference, and the presence of symptoms such as snoring, witnessed apneas, fatigue, excessive daytime sleepiness (EDS), and the presence of hypertension should prompt evaluation for OSA.

Screening instruments such as the STOP-Bang (snoring, tiredness, observed apnea, blood pressure, BMI, age, neck size, and gender)[16] and Berlin questionnaires[17] can be used for initial screening for OSA. NoSAS score (neck circumference, obesity, snoring, age, and sex) can also be used to screen for OSA in sarcoidosis patients.[6,18] ESS can be used to screen for daytime sleepiness.[19] If the patient screens as being at intermediate-to-high risk for OSA, then a confirmatory test for OSA such as a home sleep apnea test or an in-laboratory polysomnogram should be undertaken. In general, an in-laboratory polysomnogram is preferred for patients with underlying lung disease, especially those with significant hypoxemia or hypercapnia.[20] Also, patients suspected to have concomitant central sleep apnea, such as patients with neurosarcoidosis, should have in-laboratory polysomnograms as these are still considered the gold standard for the diagnosis of central sleep apnea.[21]

A morning blood gas showing hypercapnia ($P_{CO_2} > 45$ mm Hg), in the presence of obesity and no other reasons to explain the hypercapnia, would be consistent with obesity hypoventilation syndrome (OHS).[22]

CLINICAL MANIFESTATIONS AND MANAGEMENT OF OBSTRUCTIVE SLEEP APNEA-SARCOID OVERLAP SYNDROME

Several of the clinical manifestations seen in OSA and sarcoidosis as listed in **Table 2** are common to both syndromes. Hence, the recognition and treatment of both syndromes might produce greater improvement in these symptoms and improve overall quality of life.

Fatigue and Sleepiness

Fatigue is physical and/or mental exhaustion and is a subjective complaint, which can often be difficult to differentiate from EDS. Fatigue is commonly measured in sarcoidosis using the FAS.[23] The Patient-Reported Outcome Measurement Information System (PROMIS) Fatigue Scale has also been used to assess fatigue in OSA patients.[24]

Fatigue is reported by up to 80% sarcoid patients[25] and has a profound impact on overall

Table 1
Salient recent studies evaluating obstructive sleep apnea in sarcoidosis

Study/Year	Type	n	Population	Outcome/Conclusion
Ertas Dogan et al,[71] 2020	Prospective	46	Clinically stable stage I and II sarcoidosis, not on treatment	67.8% had mild OSA; the frequency of OSA diagnosis increased with age
Mari et al,[72] 2020	Prospective	68	Sarcoidosis patients 18–85 y of age (part of SARCOIDOSAS study cohort)	OSA seen in 88.2% subjects; ESS was not reliable for OSA screening; CPAP improved fatigue and daytime sleepiness at 3 mo.
Ataoglu et al,[73] 2022	Prospective	60	Consecutive patients diagnosed with sarcoidosis	OSA seen in 70% (38/54) patients undergoing PSG; sarcoid disease stage (P = .026) was the single independent risk factor associated with increased risk of OSA
Judson et al,[74] 2022	Retrospective	2,720,396	10,512 patients with sarcoidosis and 2,709,884 controls without sarcoidosis from a US Veterans Health Administration database	No association between BMI and the rate of developing sarcoidosis; a diagnosis of OSA was protective from the development of sarcoidosis
Roeder et al,[6] 2022	Prospective	142	71 adult patients with sarcoidosis, 71 adult matched controls	Risk for mild OSA is 2.5-fold higher in sarcoidosis patients as compared to matched controls; NoSAS score can be used to screen for OSA in sarcoidosis patients; ESS, FAS, and FOSQ were not associated with AHI

Abbreviations: BMI, body mass index; CPAP, continuous positive airway pressure; ESS, Epworth Sleepiness Scale; FAS, fatigue assessment scale; FOSQ, functional outcomes of sleep questionnaire; NoSAS, neck circumference, obesity, snoring, age, and sex; OSA, obstructive sleep apnea; PSG, polysomnogram.

quality of life. Fatigue is also a common complaint in OSA patients.[26] Fatigue in sarcoidosis maybe caused by granulomatous inflammation and/or the effect of steroid therapy.[27] Fatigue in OSA is likely related to fragmented and non-restorative sleep.

EDS in OSA has been hypothesized to be due to chronic intermittent hypoxia and sleep fragmentation, resulting in oxidative injury and neuronal changes involving noradrenergic and dopaminergic neurotransmission in wake-promoting regions of the brain.[28] Neuroimaging studies have shown changes in gray matter[29] in the brains of OSA patients. Studies have also shown changes in white matter[30] in the brains of OSA patients with EDS.

While patients often find it difficult to distinguish between EDS and fatigue, there are distinct symptoms. Screening instruments and direct questions about the propensity to fall asleep can help to differentiate the 2. The Multiple Sleep Latency Test is an objective test which may also help to objectively measure the degree of sleepiness, but it lacks reproducibility.[31]

EDS is a common complaint in OSA patients but can also sometimes be reported by sarcoidosis patients.[32] Therefore, sarcoidosis patients who complain of EDS as the predominant compliant

Table 2
Common clinical manifestations of obstructive sleep apnea-sarcoidosis overlap syndrome with the screening tools used

Clinical Manifestations	Commonly Used Screening Tools
Fatigue	• PROMIS Fatigue Scale
Hypersomnolence	• Epworth Sleepiness Scale • Multiple Sleep Latency Test
Cognitive impairment	• Mini-Mental Status Examination • Montreal Cognitive Assessment • Psychomotor vigilance task (sustained attention/vigilance), • N-back task (working memory) • Wisconsin Card Sorting Test (cognitive flexibility)
Pulmonary hypertension	• Echocardiogram • Right heart catheterization
Hypoxemia and hypercapnia	• Arterial blood gas

Abbreviation: PROMIS, Patient-reported outcomes measurement information system.

or fatigue which is disproportionate to disease severity should be evaluated for OSA. This is especially important if patients present with risk factors for OSA such as an elevated BMI, enlarged neck circumference, history of snoring, witnessed apneas, and hypertension.

If OSA has been reasonably excluded, then alternative causes of fatigue should be investigated, including adrenal insufficiency (especially if the patient has received chronic corticosteroid therapy and has been recently tapered), obesity, hypothyroidism, sleep deprivation, sarcoidosis-associated PH (SAPH),[33] and psychological disturbances such as depression that are common in sarcoidosis.[34,35] Once these potential causes of fatigue have been excluded, then the patient may be considered to have sarcoidosis-associated fatigue. Despite the fact that sarcoidosis-associated fatigue is thought to be the systemic effect of inflammatory mediators released by the sarcoid granuloma, corticosteroids and other antisarcoid medications appear to be less than 50% effective for this problem.[27]

Wake-promoting drugs such as modafinil, armodafinil, pitolisant, and solriamfetol and stimulants such as methylphenidate have been used to treat OSA-related EDS.[28] Methylphenidate and modafinil have also been shown to be beneficial in sarcoid-related fatigue.[36] Corticosteroids and other antisarcoid medications appear to be less effective in treating fatigue.[27]

A suggested approach to the evaluation of fatigue in patients with sarcoidosis is shown in **Fig. 1**.

Hypoxemia and Hypercapnia

Nocturnal hypoxemia can occur both in OSA and sarcoidosis. REM sleep being an atonic state predisposes to nocturnal hypoxemia in patients with pre-existing lung disease such as sarcoidosis.

The nocturnal hypoxemia of OSA is related to respiratory events and sometimes also to sleep-related hypoventilation. Sleep-related hypoventilation can be an earlier stage of OHS,[37] which is associated with daytime hypoxemia and hypercapnia. OHS is characterized by obesity (BMI $\geq$ 30 kg/m^2) and hypoventilation (Paco$_2$ > 45 mm Hg) and is a diagnosis of exclusion.[22] Given its association with increased long-term morbidity and mortality,[38] it is important to recognize OHS and to treat it appropriately. OHS is more common in sarcoidosis due to the morbid obesity related to steroid use.[15]

The treatment for OHS is positive airway pressure (PAP). In chronic stable OHS patients with severe OSA, continuous PAP (CPAP) is the first-line treatment.[39] Patients who are hospitalized due to hypercapnic respiratory failure and are suspected to have OHS should be discharged home on noninvasive ventilation until further outpatient diagnostic testing and in-laboratory PAP titration can be done.[39] In patients with sarcoid and OHS, who have significant hypercapnia and pulmonary dysfunction, noninvasive bi-level nocturnal ventilation may be more appropriate than CPAP therapy.

Daytime arterial blood gas abnormalities are relatively rare in early sarcoidosis. With the progression of lung disease, significant hypoxemia can occur; however, hypercapnia remains relatively rare even in late-stage fibrocystic sarcoidosis.[40] This could be due to the increased hypoxic ventilatory drive maintaining normocapnia in advanced sarcoid interstitial lung disease.

The presence of significant hypercapnia in an obese sarcoid patient should prompt evaluation for OHS in addition to other potential etiologies such as medications which can cause hypoventilation.

Effect of Obstructive Sleep Apnea and Sarcoidosis on Pulmonary Artery Pressure

PH is defined as a mean pulmonary artery pressure (mPAP) greater than 20 mm Hg measured by right heart catheterization. Pulmonary vascular

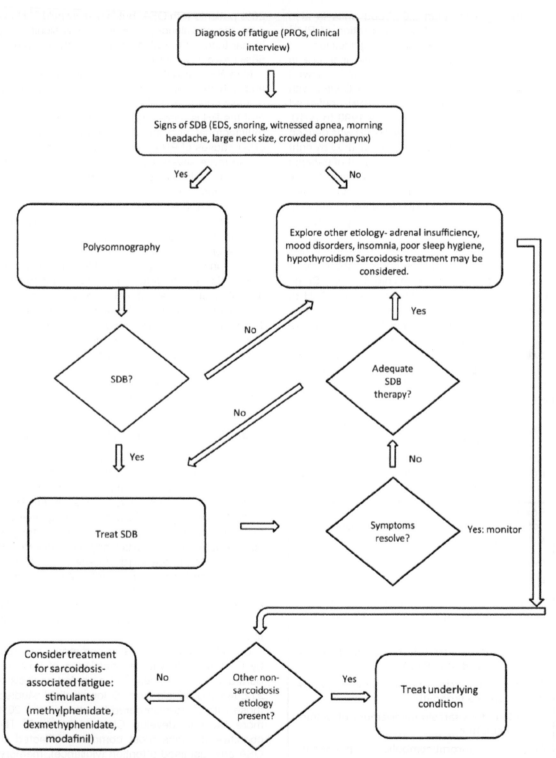

Fig. 1. Approach to fatigue in sarcoidosis. EDS, excessive daytime sleepiness; PRO, patient-reported outcome; SDB, sleep-disordered breathing. (Chitra Lal et al. Interrelationship Between Sleep-Disordered Breathing and Sarcoidosis, Chest, 148 (4), 2015, 1105-1114, https://doi.org/10.1378/chest.15-0584.)

resistance greater than 2.0 Wood units is also used for diagnosis and prognostication of PH[41] according to most recent updated guidelines.

SAPH is associated with a 7-fold increase in mortality.[42,43] Parikh and colleagues[42] followed patients at Duke University Medical Center with biopsy-proven sarcoidosis and SAPH confirmed by right heart catheterization from 1990 to 2010, for up to 11 years. In this study, SAPH was defined as mPAP $\geq$ 25 mm Hg at rest as measured by right heart catheterization. This was a cohort of patients with relatively advanced symptoms, with 70% of patients having stage IV pulmonary sarcoidosis and 77% having functional class III/IV symptoms. The mortality rate over the median 3-year follow-up was found to be 32%.

The true incidence of SAPH is unknown, and prevalence depends on the stage of the disease at which patients are assessed for PH. Some studies have reported a prevalence of SAPH of 2.9%.[44,45] There are likely ethnic differences, however, with a trend toward a higher prevalence of SAPH in non-Caucasian populations.[46,47] In advanced lung disease due to sarcoidosis, the prevalence of SAPH is much higher, with 1 study reporting a prevalence of 73.8% in a cohort of patients listed for lung transplant.[48]

Potential etiologies for SAPH are listed in **Box 1**.[15,47,49–52]

Given the significant impact of SAPH on morbidity and mortality, it is important to recognize and treat all potential causes of SAPH. PH occurs in about 20% patients with OSA, but is usually mild.[53] However, the prevalence of PH in OHS is significantly higher than in OSA alone, with 1 study reporting a 58% prevalence of PH in OHS patients.[54]

Mild PH in a patient with sarcoidosis and OSA and with no cardiac or intrinsic pulmonary vascular disease could be attributed to OSA alone. However if the PH is moderate to severe, then it is likely multifactorial and should prompt evaluation for other causes of PH as well. OHS could potentially cause more severe hemodynamic derangements due to hypoxic pulmonary vasoconstriction.

Treatment with noninvasive ventilation can improve pulmonary artery systolic pressure after 6 months of therapy in OHS patients,[55] although PAP adherence is likely an important factor in the degree of improvement seen. PH can have a significant impact on quality of life and long-term prognosis, and therefore, it is important to treat all potential causes of PH. Treatment of OSA/OHS may improve the PH seen in sarcoid patients. Therefore, patients who screen as being at high risk for OSA should be promptly evaluated for OSA and treated. Adherence to PAP therapy becomes critically important in this context.

A suggested approach to the management of SAPH is outlined in **Fig. 2**.

Cognitive Impairment in Obstructive Sleep Apnea and Sarcoidosis

Cognitive failure refers to cognitive errors in task performance which normally a person should be able to execute successfully in everyday life.[56] Cognitive failure can affect several cognitive domains including memory, concentration, and executive function. Everyday cognitive failure has been reported in one-third of general sarcoidosis patients[56] and in more than 50% of neurosarcoidosis patients.[57] Cognitive failure in sarcoidosis patients has been found to be associated with fatigue, depression, and symptoms related to small-fiber neuropathy.[56]

Cognitive deficits are also commonly reported by OSA patients with a prevalence of 25% reported in some studies.[58] In a pooled analysis of 212,943 individuals from 6 longitudinal studies, those with sleep-disordered breathing were 26% more likely to develop CI or dementia.[59] The cognitive domains most commonly affected by OSA are sustained attention (vigilance), memory, and executive function.[60] Results have been inconsistent between studies, however, due to the varying definitions of OSA used, the cognitive domains studied, variable study designs, heterogeneity of patient populations, and variable durations of longitudinal follow-up. The wealth of

---

Box 1
Potential etiologies of sarcoidosis-associated pulmonary hypertension

Interstitial lung disease (pulmonary fibrosis)

Hypoxic pulmonary vasoconstriction

Sleep-disordered breathing (OSA and OHS)

Liver involvement with porto-pulmonary hypertension

Left heart disease (sarcoid-related cardiomyopathy, diastolic dysfunction)

Extrinsic compression of pulmonary vasculature due to lymphadenopathy

Granulomatous sarcoid involvement of pulmonary vasculature

Chronic thromboembolic pulmonary hypertension

Post-capillary venule fibrosis (pulmonary veno-occlusive–like disease)

Abbreviations: OHS, obesity hypoventilation syndrome; OSA, obstructive sleep apnea.

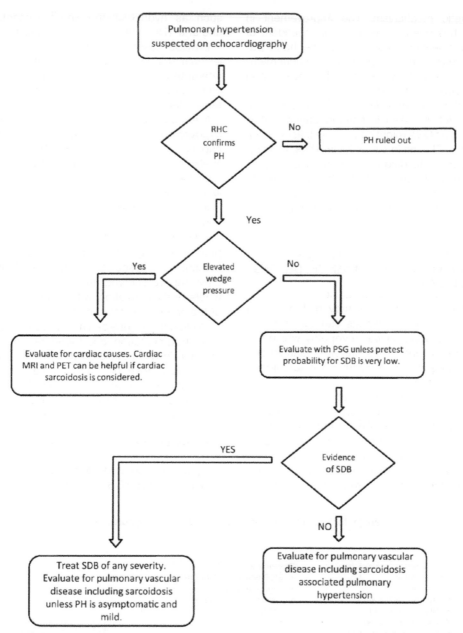

Fig. 2. Approach to pulmonary hypertension in sarcoidosis. PH, pulmonary hypertension; PSG, polysomnogram; RHC, right heart catheterization; SDB, sleep-disordered breathing. (Chitra Lal et al. Interrelationship Between Sleep-Disordered Breathing and Sarcoidosis, Chest, 148 (4), 2015, 1105-1114, https://doi.org/10.1378/chest.15-0584.)

available evidence points toward OSA as a risk factor for cognitive decline.[60]

Nocturnal hypoxemia and sleep fragmentation are likely contributory factors to the CI seen in OSA patients.[60] Neuroimaging studies in OSA patients with CI have shown gray[61,62] and white[63] matter brain changes, which may be reversed with PAP therapy.[64] Hippocampal atrophy has especially been noted in OSA patients with memory impairment.[63] Hippocampal atrophy is also seen in Alzheimer's disease (AD),[65] thus leading to the hypothesis that OSA is a modifiable risk factor for mild CI and AD. In fact, there is strong biological plausibility that the association between AD and OSA is bidirectional, but currently, data are insufficient to prove the bidirectional nature of this association.

Treatment with anti-tumor necrosis factor alpha (anti-TNF-α) drugs has been shown to improve both cognitive scores and fatigue in sarcoidosis patients,[56] which points toward a common underlying pathogenetic mechanism. The improvement in cognition has been shown to be independent of the improvement in fatigue. On the other hand, patients treated with prednisone with or without methotrexate did not show the same improvement in cognitive scores in this study.

Given the high prevalence of both OSA and cognitive deficits seen in sarcoid patients, it is very likely that OSA might cause or at least worsen some of the CI seen in sarcoidosis. Thus, it is critically important to diagnose and treat OSA early and aggressively, as a modifiable risk factor for CI. This can be an additive strategy to pharmacologic treatment for sarcoidosis in treating the CI seen in sarcoid patients.

OTHER IMPLICATIONS FOR CLINICAL MANAGEMENT OF SLEEP MANIFESTATIONS OF SARCOIDOSIS

Corticosteroids are the mainstay of therapy for sarcoidosis; however, steroids can cause weight gain and also upper airway myopathy which can worsen OSA severity. Thus, steroid-sparing therapies should be considered early on in sarcoidosis patients with OSA.[15]

SURT is strongly associated with OSA, and treatment of SURT may improve OSA severity. However, treatment of SURT requires relatively high steroid doses[66] which can cause weight gain. Thus, in such situations, attempts should be made to lower steroid dosages to the lowest dosage needed, and use steroid-sparing therapies

such as hydroxychloroquine,[10] methotrexate,[67] and anti-TNF antibodies such as infliximab.[8]

In milder cases of SURT, local therapy with intralesional steroids or upper airway surgery may be attempted,[68] instead of systemic steroids. This can help to limit the toxicity associated with systemic steroid use.

Neurosarcoidosis can also be associated with hypoventilation,[69] which can worsen the hypercapnia with concomitant OHS. Neurosarcoidosis is also a risk factor for central sleep apnea[69] and may be a secondary cause of narcolepsy[70] as well. Central sleep apnea may manifest with insomnia while narcolepsy most commonly presents with EDS, and therefore, awareness of these conditions is important. Stimulants or wake-promoting drugs can be used to treat the hypersomnolence associated with narcolepsy. One case report showed the benefit of low-dose, whole-brain irradiation with complete resolution of the narcoleptic features.[70]

Corticosteroid use can also cause insomnia and sleep fragmentation, and therefore, administering the steroid dose earlier in the morning and using the lowest dose needed can help to improve some of the sleep manifestations of steroid use.

A paradigm for the management of OSA-sarcoid overlap syndrome is shown in **Fig. 3**.

FUTURE RESEARCH QUESTIONS

Despite the magnitude of the problem, there is a paucity of data on OSA-sarcoid overlap syndrome.

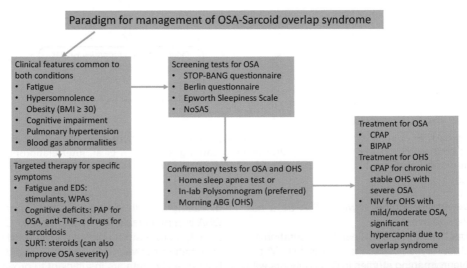

Fig. 3. Schematic representation of the management of obstructive sleep apnea-sarcoid overlap syndrome. ABG, arterial blood gas; BIPAP, bi-level positive airway pressure; BMI, body mass index; CPAP, continuous positive airway pressure; EDS, excessive daytime sleepiness; NIV, noninvasive ventilation; NoSAS, neck circumference, obesity, snoring, age, and sex; OHS, obesity hypoventilation syndrome; OSA, obstructive sleep apnea; PAP, positive airway pressure; SURT, sarcoidosis of the upper respiratory tract; TNF, tumor necrosis factor; WPAs, wake-promoting agents.

OSA and sarcoidosis both are proinflammatory states; the significance of this for long-term outcomes such as cardiovascular disease and stroke needs to be studied. Both OSA and sarcoidosis can impact cognition and with the push for AD research in patients with OSA, this association is of interest for understanding CI. Both OSA and sarcoidosis are potentially modifiable risk factors for CI, and treating both conditions might lessen the burden of mild CI and dementia in an aging population.

The impact of OSA treatment on endpoints such as PH in sarcoidosis patients also requires further study. An alternative to large-scale randomized controlled trials (RCTs), which can be costly, are large research database studies with propensity score matching. Large observational studies with propensity score matching could be a useful adjunct to RCTs.

SUMMARY

The overlap between OSA and sarcoidosis is an important association to recognize and treat. Early recognition and treatment of both conditions can improve several symptoms common to both, such as fatigue, hypersomnolence, PH, and cognitive deficits, and improve the overall quality of life of patients.

CLINICS CARE POINTS

- OSA-sarcoidosis overlap syndrome has a high prevalence
- Significant hypercapnia in an obese sarcoid patient should prompt evaluation for OHS.
- SURT is associated with a higher prevalence of OSA.
- Fatigue, hypersomnolence, PH, and cognitive complaints are common to both OSA and sarcoidosis.
- Fatigue and EDS may respond to wake-promoting drugs and stimulants, steroids and other anti-sarcoid medications appear to be less effective in treating sarcoid-related fatigue.
- Mild PH in a patient with sarcoidosis and OSA, with no cardiac or intrinsic pulmonary vascular disease, could be due to OSA alone.
- Moderate-to-severe PH in sarcoidosis patients is likely multifactorial and should prompt evaluation for other causes of PH as well.
- PAP therapy can improve PH in sarcoidosis patients with OSA/OHS.

- Everyday cognitive failure is commonly seen in sarcoidosis; anti-TNF-α drugs for sarcoidosis and PAP therapy for comorbid OSA can improve cognitive scores.
- Attempts should be made to lower steroid dosages and use steroid-sparing therapies for sarcoidosis treatment to minimize weight gain and worsening of OSA.

DISCLOSURE

Dr C. Lal is a consultant for Jazz pharmaceuticals, Chest/GSK, and Idorsia pharmaceuticals.

REFERENCES

1. Benjafield AV, Ayas NT, Eastwood PR, et al. Estimation of the global prevalence and burden of obstructive sleep apnoea: a literature-based analysis. Lancet Respir Med 2019;7(8):687–98.
2. Verbraecken J, Hoitsma E, van der Grinten CP, et al. Sleep disturbances associated with periodic leg movements in chronic sarcoidosis. Sarcoidosis Vasc Diffuse Lung Dis 2004;21(2):137–46.
3. Turner GA, Lower EE, Corser BC, et al. Sleep apnea in sarcoidosis. Sarcoidosis Vasc Diffuse Lung Dis 1997;14(1):61–4.
4. Pihtili A, Bingol Z, Kiyan E, et al. Obstructive sleep apnea is common in patients with interstitial lung disease. Sleep Breath 2013;17(4):1281–8.
5. Peppard PE, Young T, Barnet JH, et al. Increased prevalence of sleep-disordered breathing in adults. Am J Epidemiol 2013;177(9):1006–14.
6. Roeder M, Sievi NA, Schneider A, et al. The prevalence of obstructive sleep apnea in sarcoidosis and its impact on sleepiness, fatigue, and sleep-associated quality of life: a cross-sectional study with matched controls (the OSASA study). J Clin Sleep Med 2022;18(10):2415–22.
7. Shah RN, Mills PR, George PJ, et al. Upper airways sarcoidosis presenting as obstructive sleep apnoea. Thorax 1998;53(3):232–3.
8. Baughman RP, Lower EE, Tami T. Upper airway. 4: sarcoidosis of the upper respiratory tract (SURT). Thorax 2010;65(2):181–6.
9. Wilson R, Lund V, Sweatman M, et al. Upper respiratory tract involvement in sarcoidosis and its management. Eur Respir J 1988;1(3):269–72.
10. Aubart FC, Ouayoun M, Brauner M, et al. Sinonasal involvement in sarcoidosis: a case-control study of 20 patients. Medicine (Baltim) 2006;85(6):365–71.
11. Sims HS, Thakkar KH. Airway involvement and obstruction from granulomas in African-American patients with sarcoidosis. Respir Med 2007;101(11):2279–83.
12. James DG, Barter S, Jash D, et al. Sarcoidosis of the upper respiratory tract (SURT). J Laryngol Otol 1982;96(8):711–8.

13. Bingol Z, Pihtili A, Gulbaran Z, et al. Relationship between parenchymal involvement and obstructive sleep apnea in subjects with sarcoidosis. Clin Respir J 2015;9(1):14–21.

14. Troy LK, Corte TJ. Sleep disordered breathing in interstitial lung disease: a review. World J Clin Cases 2014;2(12):828–34.

15. Lal C, Medarov BI, Judson MA. Interrelationship between sleep-disordered breathing and sarcoidosis. Chest 2015;148(4):1105–14.

16. Chung F, Abdullah HR, Liao P. STOP-bang questionnaire: a practical approach to screen for obstructive sleep apnea. Chest 2016;149(3):631–8.

17. Tan A, Yin JD, Tan LW, et al. Using the berlin questionnaire to predict obstructive sleep apnea in the general population. J Clin Sleep Med 2017;13(3): 427–32.

18. Coutinho Costa J, Rebelo-Marques A, Machado JN, et al. Validation of NoSAS (Neck, Obesity, Snoring, Age, Sex) score as a screening tool for obstructive sleep apnea: analysis in a sleep clinic. Pulmonology 2019;25(5):263–70.

19. Johns MW. A new method for measuring daytime sleepiness: the Epworth sleepiness scale. Sleep 1991;14(6):540–5.

20. Kapur VK, Auckley DH, Chowdhuri S, et al. Clinical practice guideline for diagnostic testing for adult obstructive sleep apnea: an american academy of sleep medicine clinical practice guideline. J Clin Sleep Med 2017;13(3):479–504.

21. Sateia MJ. International classification of sleep disorders-third edition: highlights and modifications. Chest 2014;146(5):1387–94.

22. Balachandran JS, Masa JF, Mokhlesi B. Obesity hypoventilation syndrome epidemiology and diagnosis. Sleep Med Clin 2014;9(3):341–7.

23. De Vries J, Michielsen H, Van Heck GL, et al. Measuring fatigue in sarcoidosis: the fatigue assessment scale (FAS). Br J Health Psychol 2004;9(Pt 3):279–91.

24. Giordano NA, Pasquel FJ, Pak V, et al. Performance of PROMIS measures to assess fatigue and sleep symptom severity among african American patients newly diagnosed with obstructive sleep apnea. Clin Nurs Res 2023;32(7):1041–5.

25. Marcellis RG, Lenssen AF, Elfferich MD, et al. Exercise capacity, muscle strength and fatigue in sarcoidosis. Eur Respir J 2011;38(3):628–34.

26. Chervin RD. Sleepiness, fatigue, tiredness, and lack of energy in obstructive sleep apnea. Chest 2000; 118(2):372–9.

27. de Kleijn WP, De Vries J, Lower EE, et al. Fatigue in sarcoidosis: a systematic review. Curr Opin Pulm Med 2009;15(5):499–506.

28. Lal C, Weaver TE, Bae CJ, et al. Excessive daytime sleepiness in obstructive sleep apnea. mechanisms and clinical management. Ann Am Thorac Soc 2021; 18(5):757–68.

29. Joo EY, Tae WS, Lee MJ, et al. Reduced brain gray matter concentration in patients with obstructive sleep apnea syndrome. Sleep 2010;33(2):235–41.

30. Zhang J, Weaver TE, Zhong Z, et al. White matter structural differences in OSA patients experiencing residual daytime sleepiness with high CPAP use: a non-Gaussian diffusion MRI study. Sleep Med 2019;53:51–9.

31. Trotti LM, Staab BA, Rye DB. Test-retest reliability of the multiple sleep latency test in narcolepsy without cataplexy and idiopathic hypersomnia. J Clin Sleep Med 2013;9(8):789–95.

32. Patterson KC, Huang F, Oldham JM, et al. Excessive daytime sleepiness and obstructive sleep apnea in patients with sarcoidosis. Chest 2013;143(6): 1562–8.

33. Fleischer M, Hinz A, Brahler E, et al. Factors associated with fatigue in sarcoidosis. Respir Care 2014; 59(7):1086–94.

34. de Kleijn WP, Drent M, De Vries J. Nature of fatigue moderates depressive symptoms and anxiety in sarcoidosis. Br J Health Psychol 2013;18(2):439–52.

35. Chang B, Steimel J, Moller DR, et al. Depression in sarcoidosis. Am J Respir Crit Care Med 2001; 163(2):329–34.

36. Wagner MT, Marion SD, Judson MA. The effects of fatigue and treatment with methylphenidate on sustained attention in sarcoidosis. Sarcoidosis Vasc Diffuse Lung Dis 2005;22(3):235.

37. Boing S, Randerath WJ. Chronic hypoventilation syndromes and sleep-related hypoventilation. J Thorac Dis 2015;7(8):1273–85.

38. Berg G, Delaive K, Manfreda J, et al. The use of health-care resources in obesity-hypoventilation syndrome. Chest 2001;120(2):377–83.

39. Mokhlesi B, Masa JF, Brozek JL, et al. Evaluation and management of obesity hypoventilation syndrome. an official american thoracic society clinical practice guideline. Am J Respir Crit Care Med 2019;200(3):e6–24.

40. Bradvik I, Wollmer P, Blom-Bulow B, et al. Lung mechanics and gas exchange during exercise in pulmonary sarcoidosis. Chest 1991;99(3):572–8.

41. Maron BA. Revised definition of pulmonary hypertension and approach to management: a clinical primer. J Am Heart Assoc 2023;12(8):e029024.

42. Parikh KS, Dahhan T, Nicholl L, et al. Clinical features and outcomes of patients with sarcoidosis-associated pulmonary hypertension. Sci Rep 2019; 9(1):4061.

43. Kirkil G, Lower EE, Baughman RP. Predictors of mortality in pulmonary sarcoidosis. Chest 2018;153(1): 105–13.

44. Huitema MP, Bakker ALM, Mager JJ, et al. Prevalence of pulmonary hypertension in pulmonary sarcoidosis: the first large European prospective study. Eur Respir J 2019;54(4).

45. Pabst S, Grohe C, Skowasch D. Prevalence of sarcoidosis-associated pulmonary hypertension: cumulative analysis of two PULSAR studies. Eur Respir J 2020;55(2).

46. Alhamad EH, Idrees MM, Alanezi MO, et al. Sarcoidosis-associated pulmonary hypertension: clinical features and outcomes in Arab patients. Ann Thorac Med 2010;5(2):86–91.

47. Handa T, Nagai S, Miki S, et al. Incidence of pulmonary hypertension and its clinical relevance in patients with sarcoidosis. Chest 2006;129(5):1246–52.

48. Shorr AF, Helman DL, Davies DB, et al. Pulmonary hypertension in advanced sarcoidosis: epidemiology and clinical characteristics. Eur Respir J 2005;25(5):783–8.

49. Nunes H, Humbert M, Capron F, et al. Pulmonary hypertension associated with sarcoidosis: mechanisms, haemodynamics and prognosis. Thorax 2006;61(1):68–74.

50. Westcott JL, DeGraff AC Jr. Sarcoidosis, hilar adenopathy, and pulmonary artery narrowing. Radiology 1973;108(3):585–6.

51. Rosen Y, Moon S, Huang CT, et al. Granulomatous pulmonary angiitis in sarcoidosis. Arch Pathol Lab Med 1977;101(4):170–4.

52. Swigris JJ, Olson AL, Huie TJ, et al. Increased risk of pulmonary embolism among US decedents with sarcoidosis from 1988 to 2007. Chest 2011;140(5): 1261–6.

53. Shah FA, Moronta S, Braford M, et al. Obstructive sleep apnea and pulmonary hypertension: a review of literature. Cureus 2021;13(4):e14575.

54. Kessler R, Chaouat A, Schinkewitch P, et al. The obesity-hypoventilation syndrome revisited: a prospective study of 34 consecutive cases. Chest 2001;120(2):369–76.

55. Castro-Anon O, Golpe R, Perez-de-Llano LA, et al. Haemodynamic effects of non-invasive ventilation in patients with obesity-hypoventilation syndrome. Respirology 2012;17(8):1269–74.

56. Elfferich MD, Nelemans PJ, Ponds RW, et al. Everyday cognitive failure in sarcoidosis: the prevalence and the effect of anti-TNF-alpha treatment. Respiration 2010;80(3):212–9.

57. Voortman M, De Vries J, Hendriks CMR, et al. Everyday cognitive failure in patients suffering from neurosarcoidosis. Sarcoidosis Vasc Diffuse Lung Dis 2019;36(1):2–10.

58. Antonelli Incalzi R, Marra C, Salvigni BL, et al. Does cognitive dysfunction conform to a distinctive pattern in obstructive sleep apnea syndrome? J Sleep Res 2004;13(1):79–86.

59. Leng Y, McEvoy CT, Allen IE, et al. Association of sleep-disordered breathing with cognitive function and risk of cognitive impairment: a systematic review and meta-analysis. JAMA Neurol 2017;74(10): 1237–45.

60. Lal C, Ayappa I, Ayas N, et al. The link between obstructive sleep apnea and neurocognitive impairment: an official american thoracic society workshop report. Ann Am Thorac Soc 2022;19(8):1245–56.

61. Macey PM, Kumar R, Woo MA, et al. Brain structural changes in obstructive sleep apnea. Sleep 2008; 31(7):967–77.

62. Macey PM, Henderson LA, Macey KE, et al. Brain morphology associated with obstructive sleep apnea. Am J Respir Crit Care Med 2002;166(10): 1382–7.

63. Weng HH, Tsai YH, Chen CF, et al. Mapping gray matter reductions in obstructive sleep apnea: an activation likelihood estimation meta-analysis. Sleep 2014;37(1):167–75.

64. Canessa N, Castronovo V, Cappa SF, et al. Obstructive sleep apnea: brain structural changes and neurocognitive function before and after treatment. Am J Respir Crit Care Med 2011;183(10):1419–26.

65. Hall AM, Moore RY, Lopez OL, et al. Basal forebrain atrophy is a presymptomatic marker for Alzheimer's disease. Alzheimers Dement 2008;4(4):271–9.

66. Panselinas E, Halstead L, Schlosser RJ, et al. Clinical manifestations, radiographic findings, treatment options, and outcome in sarcoidosis patients with upper respiratory tract involvement. South Med J 2010;103(9):870–5.

67. Zeitlin JF, Tami TA, Baughman R, et al. Nasal and sinus manifestations of sarcoidosis. Am J Rhinol 2000; 14(3):157–61.

68. Kay DJ, Har-El G. The role of endoscopic sinus surgery in chronic sinonasal sarcoidosis. Am J Rhinol 2001;15(4):249–54.

69. Kim H, Bach JR. Central alveolar hypoventilation in neurosarcoidosis. Arch Phys Med Rehabil 1998; 79(11):1467–8.

70. Rubinstein I, Gray TA, Moldofsky H, et al. Neurosarcoidosis associated with hypersomnolence treated with corticosteroids and brain irradiation. Chest 1988;94(1):205–6.

71. Ertas Dogan M, Bingol Z, Aydemir L, et al. Frequency of obstructive sleep apnea in stage i and ii sarcoidosis subjects who had no corticosteroid therapy. Turk Thorac J 2020;21(5):296–302.

72. Mari PV, Pasciuto G, Siciliano M, et al. Obstructive sleep apnea in sarcoidosis and impact of cpap treatment on fatigue. Sarcoidosis Vasc Diffuse Lung Dis 2020;37(2):169–78.

73. Ataoglu O, Annakkaya AN, Arbak PM, et al. Clinical and polysomnographic evaluation of sleep-related breathing disorders in patients with sarcoidosis. Sleep Breath 2022;26(4):1847–55.

74. Judson MA, Tiwari A, Gemoets DE. The relationship of obesity and OSA to the development of sarcoidosis: a large retrospective case-control US veterans administration analysis. Chest 2022;162(5):1086–92.

Obstructive Sleep Apnea, Obesity Hypoventilation Syndrome, and Pulmonary Hypertension
A State-of-the-Art Review

Sarah Bjork, MD[a], Deepanjali Jain, MD[a], Manuel Hache Marliere, MD[a], Sanda A. Predescu, PhD[a], Babak Mokhlesi, MD, MSc[a],*

KEYWORDS

- Pulmonary hypertension • Obstructive sleep apnea • Obesity hypoventilation syndrome
- Positive airway pressure therapy • CPAP • Noninvasive ventilation • Bilevel PAP
- Pulmonary arterial hypertension • Right heart catheterization • Echocardiogram
- Pulmonary artery systolic pressure • Right ventricular systolic pressure • Hypoxemia • Hypercapnia
- Sleep disordered breathing

KEY POINTS

- Sleep-disordered breathing (SDB) is a common disease that can lead to pulmonary hypertension (PH).
- There are several mechanisms by which SDB can lead to or worsen PH, including intrathoracic pressure swings, sustained and intermittent hypoxemia, hypercapnia, and obesity.
- Treatment of SDB can improve hypoxemia and pulmonary vascular hemodynamics as well as symptoms of patients with PH.
- Further research is needed to establish better screening approaches as well as developing a multidisciplinary approach to PH that includes providers with expertise in not only PH but also in cardiology, sleep medicine, and weight management/bariatric surgery.

INTRODUCTION

Pulmonary hypertension (PH) is a heterogeneous disorder with varying outcomes across different PH groups. The prevalence of sleep-disordered breathing (SDB) and obstructive sleep apnea (OSA) varies among PH groups, and its impact on survival differs, whether by intrinsic injury or by comorbidity metabolic profile. There is a complex pathophysiological interplay between SDB and PH. In this review, we explore the impact of SDB and its downstream consequences (ie, intrathoracic pressure changes, sustained and intermittent hypoxemia, hypercapnia, and obesity) on the pulmonary artery (PA) vasculature in the context of PH. We also discuss challenges in diagnosing PH in patients with SDB, particularly in the severely obese population, underscore the need for refined diagnostic criteria and screening approaches. Lastly, we will review treatment strategies in patients with PH and comorbid SDB, including obesity hypoventilation syndrome (OHS).

---

[a] Division of Pulmonary, Critical Care and Sleep Medicine, Department of Internal Medicine, Rush University Medical Center, 1750 W. Harrison Street, Jelke 297, Chicago, IL 60612, USA
* Corresponding author. Division of Pulmonary, Critical Care and Sleep Medicine, Department of Internal Medicine, Rush University Medical Center, 1750 W. Harrison Street, Jelke 213, Chicago, IL 60612.
E-mail address: babak_mokhlesi@rush.edu

Sleep Med Clin 19 (2024) 307–325
https://doi.org/10.1016/j.jsmc.2024.02.009
1556-407X/24/© 2024 Elsevier Inc. All rights reserved.

EPIDEMIOLOGY

SDB includes multiple distinct disorders. The most prevalent form of SDB is OSA. Other important forms of SDB include central sleep apnea (CSA) with and without Cheyne–Stokes breathing pattern, sleep-related hypoventilation, sleep-related hypoxemia, and OHS. The prevalence of OSA varies widely based on how hypopneas are classified and what threshold of the apnea–hypopnea index (AHI) is considered pathologic. Population-based studies suggest that the prevalence of OSA is increasing in the United States.[1,2] In 2015, a Swiss population-based study reported a prevalence of moderate-to-severe OSA (AHI $\geq$15/h) of 23.4% in women and 49.7% in men.[3] This high prevalence of moderate-to-severe OSA could be in part attributable to the increased sensitivity of current polysomnographic technology and hypopnea scoring criteria when compared to prior population-based studies such as the Wisconsin Sleep Cohort. The global burden of OSA has been estimated at 936 million men and women aged 30 to 69 years having any OSA (AHI >5/h) and 425 million people estimated to have moderate-to-severe OSA (AHI $\geq$15/h).[4]

Two important risk factors for SDB include aging and obesity. As the global prevalence of obesity continues to increase in an aging population, the prevalence of SDB is bound to increase.[1,5–7] SDB, particularly severe OSA, is independently associated with increased likelihood of developing systemic hypertension,[8] heart failure,[9] coronary artery disease,[10] stroke,[11–13] arrhythmias,[14] and overall mortality.[10,15–17]

Although the precise prevalence of PH is unknown, it has been estimated that 1% of the global population or 80 million people have PH.[18] Cardiac disorders (group 2 PH) and pulmonary disorders/hypoxia (group 3 PH) are the leading causes of PH with a significantly higher prevalence in persons aged above 65 years.[18] Individuals with group 2 and group 3 PH are more likely to have comorbid OSA and/or obesity given that they are more likely to be older and male. In contrast, the prevalence of OSA in patients with pulmonary arterial hypertension (PAH) is lower as these patients are younger, less obese, and predominantly female.[19] Despite the lower risk, on average OSA was present in 23.5% of patients with PAH (**Table 1**). As multimodal therapeutic approaches improve patient survival in PAH,[20] the prevalence of OSA is bound to increase due to aging and increased prevalence of obesity.[21]

Prevalence of PH in OSA and OHS

A few studies have investigated the prevalence of PH in patients with OSA. Smaller studies that were limited by selection bias reported a prevalence ranging from 19% to 42%.[22–24] However, larger studies have reported higher prevalence. One of the largest studies had a cohort of 220 patients with diagnosed severe OSA who underwent right heart catheterization (RHC) regardless of underlying clinical suspicion of comorbid PH.[25] Seventeen percent of these patients had a mean pulmonary artery pressure (mPAP) greater than 20 mm Hg and therefore met the definition of PH. In this cohort, patients with PH had significantly higher body mass index (BMI; 34 vs 31 kg/m^2), higher prevalence of obstructive lung disease and lower daytime PaO_2 (64.4 vs 74.7 mm Hg). They also had a higher mean AHI (100 vs 73/h) and higher percentage of sleep time with oxygen saturation less than 90 (T90; 38.4 vs 11.9 min/h). In univariate and multivariate analyses, higher mPAP was associated with lower mean nocturnal oxygen saturation, higher BMI, and higher AHI.

In a smaller study of 83 patients with OSA who underwent RHC, 58 (70%) had PH defined by mPAP greater than 25 mm Hg; 18 out of 58 (31%) had precapillary PH.[26] In contrast to the earlier, larger study,[25] there was no difference in AHI between patients with and without PH (29.1 vs 34.6, respectively). However, patients with PH and OSA had a significantly higher T90 (20.5% vs 7.4% of total sleep time, respectively).[26]

Studies have also shown a high prevalence of exercise-induced PH in patients with OSA.[27–29] In one study, patients diagnosed with OSA (AHI >5/h) underwent RHC at rest and during exercise. PH at rest was present in 13 out of 65 (20%) patients. Exercise-induced PH was present in an additional 31 patients.[28]

The prevalence of PH in patients with OHS has been described in a large, randomized controlled trial as well as in smaller observational studies, and it ranges between 50% and 69%.[30–33] In the Pickwick study, which enrolled 246 patients with a diagnosis of OHS, over 50% of patients had echocardiographic evidence of PH (right ventricular systolic pressure or RVSP $\geq$40 mm Hg) at the time of study enrollment. Patients with comorbid OHS and PH had significantly higher BMI (43.6 vs 39.1 kg/m^2) at baseline. In multivariate analysis, higher BMI and lower daytime PaO_2 were predictors for PH. AHI and $PaCO_2$ were not predictors for PH.[34]

PATHOPHYSIOLOGY

The pathophysiology of SDB and PH is complex. For the purposes of this review, we will focus on 4 mechanistic pathways by which the downstream consequences of SDB can impact PA hemodynamics: (1) intrathoracic pressure swings during

Table 1
Prevalence of obstructive sleep apnea in precapillary/group 1 pulmonary hypertension diagnosed by right heart catheterization

	N	Age (years)	% Female	BMI or Obesity Prevalence	OSA Dx Criteria	OSA Prevalence (%)
REVEAL 2013[111] US Cohort	2959	52.7	79	32%	Medical record	599/2959 (20)
Dumitrascu et al,[112] 2013 German Cohort	28	51.1 ± 17.2	75	25.9 ± 5.6	RP AHI >10	2/28 (7)
PVDOMICS 2022[19] US Cohort	185	48.4	70	27.4[a] [23.7–32.9]	RP AHI ≥5	92/185 (49.7)
Huang et al,[84] 2023 Chinese Cohort	394	44[a] [33.0–62.2]	55	23.6 ± 8.5	RP AHI3% ≥5	114/394 (29)
Murta et al,[113] 2022 Brazilian Cohort	36	38.2[a] [38.2–57.0]	69.4	25.5[a] [20.7–28.9]	RP AHI4% ≥5	26/36 (75)
Nagaoka, et al,[114] 2018 Japanese Cohort	151	44 ± 16	75.5	21.7 ± 4.5	RP AHI3% ≥5	29/151(19.2)
Minic,[115] 2014 Canadian Cohort	52	53 ± 15	57.7	29.6 ± 9.2	AHI ≥5	29/52 (55.7)
Simonson et al,[116] 2022 US Cohort	49	56[a] [42–65]	78	30 (26–33)	AHI ≥5	13/37 (35)
OSA prevalence for all cohorts combined						904/3842 (23.5)

Abbreviations: AHI, apnea hypopnea index; OSA, obstructive sleep apnea; RP, respiratory polygraphy.
[a] Median [25–75 percentile].

obstructive apneas and hypopneas, (2) sustained and intermittent hypoxemia, (3) hypercapnia and acidosis, and (4) obesity. **Fig. 1** illustrates this complex relationship.

PH is defined by an mPAP of greater than 20 mm Hg on assessment by RHC. Precapillary PH is further defined as mPAP greater than 20 mm Hg, pulmonary artery wedge pressure (PAWP) 15 mm Hg or lesser, and pulmonary vascular resistance (PVR) greater than 2 Wood units. Combined precapillary and postcapillary PH includes patients with a PAWP greater than 15 mm Hg and PVR greater than 2 Wood units.[18]

Intrathoracic Pressure Swings

Obstructive events cause large swings in intrathoracic pressure. During obstructive apneas and hypopneas, thoracic pressure becomes more negative, which can cause an increase in right ventricular (RV) filling pressures, leftward septal deviation, reduced left ventricular function, and increased PAWP. Measuring changes in mPAP in human subjects during sleep when obstructive apneic events occur is challenging.[35] For an accurate assessment of changes in mPAP, concomitant esophageal manometry becomes critically

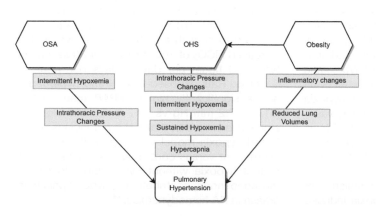

Fig. 1. Proposed pathophysiological mechanisms by which SDB can lead to PH. OHS, obesity hypoventilation syndrome; OSA, obstructive sleep apnea.

important since swings in intrapleural pressures will need to be quantified to accurately measure transmural PA pressures.[36]

Although the long-term effect of frequent and profound intrathoracic pressure swings on the pulmonary vasculature has not been fully elucidated, canine and primate models have attempted to dissect the impact of intrathoracic pressure swings versus intermittent hypoxemia on pulmonary hemodynamics. These studies are limited by the fact that they last only a few hours. Notwithstanding this important limitation, the data suggest that intermittent hypoxemia, not swings in intrathoracic pressure, lead to an acute increase in mPAP. Correction of hypoxemia with supplemental oxygen led to normalization of mPAP despite recurrent obstructive apneas with large swings in intrathoracic pressures.[37] Moreover, repetitive exposure to hypoxic gas lasting 45 to 60 seconds (4%–6% Fio_2 with 5% CO_2) without any upper airway obstruction led to similar increases in PA pressure.[37] In a primate model, central apneas that led to no changes in intrathoracic pressure also led to an increase in PA pressures due to ensuing hypoxemia.[38] The data in humans are even more limited. In one study of spontaneously breathing subjects with OSA undergoing simultaneous esophageal manometry and measurement of pulmonary hemodynamics using RHC, the degree of hypoxemia from recurrent obstructive apneas and hypopneas had a stronger relationship with the rise in transmural pulmonary artery systolic pressure (PASP) than the swings in intrathoracic pressure.[36] Collectively, these animal models and the limited human studies suggest that hypoxemia, and not intrathoracic pressure swings, is the larger driving factor in SDB leading to an acute increase in PA pressure. However, it remains unclear whether years of untreated OSA with repetitive swings in intrathoracic pressure plays an active role in the development of PH.

Hypoxemia

The impact of hypoxemia on PA pressures and RV dysfunction has been extensively studied. Animal models have explored both intermittent and sustained hypoxia to mimic the patterns of hypoxemia in human disease and its subsequent effects on PA hemodynamics. Chronic sustained hypoxia has consistently led to increased pulmonary vasoconstriction causing acute and chronic PH in various animal models. In fact, chronic sustained hypoxia has served as a reliable way to create an animal model to study PH.[39]

One of the primary proposed mechanisms for vascular remodeling is due to hypoxia-induced production of oxygen radicals such as superoxide and increased nicotinamide adenine dinucleotide phosphate (NADPH) oxidase, leading to smooth muscle proliferation and endothelial dysfunction by reduced nitric oxide bioavailability. More so, these changes were shown in mice models that were subjected to chronic intermittent hypoxia (CIH), which was defined as fractional oxygen concentration (Fio_2) cycling between 21% and 10%, 45 times per hour in a closed chamber for 8 hours per day, 5 days per week for 8 weeks.[40] This closely resembles SDB with cycling hypoxemia, and yet, it does not account for intermittent rise in CO_2 levels during apneas or the hemodynamic effects related to physiologic pressure swings due to breathing against increased upper airway resistance during obstructive apneas and hypopneas. When comparing normoxia to CIH settings, this led to modest increases in RVSP from 26.3 to 32.4 mm Hg. Interestingly, knockout mice lacking gp91phox, a NADPH oxidase subunit, showed attenuated RV hypertrophy changes under CIH compared to the wild-type mice.[40]

Hypoxic-driven NADPH oxidase-dependent regulated changes in pulmonary vasculature have also been shown in murine models under sustained hypoxic conditions (Fio_2% 10 for 3 weeks).[41] In another murine model of intermittent hypoxia, mice were exposed to 3 experimental conditions: normoxia, continuous hypoxia, and intermittent hypoxia. In the intermittent hypoxia condition, mice were exposed to air with 10% oxygen for 2 minute intervals for 9 hours a day for 28 days. RVSP and RV mass was highest in mice exposed to continuous hypoxia (44.2 mm Hg and 0.34 g, respectively) compared to normoxia (29.5 mm Hg and 0.22 g, respectively). Compared to normoxia, mice exposed to intermittent hypoxia had significantly higher RVSP (36 mm Hg) and RV mass (0.27 g).[42] Similar findings were replicated in a rat model, although this model included hypercapnia to better simulate blood gas changes that occur in OSA. Rats were exposed to 2 conditions: a control group and CIH and hypercapnia group. In the CIH and hypercapnia group, rats were exposed to air with an Fio_2 of 6% to 8% and an increased $FiCO_2$ of 10% to 14% for 30 second intervals, 8 hours per day, 5 days per week for 5 weeks. Rats exposed to CIH and hypercapnia had a significantly higher mPAP than controls (31.3 ± 7.2 mm Hg vs 20.7 ± 6.8 mm Hg). This study was limited in that it did not include a sustained hypoxia model to compare the effects of intermittent versus continuous exposure or intermittent hypoxia without hypercapnia to dissect the independent contribution of hypercapnia to increase in PA hemodynamics.[43]

Murine models have also been developed to study the effect of intermittent plus sustained hypoxia, or the so-called overlap hypoxia. In a series of experiments, mice were exposed to 4 conditions: sustained hypoxia (constant Fio_2 of 10%), intermittent hypoxia (1 minute bursts of 6% Fio_2 alternating with Fio_2 of 21% for 12 hours), overlap hypoxia, and room air. Overlap hypoxia was unique in this study and was a combination of sustained and intermittent hypoxia (Fio_2 fluctuating between 13% and 6% once per minute, for 12 hours and Fio_2 of 13% for 12 hours). The investigators found that RVSP did not change in mice exposed to intermittent hypoxia. However, a significant increase in the RVSP was noted with sustained hypoxia and overlap hypoxia when compared to mice exposed to room air. There was a 52% increase in the RVSP in the sustained hypoxia group and a 20% increase in the overlap hypoxia group.[44]

The overlap hypoxia model can be used for human conditions in which both sustained and intermittent hypoxemia coexist: that is, chronic obstructive pulmonary disease with comorbid OSA, PH with comorbid SDB, and OHS with comorbid OSA. Sustained hypoxemia during sleep can occur due to hypoventilation or PH. The addition of intermittent hypoxemia due to OSA leads to an overlap phenomenon. Patients with OSA and comorbid PH have a heightened pulmonary vasoconstrictor response to hypoxia when compared to patients without comorbid PH.[45] Therefore, the presence of SDB may lead to worsening right-sided pressures in existing PH or could lead to PH over time if untreated.

The relationship between hypoxia, OSA and PH has also been explored in canine models as well as in primates and human subjects. By its complex nature, these physiologic studies are limited by small sample sizes and duration of only a few hours. In the primate and canine models, animals were endotracheally intubated under anesthesia. Under these conditions, obstructive and central apneas were induced during RHC. These studies have consistently shown that hypoxemia induced by both central and obstructive apneas increase transmural PA pressures without any change in PAWP, and the degree of PH was directly related to the extent of hypoxemia.[37,38,46] The mPAP increased by approximately 200% when dogs were exposed to recurrent apneas lasting 45 to 60 seconds leading to intermittent drops in arterial oxygen saturation (SaO_2) from above 95% to 50%.[37] Similar increases in PASP were observed in baboons exposed to obstructive and central apneas lasting 30 to 60 seconds leading to reductions in SaO_2 from above 90% to approximately 60%.[38] When supplemental oxygen was provided

to blunt the hypoxemia during recurrent obstructive apneas in the canine model, PA hemodynamics remained normal, providing additional evidence that intermittent hypoxemia is the main driver of worsening PA hemodynamics.[37]

Although animal models have been criticized for long apneas leading to profound hypoxemia, in clinical practice, patients with very severe OSA and/or with OHS can experience similar durations of apneas leading to similar levels of intermittent hypoxemia. In one study of 4 patients with severe OSA undergoing simultaneous esophageal manometry and measurement of pulmonary hemodynamics using RHC, obstructive apneas that lasted on average 40 seconds and led to a greater degree of hypoxemia (from an average oxygen saturation by pulse oximetry (SpO_2) of 96% to 64%) led to a significant rise in transmural PASP, from an average baseline of 26 mm Hg to nearly 50 mm Hg.[47] This finding suggests that similar to animal models, patients with severe OSA (or OHS) can also experience obstructive apneas that are similar in duration leading to significant hypoxemia.

Obesity

The basic mechanisms by which obesity can lead to PH is an area of active investigation and remains to be fully elucidated. There are several noteworthy pathophysiological mechanisms by which obesity could worsen pulmonary hemodynamics, independent of SDB.

Excess adiposity increases the risk of cardiovascular disease independent of other cardiovascular risk factors such as type 2 diabetes, dyslipidemia, and SDB. Obesity leads to increased blood volume and hyperdynamic circulation, thereby exerting excess load on the cardiovascular system. Obesity can increase preload as well as left ventricular afterload. This increase in left ventricular afterload can eventually lead to concentric left ventricular hypertrophy and left ventricular diastolic dysfunction and over time to postcapillary PH and RV dysfunction.[48,49] In a study of 3790 echocardiographically normal individuals studied over a decade, there was a significant linear association between higher BMI and higher PASP. In subjects with BMI less than 25 kg/m², the mean PASP was 27 to 28 mm Hg. In contrast, in subjects with BMI greater than 35 kg/m², the mean PASP was 30 to 31 mm Hg.[50]

Another proposed mechanism by which obesity can worsen pulmonary hemodynamics is the accumulation of fat in the perivascular tissue. Although the complex pathophysiology of perivascular fat-induced microvascular dysfunction is not fully understood, a few mechanisms have been proposed and studied. Perivascular fat deposition can mechanically decrease the size of the vasculature.[51] Indirectly, this perivascular fat can induce an inflammatory cascade leading to endothelial dysfunction. Studies have reported that an increase in tumor necrosis factor-α by perivascular adipose tissue in small arteries leads to an increase in vascular endothelin-1 and endothelin-1 A receptor expression. Adipocytes also secrete inflammatory molecules that impair healthy endothelial function with diminished generation of nitric oxide, a known vasodilator with anti-inflammatory properties.[52] The interaction of hypoxia with adipose tissue further complicates the pathophysiological mechanisms. In-vitro cultures of human adipocytes exposed to hypoxic conditions (Fio_2 1%, 2.5%, and 5%) induces an upregulation of proinflammatory cytokines including IL-1.[53] In rat models, IL-1 has been shown to be a mediator of PH.[54] Furthermore, aggressive treatment of obesity with bariatric surgery has been shown to reduce perivascular adipose tissue after weight loss to the level similar to nonobese controls.[55]

Another mechanism by which obesity can worsen pulmonary hemodynamics is related to reduction in lung volumes due to body habitus with a U-shaped relationship between lung volumes and PVR, with PVR being at its lowest at functional residual capacity. However, with increasing body mass, the expiratory reserve volume decreases and resting lung volume moves toward residual volume. This leads to an increase in PVR since lower lung volumes progressively decrease the caliber of the pulmonary arteries. Given that vascular resistance is inversely proportional to the radius of a vessel to the power of 4, slight changes in the radius of extra-alveolar vessels can lead to an exponential increase in PVR.[56,57]

Histopathological studies have reported that severe obesity and untreated comorbid OHS can lead to PA muscularization, presumably due to chronic hypoxemia, and biventricular cardiac dysfunction that can ultimately lead to a combination of group 2 and group 3 PH.[58] Whether obesity leads to histopathological changes observed in group 1 PA hypertension was assessed in an autopsy study of 76 obese subjects (46 with class III obesity or BMI $\geq$40 kg/m^2) compared to 46 age-matched nonobese controls. Pulmonary hypertensive disease was present in 72% of obese subjects compared to 6% of the nonobese controls. Strikingly, pulmonary capillary hemangiomatosis (defined as diffuse or localized proliferation of alveolar capillaries on both sides of the alveolar walls, with formation of glomeruloid tufts or nodules), a histologic feature that is typically seen in patients with group 1 PAH was present in 2% of nonobese, 39% of those with BMI between 30 and 40 kg/m^2,

and 61% of severely obese subjects with a BMI of 40 kg/m^2 or greater.[59] It remains unclear whether the high prevalence of pulmonary capillary hemangiomatosis observed in the severely obese was due to chronic hypoxemia or some other angiogenic stimulus. Importantly, none of these subjects had a premortem history of pulmonary vascular disease suggesting that pulmonary vascular histologic changes may precede clinical recognition and diagnosis of PH.

Evidence shows that obesity plays an intrinsic role in the development of PH. This role is not exclusively related to mechanical load of excess body fat causing restrictive ventilatory limitations with subsequent hypoventilation and hypoxemia. In a study of obesity-prone rats that were subjected to a high-fat diet, there was evidence of oxidative stress in the PA wall, leading to subsequent PA wall remodeling and thickening when compared to low-fat-fed rats.[60] In a different rat model, where PH was induced with single subcutaneous injection of monocrotaline, calorie restriction resulted in a lower mPAP and reduced vascular remodeling and RV hypertrophy.[61]

Further evidence linking obesity to PH comes from the post hoc, cross-sectional analysis of the Pickwick trial that included 246 patients with OHS with a prevalence of PH of 50%. In this cohort, the severity of obesity, measured by the BMI, and daytime hypoxemia were independently associated with PH.[34] Collectively, the murine model studies and the analysis of the Pickwick study suggest that obesity per se is implicated in the pathogenesis of PH. These findings provide incremental evidence that obesity can be implicated in the causal pathway of PH independent of hypoxemia and SDB.

Hypercapnia

Much like obesity, the role of hypercapnia in PH has not been fully elucidated. Part of the challenge in assessing the independent contribution of hypercapnia to the development of PH is that hypoventilation in disease states also leads to hypoxemia. Rats develop a rise in pulmonary arterial pressure and RV hypertrophy as early as 1 week after exposure to chronic hypoxia with Fio_2 of 10%. However, rats exposed to 3 weeks of hypercapnia alone (without hypoxia) did not experience any significant changes in pulmonary hemodynamics compared to control. Interestingly, when hypercapnia was added to the hypoxic condition (Fio_2 10% and $FiCO_2$ 10%), the deleterious effect of hypoxia on the pulmonary vasculature was attenuated compared to hypoxia alone.[62] Similarly, in newborn rats that were chronically exposed to hypoxic conditions (Fio_2 13%), higher concentrations of CO_2

($FiCO_2$ 10%) normalized RV performance, limited oxidant stress, and prevented upregulation of endothelin-1.[63] These animal studies demonstrate that hypercapnia in isolation may not lead to PH. This is consistent with human data demonstrating that in patients with OHS, hypercapnia was not independently associated with PH after adjusting for hypoxemia and obesity.[34]

In a large, retrospective single-center study of 491 patients with compensated hypercapnia, there was an association between hypercapnia and worse outcomes, including mortality.[64] However, the limitation of this study was that the association of hypercapnia with outcomes was not adjusted for concomitant hypoxemia. Hypercapnia may have other downstream deleterious effects unrelated to its effect on the pulmonary vasculature. Accumulating evidence in various animal models suggests that hypercapnia without concomitant hypoxemia leads to a reduction in innate immune response.[65–67] In summary, although hypercapnia may not be pathophysiologically linked to PH, it may have other deleterious effects and should be treated accordingly.

CHALLENGES
Challenges with Echocardiography

There are several technical challenges in correctly diagnosing and classifying PH in patients with OHS and/or severe OSA who are severely obese. Transthoracic echocardiography is an excellent screening tool and the recommended first step to assess for PH.[18] RVSP is considered a reasonable surrogate of PASP in the absence of pulmonic stenosis or RV tract obstruction. RVSP is calculated by the modified Bernoulli formula: $RVSP = 4(peak\ tricuspid\ regurgitation\ velocity)^2 + right\ atrial\ pressure$.[68] However, it is not possible to obtain a reliable tricuspid regurgitation (TR) velocity to estimate the RVSP in up to 40% to 50% of patients.[69–73] This technical challenge is even more prevalent in severely obese patients due to difficulty obtaining adequate views during echocardiography. Additionally, in high-output cardiac states, the TR velocity may overestimate pressure gradients. Conversely, TR can underestimate pressure gradients. Both these scenarios lead to inaccuracies of RVSP estimation.[18]

Another limitation of echocardiography is that the echocardiographer must estimate the right atrial pressure by determining the diameter of the inferior vena cava and the percentage of collapse during inspiration. This partly subjective estimation of right atrial pressure adds to inaccuracies of calculating RVSP or PASP by echocardiography. Most commonly, the right atrial pressure is assumed to be 5 to 10 mm Hg.[69] Although

guidelines caution against relying solely on RVSP as described above,[18] accumulating evidence suggest that RVSP measured by echocardiography is strongly associated with mortality.[69,70,74] Additional echocardiographic parameters of such as RV outflow tract acceleration time less than 105 milliseconds and tricuspid annular plane systolic excursion (TAPSE)/PASP ratio less than 0.55 mm/mm Hg can provide further confirmation of PH.[18] In summary, even though echocardiography is considered to be an extremely useful screening tool for PH, RHC remains the gold standard to accurately diagnose and classify PH.

Significance of Elevated Pulmonary Artery Systolic Pressure on Echocardiography

It is important to note that despite the above-mentioned limitations of echocardiography in assessing PH, elevated RVSP (or PASP) has a strong association with patient outcomes. In the National Echocardiography Database of Australia cohort (n = 313,492), RVSP could be calculated in 50% of patients. In this subgroup, 19% had elevated PASP defined as 40 mm Hg or greater. Adjusted 5 year all-cause mortality incrementally increased with higher PASP, from 20% in those with PASP less than 40 mm Hg to 55.6% in mild PH (PASP 40–49.9 mm Hg), 69% in moderate PH (50–59.9 mm Hg) to 78% in severe PH (PASP ≥60 mm Hg).[69] In fact, even mildly elevated PASP on echocardiography, defined as 30 to less than 40 mm Hg, has been associated with increased mortality.[69,70,74] Therefore, patients with SDB who are found to have mild PH on echocardiography may benefit from additional evaluation and treatment of PH. This is particularly relevant in patients with OHS because of persistent PH despite positive airway pressure therapy.[31,75] In the Pickwick trial, the prevalence of PH, defined as PASP greater than or equal to 40 mm Hg, decreased significantly after 3 years of positive airway pressure therapy. However, despite improvements in pulmonary hemodynamics, nearly a quarter of patients had PASP greater than 40 mm Hg.[31] In a smaller study of 21 patients with successfully treated OHS after 3 months of home noninvasive ventilation, 9 patients (43%) had persistent PH on RHC, with 6 out of these 9 patients having only precapillary PH.[75] Consequently, clinicians should consider additional evaluation and treatment of PH in patients with SDB/OHS who continue to have elevated PASP despite initial improvement with adherent positive airway pressure therapy. It is important to ascertain whether this residual PH is precapillary in nature and would benefit from pharmacotherapy.

Challenges with Right Heart Catheterization

RHC also has limitations, particularly in the severely obese patients. In this patient population, respiratory effort and swings in pleural pressure while in the supine position can be significant and can make the interpretation of pressure waveforms quite challenging. Moreover, in severely obese patients, there can be a clinically significant level of intrinsic positive end expiratory pressure (PEEP) while in the supine position.[76] Without concomitant esophageal manometry, the interpretation of cardiac waveforms can become very challenging. Clinicians performing RHC in patients who have significant respiratory excursion due to obesity and/or dyspnea use a variety of techniques to try to obtain reliable PA pressures and PAWP. One of these maneuvers consists of averaging pressures measured across several respiratory cycles. Another approach is to ask the patient to momentarily hold their breath at functional residual capacity in order to measure mPAP and PAWP while there is no respiratory effort. However, these approaches do not take into account the intrinsic PEEP and/or significant swings in pleural pressure that is frequently present in spontaneously breathing severely obese patients while in the supine position. These oversights can lead to misclassification of PH, potentially delaying or preventing appropriate treatment.

To more accurately assess and overcome these limitations, Khirfan and colleagues examined 53 severely obese patients with mPAP greater than 20 mm Hg and PAWP greater than or equal to 12 mm Hg.[77] Esophageal manometry was performed to account for dynamic respiratory fluctuations in intrathoracic pressures and intrinsic PEEP at end expiration in the supine position. Accurate transmural pressures were obtained by subtracting esophageal pressure from mPAP and PAWP and these values were compared to measurements obtained at the end of exhalation or obtained by averaging pressures across several respiratory cycles. Assessment of pulmonary hemodynamics using esophageal manometry was superior to the other 2 methods. Postcapillary PH decreased from 32 out of 53 (60%) to 4 out of 53 (7.5%) patients. At the same time, precapillary PH increased from 1 out of 53 (2%) to 13 out of 53 (24.5%) patients. Notably, 12 out of 53 (23%) patients no longer classified as having PH following this adjustment.[77]

Performing measurements in the sitting position can significantly decrease intrinsic PEEP and reduce intrathoracic pressure swings in severely obese subjects.[76] When patients undergoing RHC were transitioned from supine to the sitting position, there was a significant decrease in right atrial pressure, mPAP, PAWP, and cardiac output. In fact, the accuracy of pulmonary hemodynamics with the head of the bed elevated was very similar to adjusted measurements using esophageal manometry.[77] These findings underscore the potential for misclassification and misdirected treatment strategies in symptomatic patients with PH due to inaccurate PH phenotyping. As such, it is important for clinicians caring for severely obese patients with SDB/OHS to recognize that RHC has significant limitations. It is our opinion that pulmonologists and sleep specialists need to discuss RHC techniques with experts who perform RHC to ensure a more accurate diagnosis and classification of PH and not assume that all patients with SDB/OHS have group 3 PH.

Pulmonary Hemodynamic Assessment During Wake Versus Sleep

Another important limitation of RHC (or echocardiography) is that it is performed during wakefulness when patients with SDB are not experiencing repetitive apneas and/or hypopneas, hypoxemia/hypercapnia, and significant intrathoracic pleural pressure swings while breathing against an occluded upper airway. This might be more relevant when dynamic, reversible, and treatable changes can occur before actual PA remodeling takes place, which ultimately leads to less-reversible RV failure.

A few studies have investigated performing pulmonary hemodynamics in patients with SBD during sleep.[35,36,78,79] Kang and colleagues performed awake and sleep RHC in 6 patients with known OSA and PH. The rise in mPAP was significantly higher in rapid eye movement (REM) vs non-REM sleep (11.6 vs 6.9 mm Hg). However, the degree of oxygen desaturation with apneic events was also greater during REM sleep (23% vs 14%).[78] In a follow-up study by the same group, they were able to demonstrate that for the same level of hypoxemia, obstructive events during REM sleep led to a larger increase in mPAP than non-REM sleep.[79] This phenomenon has also been described in the context of systemic hypertension.[80,81] Therefore, it is plausible that similar to systemic blood pressure, PA vascular tone is more elevated in REM sleep, and therefore, any degree of hypoxemia leads to a higher increase in PA pressures compared to non-REM sleep.

Exercise-induced Pulmonary Hypertension

In addition to proper patient positioning, incorporating an exercise component into RHC can lead to a more accurate diagnosis of PH in patients with SDB. Studies have shown that adding exercise RHC can increase the detection rate of PH in OSA by up to 55%.[27–29] This highlights the importance of exercise RHC in identifying occult PH that may be missed during a resting RHC procedure—especially in a population where the contribution of SDB to PH development is being debated as negligible. A pathologic increase in PA pressure with exertion has been associated with impaired prognosis in patients with unexplained exercise dyspnea.[18] It remains unclear whether more aggressive treatment of SDB will improve outcomes in patients with exercise-induced PH.

TREATMENT

The effective treatment of PH in the setting of SDB and OHS involves (1) screening of patients with diagnosed PH for SDB; (2) screening of patients with SDB and obesity for PH; (3) utilization of positive airway pressure therapy for patients with PH and OSA/OHS and supplemental oxygen for patients who only have sleep hypoxemia; and (4) multidisciplinary efforts to address obesity and optimize left heart disease, if present (**Fig. 2**).

Screening Patients with PH for SDB and Nocturnal Hypoxemia

Several studies have reported a prevalence of OSA ranging from 7% to 55% in patients with precapillary PH (see **Table 1**). There are also studies to suggest that in patients with PH, comorbid OSA leads to worsening PA pressures, likely

mediated by nocturnal hypoxemia. In patients diagnosed with PAH, nocturnal hypoxemia can be present despite normoxia during daytime and even with exertion. In a cross-sectional study of 43 patients with PAH, 69.7% had significant nocturnal hypoxemia (T90 > 10%) and of those with nocturnal oxygen desaturation, 87% had a T90 of greater than 20%. These patients, however, did not consistently have concomitant daytime hypoxemia. Patients experiencing nocturnal hypoxemia had higher mPAP on RHC compared to those who did not (53.7 ± 16.5 vs 45 ± 13.6 mm Hg, respectively).[82] This brings to light the population of patients with PAH with a missed diagnosis of SDB and/or nocturnal hypoxemia.

In patients with precapillary group 1 PH, pulmonary vascular disease phenomics (PVDOMICS) data suggest there is a significant burden of OSA and nocturnal hypoxemia in patients with group 1 PH.[19] Out of 186 participants who underwent home respiratory polygraphy, the prevalence of OSA defined as AHI of greater than or equal to 5/h was 49.7%. Moderate-or-severe OSA (AHI ≥15/h) was 22%.[83] Even though 39.8% of these patients underwent home respiratory polygraphy while on therapy (ie, oxygen, positive airway pressure therapy, or both), the median T90 was 37% of the total recording time, consistent with a significant burden of hypoxemia.[19,83] It remains unclear whether such high burden of hypoxemia was due to OSA or PH. A large, single-center, retrospective study from China was able to address this question.[84] These investigators obtained respiratory polygraphy in 627

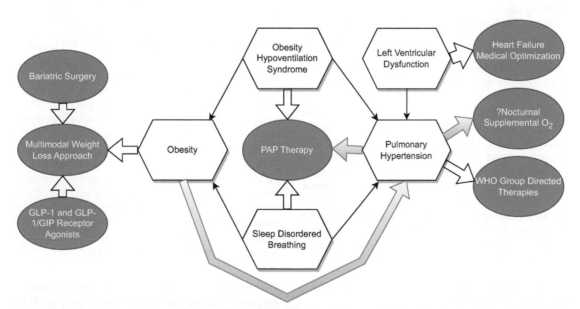

Fig. 2. Treatment approach algorithm for SDB and PH. GIP, glucose-dependent insulinotropic polypeptide; GLP-1, glucagon-like peptide 1; PAP, positive airway pressure; WHO, World Health Organization; Gray arrow, proposed mechanism and treatment pathway; White arrow, accepted treatment pathway.

patients undergoing evaluation for PH with RHC. Of these, 434 had PH and 90% were classified as pre-capillary in nature. PH with comorbid OSA was present in 134 (30%) of the patients. Nocturnal hypoxemia was assessed by T90. In this cohort, patients with PH and comorbid OSA experienced significantly greater degree of nocturnal hypoxemia compared to patients with only PH (median T90 of 9.4% vs 0.3%, respectively) despite having less severe elevation of PH (median mPAP of 43 vs 51 mm Hg, respectively).[84] Despite its retrospective nature, a major strength of this study is that it provides data on patients with PH without OSA to address the chicken and egg conundrum: is hypoxemia in patients with PH predominantly due to PH or to comorbid SDB? The data suggest that SDB is an important contributor to nocturnal hypoxia in patients with pre-capillary PH, and as such, it is appropriate to screen all patients with precapillary PH for SDB and nocturnal hypoxemia.[85]

Screening of Patients with SDB and Obesity for PH

Current PH or SDB guidelines do not provide specific recommendations on whether patients with SDB should be screened for PH. Screening all patients with SDB for PH would be impractical. However, there may be a subset of patients with SDB who would benefit from being screened for PH with echocardiography. These include those who have significant burden of hypoxemia during sleep, have evidence of daytime hypoxemia or hypercapnia, have unexplained dyspnea, and are severely obese. In patients enrolled in the Registry to Evaluate Early and Long-term PAH Disease Management (REVEAL), OSA and obesity were associated with delays in diagnosing PAH.[86] In a retrospective analysis of 8940 patients undergoing RHC, obesity was associated with greater prevalence of postcapillary, mixed, and precapillary PH.[87] For every 5 unit increment in the BMI, the odds ratio for precapillary PH increased significantly by 1.18. In fact, the cohort included 659 severely obese patients, and this group was at highest risk for PH, with a prevalence of precapillary PH of 14%.[87] As such, in severely obese who are symptomatic, it is important to consider PH as a diagnosis and not attribute all symptoms to severe obesity and/or SDB, particularly that a proportion of these patients may have group 1 PH and may benefit from pharmacotherapy.[88]

Positive Airway Pressure Therapy in PH with Comorbid OSA or OHS

Despite the high prevalence of comorbid SDB in patients with PH and the extensive pathophysiologic mechanisms linking SDB and nocturnal hypoxemia with PH, there are limited data examining the impact of positive airway pressure therapy on pulmonary hemodynamics. Most studies are limited by being observational in nature, having small sample sizes with various follow-up periods, and using different techniques to measure pulmonary hemodynamics. It is important to note that to more accurately assess the effect of positive airway pressure therapy on pulmonary hemodynamics, it is imperative to examine studies that only include patients who have PH at baseline. This approach can explain the discrepancy between 2 meta-analyses, one that included all patients (including those who did not have PH at baseline) leading to a very small effect size of positive airway pressure therapy in reducing PA pressures (1.34 mm Hg, 95% CI 0.34–2.33)[89] versus another meta-analysis that only included patients with PH at baseline (13.3 mm Hg, 95% CI 12.7–14.0).[90] Importantly, both these meta-analyses did not include patients with OHS. In **Table 2**, we summarize 11 studies that include patients with predominantly severe OSA or OHS and PH at baseline, were treated with positive airway pressure therapy, and had adequate adherence to therapy (n = 262). The improvement in PA pressures ranged from 4 to 17.6 mm Hg, with a weighted average of 10.5 mm Hg. The effect of positive airway pressure therapy was similar in OSA and OHS. Moreover, in the Pickwick trial, there was no significant difference between noninvasive ventilation (NIV) and continuous positive airway pressure (CPAP) in the degree of improvement of PH in patients with OHS who had comorbid severe OSA.[31]

As illustrated in **Table 2**, persistent PH is not an uncommon finding despite initial improvements in pulmonary hemodynamics with adherent positive airway pressure therapy, particularly in patients with OHS.[31,75] Even mildly elevated PASP on echocardiography is associated with increased mortality.[69,70,74] As such, we recommend that if patients with OSA and/or OHS have persistently elevated PASP on echocardiography after 6 to 12 months of adherent positive airway pressure therapy, clinicians should consider referring these patients to multidisciplinary PH clinics for consideration of RHC. It is important to determine if the residual PH is precapillary in nature and whether it would benefit from medications for PAH.

Potential Adverse Effects of Positive Airway Pressure Therapy in Pulmonary Hypertension

One area of concern is whether positive airway pressure therapy can adversely affect RV function

Table 2
Effect of positive airway pressure therapy on right-sided heart pressures in patients with pulmonary hypertension at baseline

Author	Study Design	Total Sample (n)	PH Treated with PAP (n)	SDB Type	BMI (kg/m²)	OSA Severity (AHI)	PAP Usage (h/night)	Therapy Duration (months)	Baseline Right-sided Pressure	Follow-up Right-sided Pressure
Chaouat et al,[117] 1997	Obs RHC	65	11	OSA	33±6[a]	87 ± 33[a]	CPAP 5.2[a,f]	64 ± 6	24±5[b]	20±7[b]
Alchanatis et al,[118] 2001	CC TTE	29	6	OSA	41 ± 7	63 ± 18	CPAP 5.4[a,f]	6	25.6 ± 4.0[c]	19.5 ± 1.5[c]
Sajkov et al,[119] 2002	Obs RHC	20	5	OSA	32 ± 3.6[a]	48.6 ± 23.3[a]	CPAP 5.1[a,f]	4	24.4 ± 5.0[b,g]	15.2 ± 2.8[b,g]
Arias et al,[120] 2006	RCT-CO TTE	21	11	OSA	33.6 ± 4.4	68.7 ± 24.9	CPAP 6.2[a,f]	3	38.3 ± 5.4[c,g]	29.8 ± 2.6[c,g]
Colish et al,[121] 2012	Obs TTE	47	47	OSA	38 ± 9	63 ± 30	CPAP >4.5[a]	12	54±6[d]	39±5[d]
Shehata et al,[122] 2013	CC TTE	24	10	OSA	32.2 ± 4	84[e]	CPAP >6[a]	6	35[c,e]	26[c,e]
Marvisi et al,[123] 2015	CC TTE	25	17	OSA	32 ± 6	59.3 ± 24	CPAP >4[a]	9	39.8 ± 4.1[c]	22.2±3[c]
Sharma et al,[124] 2019	RCT TTE	21	10	OSA	28.8 ± 5.8[a]	31.8 ± 8.0	AutoPAP Total 29.7 h[f]	48 h	58.6 ± 2.5[d]	42.8 ± 2.7[d]
Chu et al,[125] 2020 High altitude	CC TTE	71	45	OSA	26.0 ± 2.4[a]	44.3 ± 17.2[e]	CPAP "compliant"	6	44.6 ± 8.0[d]	37.9 ± 6.9[d]

(continued on next page)

Table 2
(continued)

Author	Study Design	Total Sample (n)	PH Treated with PAP (n)	SDB Type	BMI (kg/m²)	OSA Severity (AHI)	PAP Usage (h/night)	Therapy Duration (months)	Baseline Right-sided Pressure	Follow-up Right-sided Pressure
Castro-Añón et al,[126] 2012	CC TTE	30	13	OHS + OSA	43.3 ± 9.8	37.1 ± 23.0	NIV ≥4[a]	6	58 ± 11[d]	44 ± 12[d]
Masa et al,[31] 2020	RCT/post-hoc TTE	94	49	OHS + OSA	43.1[a,e]	69.3[a,e]	NIV 6[a,e]	36	48.8 ± 10.5[d]	40.0 ± 9.5[d]
Masa et al,[31] 2020	RCT/post-hoc TTE	102	38	OHS + OSA	42.5[a,e]	69[a,e]	CPAP 6[a,e]	36	53.9 ± 10.5[d]	43.2 ± 8.7[d]
Improvement in right-sided pressures[h]										10.5 mm Hg

Abbreviations: Obs, observational; CC, case control; NIV, noninvasive ventilation; RCT-CO, randomized controlled trial crossover; RHC, right heart catheterization; TTE, transthoracic echocardiogram.
Patients with PH alone.
[a] Entire cohort.
[b] mPAP via RHC.
[c] mPAP via TTE Doppler.
[d] RVSP via TTE Doppler.
[e] Median.
[f] Mean.
[g] Calculated from raw data provided in the article.
[h] Weighted average excluding study by Sharma given that duration of therapy was short.

by decreasing preload in patients with PH, particularly in those with milder forms of OSA who do not experience significant sleep hypoxemia. Although more research is needed in this area, one small study found an improvement in RV ejection fraction measured by cardiac magnetic resonance after 6 months of adherent CPAP therapy in 15 patients with mild-to-moderate OSA (right ventricular ejection fraction increased from 52.8 ± 4.1–59.4 ± 8.3, P = .014).[91]

Another area of concern is whether positive airway pressure therapy can lead to excessive increase in lung volumes and thereby adversely impacting endothelial function. In one study, investigators measured levels of several biomarkers, including circulating angiopoietin-2 at baseline and after 3 months of adherent CPAP therapy in 77 participants with moderate-to-severe OSA and no parenchymal lung disease.[92] Angiopoietin-2 is a biomarker of lung injury and an amplifier of inflammation and endothelial injury and its level correlates with the severity of OSA and sleep hypoxemia. Surprisingly, there was a slight, yet statistically significant increase in angiopoietin-2 with CPAP therapy. Even though CPAP resolved intermittent hypoxemia, it may have led to endothelial injury by a different mechanism. The authors speculated that it could be related to excess lung inflation with CPAP.[92] Although the effect of CPAP on functional residual capacity has not been tested during sleep in obese persons with OSA, CPAP of 5 to 10 cm H_2O pressure can increase the functional residual capacity by more than 1000 cc in healthy adults.[93] However, in an obese subject with a low expiratory reserve volume while supine, CPAP levels typically used to treat OSA may simply raise the expiratory lung volume and functional residual capacity to normal levels, without leading to lung overdistention. Clearly, further research is needed to ensure CPAP can be safely used in patients with PH and comorbid OSA, particularly those with milder forms of SDB.

Treatment of Obesity

As obesity plays a significant role in SDB and PH, an aggressive and multimodal approach to weight loss should be pursued. Bariatric surgery has been shown to improve pulmonary hemodynamics in severely obese patients with PH, with resolution of PH in some patients.[94–97] Bariatric surgery in patients with OHS can also lead to significant improvement in PA pressures, although it is unclear if this improvement is due to improvement in gas exchange, OSA, lung mechanics or a combination of these changes. In 17 patients with OHS and PH, a mean weight loss of 42% led to a significant decrease in mPAP by RHC from 36 ± 14 to 23 ± 7 mm Hg. However, PH persisted in 10 out of 17 (59%) patients.[97,98]

Randomized controlled trials of subcutaneous glucagon-like peptide-1 (GLP-1) receptor agonists (semaglutide 2.4 mg/wk) for 68 weeks or GLP-1/glucose-dependent insulinotropic polypeptide (GIP) receptor agonists (tirzepatide 15 mg/wk) for 72 weeks have shown significant reductions in body weight of 15% (~16 kg) and 21% (~22 kg), respectively.[99,100] This degree of weight loss, if sustained, can lead to significant improvement in SDB/hypoxemia in patients with OSA or OHS.[101,102] Weight loss induced by semaglutide can also lead to improvements quality of life and exercise capacity in obese patients with heart failure with preserved ejection fraction.[103] It remains unclear whether these medications improve pulmonary hemodynamics by mechanisms other than weight loss, such as reducing inflammation, vascular remodeling, and metabolic improvements.[104,105]

Supplemental Oxygen in Pulmonary Hypertension and Nocturnal Hypoxemia

There is accumulating evidence that sleep-related hypoxemia is a more important contributor to patient outcomes in PH than the AHI.[106] In the PVDOMICS cohort of patients with PAH who completed home respiratory polygraphy, elevated T90 was associated with elevated mPAP on RHC and RVSP on echocardiogram. For every 10% increment in T90, mPAP increased by 1.86 mm Hg and RVSP increased by 2.49 mm Hg. In contrast, AHI was not associated with mPAP or RVSP.[83] A median T90 threshold greater than 37% and mean SpO_2 less than 90% were associated with decreased transplant-free survival. For each 10% increase in T90, the risk for transplantation or death increased by 12%.[83]

Despite the association between sleep hypoxemia and patient outcomes, there is a paucity of data on whether the treatment of sleep hypoxemia with supplemental oxygen improves outcomes in patients with PH with or without comorbid SDB. In the REVEAL registry study, group 1 patients with PAH were categorized into two groups: those receiving supplemental oxygen and those who did not.[107] Only patients with severe reduction in diffusing capacity for carbon monoxide (DLCO) had a survival benefit with supplemental oxygen therapy. The limitation of this study is that it did not assess oxygen supplementation during sleep. In a randomized, cross-over trial that assessed 23 patients with precapillary PH and SDB (mean nocturnal SpO_2 <90% or 3% oxygen saturation index >10/h) but without significant daytime hypoxemia, treatment with 3 L/min nocturnal oxygen led to improvements in certain RV parameters, nocturnal O_2 saturation, and 6 minute walk distance.[108]

Further studies are needed to assess whether treatment should focus only on treating nocturnal hypoxemia with supplemental oxygen during sleep versus treatment of comorbid SDB with positive airway pressure therapy.

Multidisciplinary Clinics to Treat PH and SDB

Current PH guidelines recommend that PH centers provide care by a multidisciplinary team with providers from a broad spectrum of medical disciplines (pulmonologists, cardiologists, radiologists, and rheumatologists), as well as those with an expertise in providing psychological and social support.[18] Studies that describe an established multidisciplinary approach in a health system suggest that this approach leads to a more efficient and comprehensive diagnostic workup for patients with PH.[109,110] We propose that multidisciplinary clinics that include medical experts in sleep and weight loss, in addition to the more traditional disciplines involved in the management of patients with PH, may improve outcomes. However, further studies are needed to assess whether multidisciplinary PH clinics lead to improved patient-centered outcomes.

GAPS OF KNOWLEDGE

Despite advances in the field, important gaps of knowledge persist. Here, we list a few areas that in our opinion require further investigation.

1. What is the contribution of untreated sleep hypoxemia due to SDB in PAH (group 1 PH) and does it worsen patient outcomes?
2. Should hypoxemia due to SDB be treated with oxygen or positive airway pressure therapy?
3. Does treatment of sleep hypoxemia in PAH improve patient-centric outcomes?
4. Does untreated SDB diminish response to approved pharmacotherapy in patients with PAH or pulmonary hypertension associated with interstitial lung disease (PH-ILD)?
5. What is the contribution of obesity to PAH, independent of SDB?
6. Does treatment of obesity with GLP-1 receptor agonists and GLP-1/GIP receptor agonists (eg, semaglutide and tirzepatide) improve pulmonary hemodynamics in obese patients with PH or PAH?
7. Does echocardiographic improvement in PASP/RVSP with positive airway pressure therapy (or oxygen) lead to improvement in patient-centered outcomes?
8. What are the best practices for RHC in severely obese patients to avoid misclassification of PH?
9. Should severely obese patients with SDB who have persistent PH despite positive airway pressure therapy be evaluated for precapillary PH by RHC?
10. Do patients with OSA or OHS who are adherent to positive airway pressure therapy and are found to have comorbid precapillary PH benefit from PAH-specific pharmacotherapy?

CLINICS CARE POINTS

- Sleep-disordered breathing and sleep hypoxemia are prevalent in patients with pulmonary hypertension.
- In patients with pulmonary hypertension, sleep hypoxemia is associated with worse outcomes.
- Patients with pulmonary hypertension should be screened for sleep-disordered breathing and sleep hypoxemia.
- Positive airway pressure therapy (CPAP or NIV) during sleep improves sleep hypoxemia due to sleep-disordered breathing.
- Limited data suggests that treatment of obstructive sleep apnea and obesity hypoventilation syndrome with positive airway pressure therapy improves pulmonary hypertension.

ACKNOWLEDGMENTS

The authors acknowledge the contribution of Dr Mona T. Vashi, MD (Assistant Professor of Medicine) while writing this article.

DISCLOSURE

None of the authors have any conflicts of interest to declare.

REFERENCES

1. Peppard PE, Young T, Barnet JH, et al. Increased prevalence of sleep-disordered breathing in adults. Am J Epidemiol 2013;177(9):1006–14.
2. Young T, Palta M, Dempsey J, et al. The occurrence of sleep-disordered breathing among middle-aged adults. N Engl J Med 1993;328(17):1230–5.

3. Heinzer R, Vat S, Marques-Vidal P, et al. Prevalence of sleep-disordered breathing in the general population: the HypnoLaus study. Lancet Respir Med 2015;3(4):310–8.

4. Benjafield AV, Ayas NT, Eastwood PR, et al. Estimation of the global prevalence and burden of obstructive sleep apnoea: a literature-based analysis HHS Public Access. Lancet Respir Med 2019;7(8):687–98.

5. Newman AB, Foster G, Givelber R, et al. Progression and regression of sleep-disordered breathing with changes in weight: the sleep heart health study. Arch Intern Med 2005;165(20):2408–13.

6. Peppard PE, Young T, Palta M, et al. Longitudinal study of moderate weight change and sleep-disordered breathing. JAMA 2000;284(23):3015–21.

7. Young T, Shahar E, Nieto FJ, et al. Predictors of sleep-disordered breathing in community-dwelling adults: the sleep heart health study. Arch Intern Med 2002;162(8):893–900.

8. Peppard PE, Young T, Palta M, et al. Prospective study of the association between sleep-disordered breathing and hypertension. N Engl J Med 2000; 342(19):1378–84.

9. Yeghiazarians Y, Jneid H, Tietjens JR, et al. Obstructive sleep apnea and cardiovascular disease: a scientific statement from the american heart association. Circulation 2021;144(3):e56–67.

10. Punjabi NM, Caffo BS, Goodwin JL, et al. Sleep-disordered breathing and mortality: a prospective cohort study. PLoS Med 2009;6(8):e1000132.

11. Arzt M, Young T, Finn L, et al. Association of sleep-disordered breathing and the occurrence of stroke. Am J Respir Crit Care Med 2005;172(11):1447–51.

12. Valham F, Mooe T, Rabben T, et al. Increased risk of stroke in patients with coronary artery disease and sleep apnea: a 10-year follow-up. Circulation 2008; 118(9):955–60.

13. Yaggi HK, Concato J, Kernan WN, et al. Obstructive sleep apnea as a risk factor for stroke and death. N Engl J Med 2005;353(19):2034–41.

14. Mehra R, Benjamin EJ, Shahar E, et al. Association of nocturnal arrhythmias with sleep-disordered breathing: the sleep heart health study. Am J Respir Crit Care Med 2006;173(8):910–6.

15. Campos-Rodriguez F, Martinez-Garcia MA, de la Cruz-Moron I, et al. Cardiovascular mortality in women with obstructive sleep apnea with or without continuous positive airway pressure treatment: a cohort study. Ann Intern Med 2012;156(2):115–22.

16. Marin JM, Carrizo SJ, Vicente E, et al. Long-term cardiovascular outcomes in men with obstructive sleep apnoea-hypopnoea with or without treatment with continuous positive airway pressure: an observational study. Lancet 2005;365(9464):1046–53.

17. Young T, Finn L, Peppard PE, et al. Sleep disordered breathing and mortality: eighteen-year follow-up of the Wisconsin sleep cohort. Sleep 2008;31(8):1071–8.

18. Humbert M, Kovacs G, Hoeper MM, et al. 2022 ESC/ERS Guidelines for the diagnosis and treatment of pulmonary hypertension. Eur Respir J 2023;61(1):2200879.

19. Hemnes AR, Leopold JA, Radeva MK, et al. Clinical characteristics and transplant-free survival across the spectrum of pulmonary vascular disease. J Am Coll Cardiol 2022;80(7):697–718.

20. Chang KY, Duval S, Badesch DB, et al. Mortality in pulmonary arterial hypertension in the modern Era: early insights from the pulmonary hypertension association registry. J Am Heart Assoc 2022;11: 24969.

21. Min J, Feng R, Badesch D, et al. Obesity in pulmonary arterial hypertension the pulmonary hypertension association registry. Ann Am Thorac Soc 2021; 18(2):229–37.

22. Krieger J, Sforza E, Apprill M, et al. Pulmonary hypertension, hypoxemia, and hypercapnia in obstructive sleep apnea patients. Chest 1989; 96(4):729–37.

23. Laks L, Lehrhaft B, Grunstein RR, et al. Pulmonary hypertension in obstructive sleep apnoea. Eur Respir J 1995;8(4):537–41.

24. Sanner BM, Doberauer C, Konermann M, et al. Pulmonary hypertension in patients with obstructive sleep apnea syndrome. Arch Intern Med 1997; 157(21):2483–7.

25. Chaouat A, Weitzenblum E, Krieger J, et al. Pulmonary hemodynamics in the obstructive sleep apnea syndrome. Results in 220 consecutive patients. Chest 1996;109(2):380–6.

26. Minai OA, Ricaurte B, Kaw R, et al. Frequency and impact of pulmonary hypertension in patients with obstructive sleep apnea syndrome. Am J Cardiol 2009;104:1300–6.

27. Hetzel M, Kochs M, Marx N, et al. Pulmonary hemodynamics in obstructive sleep apnea: frequency and causes of pulmonary hypertension. Lung 2003;181(3):157–66.

28. Podszus T, Bauer W, Mayer J, et al. Sleep apnea and pulmonary hypertension. Klin Wochenschr 1986;64(3):131–4.

29. Weitzenblum E, Krieger J, Apprill M, et al. Daytime pulmonary hypertension in patients with obstructive sleep apnea syndrome. Am Rev Respir Dis 1988;138(2):345–9.

30. Masa JF, Mokhlesi B, Benítez I, et al. Long-term clinical effectiveness of continuous positive airway pressure therapy versus non-invasive ventilation therapy in patients with obesity hypoventilation syndrome: a multicentre, open-label, randomised controlled trial. Lancet 2019;393(10182):1721–32.

31. Masa JF, Mokhlesi B, Benítez I, et al. Echocardiographic changes with positive airway pressure

therapy in obesity hypoventilation syndrome. long-term pickwick randomized controlled clinical trial. Am J Respir Crit Care Med 2020;201(5):586–97.

32. Almeneessier AS, Nashwan SZ, Al-Shamiri MQ, et al. The prevalence of pulmonary hypertension in patients with obesity hypoventilation syndrome: a prospective observational study. J Thorac Dis 2017;9(3):779–88.

33. Alawami M, Mustafa A, Whyte K, et al. Echocardiographic and electrocardiographic findings in patients with obesity hypoventilation syndrome. Intern Med J 2015;45(1):68–73.

34. Masa JF, Benítez ID, Javaheri S, et al. Risk factors associated with pulmonary hypertension in obesity hypoventilation syndrome. J Clin Sleep Med 2022; 18(4):983–92.

35. Tilkian AG, Guilleminault C, Schroeder JS, et al. Hemodynamics in sleep induced apnea. Studies during wakefulness and sleep. Ann Intern Med 1976;85(6):714–9.

36. Marrone O, Bonsignore MR, Romano S, et al. Slow and fast changes in transmural pulmonary artery pressure in obstructive sleep apnoea. Eur Respir J 1994;7(12):2192–8.

37. Iwase N, Kikuchi Y, Hida W, et al. Effects of repetitive airway obstruction on O2 saturation and systemic and pulmonary arterial pressure in anesthetized dogs. Am Rev Respir Dis 1992; 146(6):1402–10.

38. Fletcher EC, Goodnight-White S, Munafo D, et al. Rate of oxyhemoglobin desaturation in obstructive versus nonobstructive apnea. Am Rev Respir Dis 1991;143(3):657–60.

39. Stenmark KR, Meyrick B, Galie N, et al. Animal models of pulmonary arterial hypertension: the hope for etiological discovery and pharmacological cure. Am J Physiol Lung Cell Mol Physiol 2009;297(6):1013–32.

40. Nisbet RE, Graves AS, Kleinhenz DJ, et al. The role of NADPH oxidase in chronic intermittent hypoxia-induced pulmonary hypertension in mice. Am J Respir Cell Mol Biol 2009;40(5):601–9.

41. Mittal M, Roth M, König P, et al. Hypoxia-dependent regulation of nonphagocytic NADPH oxidase subunit NOX4 in the pulmonary vasculature. Circ Res 2007;101(3):258–67.

42. Fagan KA. Selected Contribution: pulmonary hypertension in mice following intermittent hypoxia. J Appl Physiol 2001;90(6):2502–7.

43. Mcguire M, Bradford A, Mcguire AMB. Chronic intermittent hypercapnic hypoxia increases pulmonary arterial pressure and haematocrit in rats. Eur Respir J 2001;18:279–85.

44. Zhen X, Moya EA, Gautane M, et al. Combined intermittent and sustained hypoxia is a novel and deleterious cardio-metabolic phenotype. Sleep 2022;45(6):zsab290.

45. Sajkov D, McEvoy RD. Obstructive sleep apnea and pulmonary hypertension. Prog Cardiovasc Dis 2009;51(5):363–70.

46. Fletcher EC, Proctor M, Yu J, et al. Pulmonary edema develops after recurrent obstructive apneas. Am J Respir Crit Care Med 1999;160(5 Pt 1):1688–96.

47. Schäfer H, Hasper E, Ewig S, et al. Pulmonary haemodynamics in obstructive sleep apnoea: time course and associated factors. Eur Respir J 1998; 12:679–84.

48. Vasan RS. Cardiac function and obesity. Heart 2003;89(10):1127–9.

49. Powell-Wiley TM, Poirier P, Burke LE, et al. Obesity and cardiovascular disease: a scientific statement from the american heart association. Circulation 2021;143(21).

50. McQuillan BM, Picard MH, Leavitt M, et al. Clinical correlates and reference intervals for pulmonary artery systolic pressure among echocardiographically normal subjects. Circulation 2001;104(23):2797–802.

51. Ayinapudi K, Singh T, Motwani A, et al. Obesity and pulmonary hypertension. Curr Hypertens Rep 2018;20(12):99.

52. Virdis A, Duranti E, Rossi C, et al. Tumour necrosis factor-alpha participates on the endothelin-1/nitric oxide imbalance in small arteries from obese patients: role of perivascular adipose tissue. Eur Heart J 2015;36(13):784–94.

53. Snodgrass RG, Boß M, Zezina E, et al. Hypoxia potentiates palmitate-induced pro-inflammatory activation of primary human macrophages. J Biol Chem 2016;291(1):413–24.

54. Voelkel NF, Tuder RM, Bridges J, et al. Interleukin-1 receptor antagonist treatment reduces pulmonary hypertension generated in rats by monocrotaline. Am J Respir Cell Mol Biol 1994; 11(6):664–75.

55. Aghamohammadzadeh R, Greenstein AS, Yadav R, et al. Effects of bariatric surgery on human small artery function: evidence for reduction in perivascular adipocyte inflammation, and the restoration of normal anticontractile activity despite persistent obesity. J Am Coll Cardiol 2013;62(2):128–35.

56. Kellow NH, Scott AD, White SA, et al. Comparison of the effects of propofol and isoflurane anaesthesia on right ventricular function and shunt fraction during thoracic surgery. Br J Anaesth 1995; 75(5):578–82.

57. Fischer LG, Aken H Van, Bürkle H. Management of pulmonary hypertension: physiological and pharmacological considerations for anesthesiologists. Anesth Analg 2003;96(6):1603–16.

58. Ahmed Q, Chung-Park M, Tomashefski JF. Cardiopulmonary pathology in patients with sleep apnea/obesity hypoventilation syndrome. Hum Pathol 1997;28(3):264–9.

59. Haque AK, Gadre S, Taylor J, et al. Original articles pulmonary and cardiovascular complications of obesity an autopsy study of 76 obese subjects. Arch Pathol Lab Med 2008;132(9):1397–404.
60. Irwin DC, Garat CV, Crossno JT, et al. Obesity-related pulmonary arterial hypertension in rats correlates with increased circulating inflammatory cytokines and lipids and with oxidant damage in the arterial wall but not with hypoxia. Pulm Circ 2014;4(4):638–53.
61. Ding M, Lei J, Qu Y, et al. Calorie restriction attenuates monocrotaline-induced pulmonary arterial hypertension in rats. J Cardiovasc Pharmacol 2015;65(6):562–70.
62. Ooi H, Cadogan E, Sweeney M, et al. Chronic hypercapnia inhibits hypoxic pulmonary vascular remodeling. Am J Physiol Heart Circ Physiol 2000;278(2):H331–8.
63. Kantores C, McNamara PJ, Teixeira L, et al. Therapeutic hypercapnia prevents chronic hypoxia-induced pulmonary hypertension in the newborn rat. Am J Physiol Lung Cell Mol Physiol 2006;291(5):L912–22.
64. Wilson MW, Labaki WW, Choi PJ. Mortality and healthcare use of patients with compensated hypercapnia. Ann Am Thorac Soc 2021;18(12):2027–32.
65. Helenius IT, Krupinski T, Turnbull DW, et al. Elevated CO2 suppresses specific Drosophila innate immune responses and resistance to bacterial infection. Proc Natl Acad Sci U S A 2009;106(44):18710–5.
66. Gates KL, Howell HA, Nair A, et al. Hypercapnia impairs lung neutrophil function and increases mortality in murine pseudomonas pneumonia. Am J Respir Cell Mol Biol 2013;49(5):821–8.
67. Shigemura M, Lecuona E, Angulo M, et al. Elevated CO2 regulates the Wnt signaling pathway in mammals, Drosophila melanogaster and Caenorhabditis elegans. Sci Rep 2019;9(1):18251.
68. Rudski LG, Lai WW, Afilalo J, et al. Guidelines for the echocardiographic assessment of the right heart in adults: a report from the American Society of Echocardiography endorsed by the European Association of Echocardiography, a registered branch of the European Society of Cardiology, and the Canadian Society of Echocardiography. J Am Soc Echocardiogr 2010;23(7):685–713.
69. Strange G, Stewart S, Celermajer DS, et al. Threshold of pulmonary hypertension associated with increased mortality. J Am Coll Cardiol 2019;73(21):2660–72.
70. Huston JH, Maron BA, French J, et al. Association of mild echocardiographic pulmonary hypertension with mortality and right ventricular function. JAMA Cardiol 2019;4(11):1112–21.
71. Choudhary G, Jankowich M, Wu WC. Prevalence and clinical characteristics associated with pulmonary hypertension in African-Americans. PLoS One 2013;8(12):e84264.
72. O'Leary JM, Assad TR, Xu M, et al. Lack of a tricuspid regurgitation Doppler signal and pulmonary hypertension by invasive measurement. J Am Heart Assoc 2018;7(13):e009362.
73. Taleb M, Khuder S, Tinkel J, et al. The diagnostic accuracy of Doppler echocardiography in assessment of pulmonary artery systolic pressure: a meta-analysis. Echocardiography 2013;30(3):258–65.
74. Jankowich M, Maron BA, Choudhary G. Mildly elevated pulmonary artery systolic pressure on echocardiography: bridging the gap in current guidelines. Lancet Respir Med 2021;9(10):1185–91.
75. Kauppert CA, Dvorak I, Kollert F, et al. Pulmonary hypertension in obesity-hypoventilation syndrome. Respir Med 2013;107(12):2061–70.
76. Steier J, Jolley CJ, Seymour J, et al. Neural respiratory drive in obesity. Thorax 2009;64(8):719–25.
77. Khirfan G, Melillo CA, Al Abdi S, et al. Impact of esophageal pressure measurement on pulmonary hypertension diagnosis in patients with obesity. Chest 2022;162(3):684–92.
78. Kang J, Kimura H, Niijima M, et al. [Nocturnal pulmonary hypertension in patients with obstructive sleep apnea associated with daytime pulmonary hypertension]. Nihon Kyobu Shikkan Gakkai Zasshi 1997;35(11):1173–8.
79. Niijima M, Kimura H, Edo H, et al. Manifestation of pulmonary hypertension during REM sleep in obstructive sleep apnea syndrome. Am J Respir Crit Care Med 1999;159(6):1766–72.
80. Mokhlesi B, Finn LA, Hagen EW, et al. Obstructive sleep apnea during REM sleep and hypertension. results of the Wisconsin Sleep Cohort. Am J Respir Crit Care Med 2014;190(10):1158–67.
81. Mokhlesi B, Hagen EW, Finn LA, et al. Obstructive sleep apnoea during REM sleep and incident non-dipping of nocturnal blood pressure: a longitudinal analysis of the Wisconsin Sleep Cohort. Thorax 2015;70(11):1062–9.
82. Minai OA, Pandya CM, Golish JA, et al. Predictors of nocturnal oxygen desaturation in pulmonary arterial hypertension. Chest 2007;131(1):109–17.
83. Lowery MM, Hill NS, Wang L, et al. Sleep-related hypoxia, right ventricular dysfunction, and survival in patients with group 1 pulmonary arterial hypertension. J Am Coll Cardiol 2023;82(21):1989–2005.
84. Huang Z, Duan A, Hu M, et al. Implication of prolonged nocturnal hypoxemia and obstructive sleep apnea for pulmonary hemodynamics in patients being evaluated for pulmonary hypertension: a retrospective study. J Clin Sleep Med 2023;19(2):213–23.

85. Yang JZ, Mokhlesi B, Mesarwi OA. Obstructive sleep apnea and pulmonary hypertension: the pendulum swings again. J Clin Sleep Med 2023; 19(2):209–11.

86. Brown LM, Chen H, Halpern S, et al. Delay in recognition of pulmonary arterial hypertension: factors identified from the REVEAL Registry. Chest 2011;140(1):19–26.

87. Frank RC, Min J, Abdelghany M, et al. Obesity is associated with pulmonary hypertension and modifies outcomes. J Am Heart Assoc 2020;9(5):e014195.

88. Shujaat A, Bellardini J, Girdhar A, et al. Use of pulmonary arterial hypertension-specific therapy in overweight or obese patients with obstructive sleep apnea and pulmonary hypertension. Pulm Circ 2014;4(2):244–9.

89. Sun X, Luo J, Xiao Y. Continuous positive airway pressure is associated with a decrease in pulmonary artery pressure in patients with obstructive sleep apnoea: a meta-analysis. Respirology 2014; 19(5):670–4.

90. Imran TF, Ghazipura M, Liu S, et al. Effect of continuous positive airway pressure treatment on pulmonary artery pressure in patients with isolated obstructive sleep apnea: a meta-analysis. Heart Fail Rev 2016;21(5):591–8.

91. Samaranayake CB, Turnbull C, Neubauer S, et al. Right ventricular responses to CPAP therapy in obstructive sleep apnea: CMR analysis of the MOSAIC randomized trial. Pulm Circ 2023;13(1): e12201.

92. Gottlieb DJ, Lederer DJ, Kim JS, et al. Effect of positive airway pressure therapy of obstructive sleep apnea on circulating Angiopoietin-2. Sleep Med 2022;96:119–21.

93. Andersson B, Lundin S, Lindgren S, et al. End-expiratory lung volume and ventilation distribution with different continuous positive airway pressure systems in volunteers. Acta Anaesthesiol Scand 2011;55(2):157–64.

94. Valera RJ, Fonnegra CB, Cogollo VJ, et al. Impact of rapid weight loss after bariatric surgery in systemic inflammatory response and pulmonary hemodynamics in severely obese subjects with pulmonary hypertension. J Am Coll Surg 2023; 236(2):365–72.

95. Salman AA, Salman MA, Shaaban HED, et al. Effect of bariatric surgery on the cardiovascular system in obese cases with pulmonary hypertension. Obes Surg 2021;31(2):523–30.

96. Sheu EG, Channick R, Gee DW. Improvement in severe pulmonary hypertension in obese patients after laparoscopic gastric bypass or sleeve gastrectomy. Surg Endosc 2016;30(2):633–7.

97. Sugerman HJ, Fairman RP, Baron PL, et al. Gastric surgery for respiratory insufficiency of obesity. Chest 1986;90(1):81–6.

98. Sugerman HJ, Baron PL, Fairman RP, et al. Hemodynamic dysfunction in obesity hypoventilation syndrome and the effects of treatment with surgically induced weight loss. Ann Surg 1988;207(5): 604–13.

99. Wilding JPH, Batterham RL, Calanna S, et al. Once-weekly semaglutide in adults with overweight or obesity. N Engl J Med 2021;384(11):989–1002.

100. Jastreboff AM, Aronne LJ, Ahmad NN, et al. Tirzepatide once weekly for the treatment of obesity. N Engl J Med 2022;387(3):205–16.

101. Mokhlesi B, Masa JF, Brozek JL, et al. Evaluation and management of obesity hypoventilation syndrome. an official american thoracic society clinical practice guideline. Am J Respir Crit Care Med 2019;200(3):e6–24.

102. Kakazu MT, Soghier I, Afshar M, et al. Weight loss interventions as treatment of obesity hypoventilation syndrome. a systematic review. Ann Am Thorac Soc 2020;17(4):492–502.

103. Kosiborod MN, Abildstrøm SZ, Borlaug BA, et al. Semaglutide in patients with heart failure with preserved ejection fraction and obesity. N Engl J Med 2023;389(12):1069–84.

104. King NE, Brittain E. Emerging therapies: the potential roles SGLT2 inhibitors, GLP1 agonists, and ARNI therapy for ARNI pulmonary hypertension. Pulm Circ 2022;12(1):e12028.

105. Morrison AM, Huang S, Annis JS, et al. Cardiometabolic risk factors associated with right ventricular function and compensation in patients referred for echocardiography. J Am Heart Assoc 2023; 12(12):e028936.

106. Samhouri B, Venkatasaburamini M, Paz H, et al. Pulmonary artery hemodynamics are associated with duration of nocturnal desaturation but not apnea-hypopnea index. J Clin Sleep Med 2020; 16(8):1231–9.

107. Farber HW, Badesch DB, Benza RL, et al. Use of supplemental oxygen in patients with pulmonary arterial hypertension in REVEAL. J Heart Lung Transplant 2018;37(8):948–55.

108. Ulrich S, Keusch S, Hildenbrand FF, et al. Effect of nocturnal oxygen and acetazolamide on exercise performance in patients with pre-capillary pulmonary hypertension and sleep-disturbed breathing: randomized, double-blind, cross-over trial. Eur Heart J 2015;36(10):615–23.

109. Vonk MC, van Dijk APJ, Heijdra YF, et al. Pulmonary hypertension: its diagnosis and management, a multidisciplinary approach. Neth J Med 2005; 63(6):193–8.

110. Jankowich M, Hebel R, Jantz J, et al. Multispecialty pulmonary hypertension clinic in the VA. Pulm Circ 2017;7(4):758–67.

111. Poms AD, Turner M, Farber HW, et al. Comorbid conditions and outcomes in patients with

pulmonary arterial hypertension: a REVEAL registry analysis. Chest 2013;144(1):169–76.

112. Dumitrascu R, Tiede H, Eckermann J, et al. Sleep apnea in precapillary pulmonary hypertension. Sleep Med 2013;14(3):247–51.

113. Murta MS, Duarte RLM, Waetge D, et al. Sleep-disordered breathing in adults with precapillary pulmonary hypertension: prevalence and predictors of nocturnal hypoxemia. Lung 2022;200(4): 523–30.

114. Nagaoka M, Goda A, Takeuchi K, et al. Nocturnal hypoxemia, but not sleep apnea, is associated with a poor prognosis in patients with pulmonary arterial hypertension. Circ J 2018;82(12): 3076–81.

115. Minic M, Granton JT, Ryan CM. Sleep disordered breathing in group 1 pulmonary arterial hypertension. J Clin Sleep Med 2014;10(3):277–83.

116. Simonson JL, Pandya D, Khan S, et al. Comparison of obstructive sleep apnoea prevalence and severity across WHO pulmonary hypertension groups. BMJ Open Respir Res 2022;9(1):e001304.

117. Chaouat A, Weitzenblum E, Kessler R, et al. Five-year effects of nasal continuous positive airway pressure in obstructive sleep apnoea syndrome. Eur Respir J 1997;10(11):2578–82.

118. Alchanatis M, Tourkohoriti G, Kakouros S, et al. Daytime pulmonary hypertension in patients with obstructive sleep apnea: the effect of continuous positive airway pressure on pulmonary hemodynamics. Respiration 2001;68(6):566–72.

119. Sajkov Dimitar, Wang Tingting, Nicholas A S, et al. Continuous positive airway pressure treatment improves pulmonary hemodynamics in patients with obstructive sleep apnea. Am J Respir Crit Care Med 2002;165:152–8.

120. Arias MA, García-Río F, Alonso-Fernández A, et al. Pulmonary hypertension in obstructive sleep apnoea: effects of continuous positive airway pressure: a randomized, controlled cross-over study. Eur Heart J 2006;27(9):1106–13.

121. Colish J, Walker JR, Elmayergi N, et al. Obstructive sleep apnea: effects of continuous positive airway pressure on cardiac remodeling as assessed by cardiac biomarkers, echocardiography, and cardiac MRI. Chest 2012;141(3):674–81.

122. Shehata MEA, El-Desoky ME, El-Razek Maaty A, et al. Pulmonary hypertension in obstructive sleep apnea hypopnea syndrome. Egyptian J Chest Dis and Tuberc 2013;62(3):459–65.

123. Marvisi M, Vento MG, Balzarini L, et al. Continuous positive airways pressure and uvulopalatopharyngoplasty improves pulmonary hypertension in patients with obstructive sleep apnoea. Lung 2015;193(2): 269–74.

124. Sharma S, Fox H, Aguilar F, et al. Auto positive airway pressure therapy reduces pulmonary pressures in adults admitted for acute heart failure with pulmonary hypertension and obstructive sleep apnea. The ASAP-HF Pilot Trial. Sleep 2019;42(7):zsz100.

125. Chu AA, Yu HM, Yang H, et al. Evaluation of right ventricular performance and impact of continuous positive airway pressure therapy in patients with obstructive sleep apnea living at high altitude. Sci Rep 2020;10(1):20186.

126. Castro-Añón O, Golpe R, Pérez-de-Llano LA, et al. Haemodynamic effects of non-invasive ventilation in patients with obesity-hypoventilation syndrome. Respirology 2012;17(8):1269–74.

Intermittent Versus Sustained Hypoxemia from Sleep-disordered Breathing
Outcomes in Patients with Chronic Lung Disease and High Altitude

Alyssa A. Self, MD, Omar A. Mesarwi, MD*

KEYWORDS

- Overlap hypoxia • Sleep apnea • Cardiometabolic outcomes • Combined hypoxia

KEY POINTS

- Sustained and intermittent hypoxemia may be superimposed in a variety of clinical scenarios.
- These combined hypoxic states may not be fully described by simple metrics of hypoxemia.
- In general, adverse outcomes in such states are related to the severity of hypoxemia.
- Treatment strategies for improving hypoxemia may include nasal continuous positive airway pressure, but there are few studies in general, and the effects of supplemental oxygen alone are underinvestigated.
- Mechanisms explaining adverse effects of combined hypoxic states may include excess burden of reactive oxygen species, pulmonary hypertension, and glucose and lipid dysregulation, but additional study is required.

INTRODUCTION

There is considerable variability in the presentation of hypoxemia in various respiratory diseases and physiologic states. Hypoxemia may be sustained—that is, present at least to some degree throughout the day, though perhaps more severe at night—or it may be intermittent, with cyclic alterations in the partial pressure of arterial oxygen (Pa_{O_2}), as in sleep-disordered breathing. Some individuals experience both of these states concurrently, such as in the chronic obstructive pulmonary disease/obstructive sleep apnea (COPD/OSA) overlap syndrome (OS) or during periodic breathing at high altitude. Understanding the effects of superimposed hypoxemic states can be challenging, particularly since other physiologic manifestations, such as hypercapnia, changes to hypoxic and hypercapnic ventilatory responses, and muscle fatigue, may be present. In this brief review, we describe the metrics of hypoxemia and some limitations and investigate physiologic and pathologic states of combined sustained and intermittent hypoxemia, with a focus on clinical outcomes.

Hypoxemia During Sleep: Metrics and Consequences

Polysomnography and type 3 home-based studies can readily report multiple parameters to convey the severity of nocturnal hypoxemia. These include the percentage of total sleep time with oxygen saturation less than 90% (T90), the oxygen desaturation index (ODI), and oxyhemoglobin saturation nadir.[1–3] OSA is associated with an increased risk of cardiovascular disease, neurocognitive disorders, and metabolic dysfunction,

Division of Pulmonary, Critical Care, and Sleep Medicine and Physiology, University of California, San Diego, 9500 Gilman Drive Mail Code 0623A, La Jolla, CA 92093, USA
* Corresponding author.
E-mail address: omesarwi@health.ucsd.edu

Sleep Med Clin 19 (2024) 327–337
https://doi.org/10.1016/j.jsmc.2024.02.011
1556-407X/24/© 2024 Elsevier Inc. All rights reserved.

though trials have been conflicting on the benefit of continuous positive airway pressure (CPAP) therapy, particularly regarding a reduction in cardiovascular events.[4–6] Studies have shown an association between various metrics of hypoxemia and cardiovascular outcomes in OSA,[7–10] though an inherent limitation of these single-variable metrics is that they do not encapsulate both the depth and duration of desaturation events and are not specific to hypoxic events resulting from OSA.[11,12]

Hypoxic Burden

Investigations have more recently turned to novel ways to characterize nocturnal hypoxia, one of which is the hypoxic burden. The hypoxic burden is calculated as the area under the oxyhemoglobin saturation curve corresponding to respiratory events.[13] When compared to single metrics such as ODI, mean saturation, and saturation nadir, the hypoxic burden reflects both the changes in the SpO_2 during sleep, the extent of SpO_2 decline, and hypoxemia duration during hypopnea and apnea events.[12] A recent study by Li and colleagues demonstrated that the hypoxic burden was positively correlated with the apnea-hypopnea index (AHI), was able to accurately distinguish OSA from non-OSA, and was able to predict the severity of OSA better than anthropometrics, lowest or mean peripheral saturation, or the Epworth Sleepiness Scale.[14]

Hypoxic burden and cardiovascular disease
Additionally, a growing body of literature supports the use of hypoxic burden to predict cardiovascular risk. Azarbarzin and colleagues reported that the hypoxic burden is associated with cardiovascular mortality after adjusting for confounding factors in 2 cohort studies: the Outcomes of Sleep Disorders in Older Men (MrOS) and the Sleep Heart Health Study (SHHS). In the MrOS cohort, hypoxic burden was associated with increased all-cause mortality, though this effect was not found in the SHHS cohort.[13,15] In both cohorts, the hypoxic burden was found to be predictive of congestive heart failure in men regardless of AHI, though the same effect was not seen in women.[16] Hypoxic burden has also been associated with an increased risk of major adverse cardiovascular events (MACE) (a composite outcome including acute myocardial infarction, all-cause mortality, unplanned coronary revascularization, and stroke) in a French cohort study of patients with newly diagnosed OSA and no known cardiovascular disease.[17] In a post hoc analysis of the ISAACC trial examining effects of nasal CPAP on cardiovascular events in patients with acute coronary syndrome, patients were categorized as having high

or low hypoxic burden relative to a median value. The study found that in the high hypoxic burden group, CPAP was associated with a significant reduction in cardiovascular events.[18] A recent retrospective chart review also showed a correlation between the hypoxic burden and both hypertension and impaired fasting glucose.[19] Further, Esmaeili and colleagues recently showed that hypoxic burden calculated from automatically scored desaturations—compared to manual scoring in previous studies—was associated with excessive daytime sleepiness, hypertension, and cardiovascular mortality with similar effect size, which could lead to integration of a more automated technology to predict clinically relevant outcomes.[20] Studies to date have primarily focused on the use of hypoxic burden to identify patients at risk of adverse cardiovascular events, though further studies are needed on whether this novel metric also correlates with neurocognitive dysfunction and metabolic disorders, both of which are known consequences of OSA. Other novel metrics of hypoxemia have been explored, though it is important to note that no single metric exists, which gives complete insight about the relative contributions of intermittent versus sustained hypoxemia to clinical outcomes. The hypoxic burden has also been critiqued slightly, insofar as it might represent in patients with OSA a surrogate of the presence of visceral adiposity.[21]

Clinical Examples of Combined Hypoxic States

There are several important clinical disease states in which sleep-disordered breathing may be superimposed upon a chronic state of mild or moderate hypoxemia. Baseline hypoxemia may be imposed by obesity, COPD or other lung disease, or living at high altitude.

Chronic obstructive pulmonary disease/ obstructive sleep apnea overlap syndrome
Perhaps the most common, and best described, an example of a disease state in which one might encounter combined sustained and intermittent hypoxemia is the COPD/OSA OS. OS is thought to be highly prevalent: COPD affects perhaps 10% of US adults,[22] and OSA is present in 20% to 30% of adults and afflicts nearly a billion adults worldwide.[23] However, the prevalence of OS may be higher than expected from these data: Epidemiologic studies describe the prevalence of OSA among those with COPD to be more than 50%,[24] and two-thirds in those with moderate-to-severe COPD.[25] Among those with significant emphysema or lung parenchymal destruction in COPD, baseline hypoxemia might be common, and intermittent hypoxemia caused by OSA can be

superimposed.[26,27] It is important to note that the spectrum of hypoxemia in OS can be highly variable, however, given the heterogeneity of disease severity in COPD and OSA, and that hypoxemia is one of many possible physiologic derangements in OS. Patients with COPD may have chronic hypercapnia, respiratory muscle weakness, impaired diffusing capacity, chronic respiratory infections due to immune dysfunction, and other issues.[28–30] Those with OSA may have intermittent hypercapnia, arousals from sleep, sympathetic nervous system activation, and intrathoracic pressure swings.[31,32] These disease effects may occur to varying degrees in OS, which adds a layer of additional complexity to our understanding of this combined disease state. Studying effects of hypoxemia in OS may therefore be challenging, and analysis limited, by such confounding issues.

Despite these limitations, we have firm data that patients with OS fare worse than patients with either COPD or OSA alone. Marin and colleagues published a seminal paper demonstrating worse longitudinal survival and COPD exacerbation-free survival in patients with OS than in those with COPD alone, and importantly, the CPAP use in patients with OS was associated with outcomes similar to those with COPD alone.[33] Adverse outcomes in those with OS have since been shown in other cohorts. Overall mortality, cardiovascular mortality, and COPD exacerbation-free mortality are all higher in those with OS than either individual OS component.[33–38] A variety of important cardiometabolic outcomes are demonstrably more common in OS than in either COPD or OSA alone.[33,36,38–51] In addition, cardiovascular comorbidities are associated with more severe nocturnal hypoxemia in OS (mean baseline saturation, nadir saturation, and T90).[34] Kendzerska and colleagues showed that Kaplan–Meier curves of cardiovascular event-free survival in OS versus OSA alone and COPD alone appeared similar when the presence of nocturnal hypoxemia (T90 $\geq$ 10 minutes/night) was used as a surrogate for OSA, suggesting that nocturnal hypoxemia may drive poor cardiovascular outcomes in OS. However, another recent publication found that nocturnal hypoxemia was a mortality risk factor in a combined group of OSA and OS patients, but not in OS specifically, though this study included a limited number of OS patients.[52] In any case, the existing data linking mortality or other endpoints in OS to hypoxemia specifically are suggestive but overall fairly limited, and higher quality data are clearly needed. Moreover, the relationship between poor outcomes in OS and physiologic effects aside from hypoxemia has received comparatively little attention in the literature.

There are currently no long-term randomized, controlled trials of any specific therapy in OS and, to our knowledge, no specific clinical guidelines in this unique population. In our experience, patients with OS are typically treated separately for COPD and OSA. CPAP has been shown in uncontrolled associative,[52–54] longitudinal,[33] and a small prospective cohort study[55] to be associated with improvements in mortality and COPD exacerbation-free mortality in OS. A recent systematic review on the subject determined that CPAP use may improve a variety of important outcomes in OS, including the rate of COPD exacerbation and overall mortality.[56] However, the authors note several limitations in interpretation of these data, including heterogeneity in the definitions of COPD and OSA, variability in CPAP use, availability of only observational trials in this space, small trial sizes, and lack of consistent adjustment for confounding variables. We also note that practice standards in COPD and OSA have both shifted considerably in the years since some of the applicable studies were published. Finally, we also observe that CPAP impacts multiple physiologic consequences of both OSA and COPD, and even prospective studies of CPAP in OS may provide little mechanistic understanding of the impact of hypoxemia specifically, let alone the respective contributions of intermittent or sustained hypoxemia. Comparisons of CPAP to noninvasive positive pressure ventilation and oxygen therapy would enhance our understanding of this disease state considerably.

Obstructive sleep apnea and other lung disease

Sleep-disordered breathing may be comorbid with other disease states besides COPD, and cross-sectional studies have shown high prevalence rates of sleep apnea in some chronic lung diseases. This combination can also result in clinically evident superimposition of sustained and intermittent hypoxemia. Patients with idiopathic pulmonary fibrosis (IPF), for example, commonly have both resting and exertional hypoxemia, and rates increase as a function of the duration of illness.[57] More than half of IPF patients have comorbid OSA,[58–60] potentially resulting in a pattern of superimposed sustained and intermittent hypoxemia similar to that seen in OS. This figure is well above what one would estimate in a matched, non-IPF population. Like COPD/OSA overlap, IPF/OSA overlap may present with myriad physiologic derangements aside from hypoxemia, and there may be considerable heterogeneity in the severity of any of these factors.[61,62] Nocturnal hypoxemia in IPF/OSA overlap is both common and likely harmful, with an association across multiple studies with excess mortality and the presence of pulmonary hypertension.[63–66] Multiple parameters of hypoxemia in sleep studies have formed the basis of these associations: AHI, ODI, nadir, and mean oxyhemoglobin saturation during sleep, and the T90 and T88 have all been associated with adverse outcomes among those with IPF and OSA. In addition, cardiovascular disease, oxidative stress, and ischemic heart disease are all more common in patients with IPF and comorbid OSA than in IPF alone.[67,68] Similar to the COPD/OSA OS, there are no large-scale randomized trials of therapy in IPF/OSA, and an understanding of the relative contributions of sustained versus intermittent hypoxemia in this combined disease state is lacking. Although IPF is far less common than COPD, prognosis is worse and treatment options are considerably more limited in IPF, highlighting the critical need for further research in this field. The effects of hypoxemia in OSA comorbid with other chronic lung diseases are also relatively underexplored.

Obesity hypoventilation syndrome

Obesity hypoventilation syndrome (OHS) is defined as the presence of daytime alveolar hypoventilation in the presence of obesity (body mass index [BMI] $\geq$30 kg/m^2) and is a diagnosis of exclusion.[69–71] Thus, other potential causes of hypoventilation should be ruled out prior to applying the label of OHS. Approximately 90% of patients with OHS have concomitant OSA,[70] and given the increasing prevalence of obesity in the general population, OHS is expected to become more common over time. Patients with combined OSA/OHS may exhibit a pattern of combined sustained and intermittent hypoxemia similar to that described in the sections earlier, despite the lack of pulmonary parenchymal disease present in other groups. This finding stems from the fact that obesity itself may lead to hypoxemia in a dose-dependent manner, leading to sustained hypoxemia, upon which intermittent hypoxemia from OSA is usually superimposed. In a series of 118 subjects, Littleton and Tulaimat found that the functional residual capacity and Pao$_2$ both decreased, and the alveolar–arterial oxygen gradient increased, with increasing BMI.[72] As one might expect, resting hypoxemia also predicts the presence of OHS,[73,74] though guidelines suggest against relying on this metric alone in determining when to obtain additional supportive data in the diagnosis of OHS.[75] It follows, then, that nocturnal hypoxemia is generally more severe in OHS/OSA than in OSA alone. Importantly, significant hypoxemia may persist even after initiation of CPAP therapy.[76]

Mortality and other important outcomes are substantially worse in OHS/OSA than in OSA alone, and hypoxemia is an independent predictor of mortality in this syndrome.[77–79] As might be expected, weight loss is a valid treatment option for OHS, although the data supporting this approach are weak, and the specific thresholds for weight loss poorly defined.[80] CPAP therapy is another important treatment modality for OHS/OSA. Recent studies have shown that nasal CPAP is as effective as bi-level ventilation at improving outcomes in OHS/OSA,[81,82] but the unique effects of oxygenation in such outcomes (and by corollary, the effects of improving oxygenation alone) are unknown.

High altitude

Over 80 million people live at high altitude (>2500 m above sea level).[83] Atmospheric pressure is inversely related to altitude (thus, the partial pressure of inspired oxygen is reduced with ascending altitude). This hypobaric hypoxia causes a reduction in arterial oxygen partial pressure of oxygen (Pao$_2$), as well as ventilatory changes—both increased minute ventilation and respiratory alkalosis—resulting in relative hypocapnia and an increase in loop gain.[84,85] As such, those at high altitude may have a predisposition to sleep-disordered breathing, including exacerbation of OSA,[85] and the appearance of central sleep apnea,[84,86–91] each of which may become more severe with time at altitude or with further ascent. Unsurprisingly then, sleep at high altitude is associated with a state of oxygenation involving both chronic sustained and superimposed intermittent hypoxemia. AHI, ODI, and resting and nadir SpO$_2$ are all worse at high altitude relative to sea level.[86] Though evidence is conflicting, some studies suggest that the effect of altitude on AHI may diminish over time,[91,92] but nonetheless, the overall burden of sleep-disordered breathing is more profound in chronic high-altitude dwellers than in those at or near sea level.

Most available data in those who live at high altitude are cross-sectional and not longitudinal. Moreover, few data exist to inform whether improving oxygenation in those who live at high altitude improves any markers of cardiometabolic disease. However, studies by Pham and colleagues,[93] and Miele and colleagues[94] of subjects living at altitude in Peru have noted that cardiac biomarkers, glycated hemoglobin, and the homeostatic model assessment for insulin resistance are all worse as a function of more severe nocturnal hypoxemia; such relationships do not consistently exist with more traditional metrics of sleep-disordered breathing severity, such as AHI. Further research on the impact of ameliorating hypoxemia in those at altitude, whether by positive airway pressure therapy or supplemental oxygen, would help clarify causal relationships.

Understanding Combined Hypoxia in Animal Models

Many groups have studied the effects of chronic intermittent and sustained hypoxia using animal models. Chronic intermittent hypoxia causes systemic hypertension,[95–97] mild pulmonary hypertension,[98–100] atherosclerosis,[101–105] dysglycemia,[106–109] and dyslipidemia.[109–112] Similarly, chronic sustained hypoxia has been extensively studied in animals. Sustained hypoxia causes significant pulmonary hypertension[113,114] and improvements in glucose metabolism,[115,116] though without significant changes to systemic blood pressure.[117] Of note, however, there are often varying exposure severities under the umbrella of "intermittent" and, to a lesser degree, "sustained" hypoxia, and there is some variability in the above outcomes as well. A full understanding of chronic effects of sustained or intermittent hypoxia in animals depends heavily on exposure

types, specifics about the disease model (such as the specific animals, diet, and experimental conditions used), and organ systems being studied. There have been relatively few experiments directly comparing sustained versus intermittent hypoxia, or different frequencies, rates of desaturation and resaturation, and nadir oxygen concentration, in intermittent hypoxia. As such, there is room for considerable additional work to understand the dynamic effects of hypoxia modeling human disease.

One clear area of need for additional input is an understanding of general and specific effects of sustained and intermittent hypoxia on lung parenchyma and susceptibility to further disease. Intermittent hypoxia appears to increase pulmonary inflammatory cell infiltration and pro-inflammatory cytokine expression,[118] endoplasmic reticulum stress, profibrotic mediators, apoptosis,[119] and oxidative stress[120,121]; sensitizes to bleomycin-induced lung injury[122,123]; and alters pulmonary gene expression profiles.[124] However, as discussed earlier, comparative studies are sparse, and understanding these effects in the context of various models of human disease is often lacking. Sustained hypoxia may contribute to activation of some of the same pathways, including pulmonary

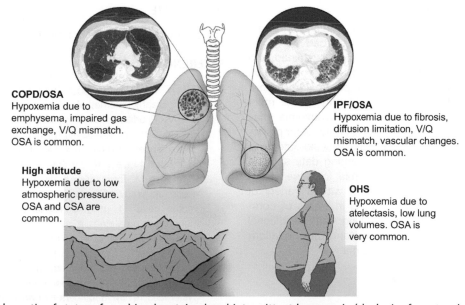

Fig. 1. Schematic of states of combined sustained and intermittent hypoxemia (clockwise from top *left*). In patients with chronic lung disease, sustained hypoxemia may manifest due to emphysema (enlargement of the air-filled spaces in the lung, causing impaired gas exchange and ventilation–perfusion mismatch), or pulmonary fibrosis (scarring in the lung tissue leading to diffusion limitations, ventilation–perfusion mismatch, and alterations in the pulmonary vasculature). Obesity hypoventilation syndrome is marked by chronic sustained hypoxemia due to pulmonary atelectasis and low lung volumes. In each of these states, obstructive sleep apnea is highly prevalent, leading to superimposed intermittent hypoxemia. At high altitude, chronic hypoxemia results from a reduction in the partial pressure of inspired oxygen, and both obstructive and central sleep apnea are common. V/Q, ventilation to perfusion ratio; CSA, central sleep apnea.

inflammatory injury[125] (reviewed in Refs.[126–128]) and oxidative stress,[129] and may sensitize to further lung injury from lipopolysaccharide.[130] However, there are still substantive gaps in our knowledge of adaptive and maladaptive effects of both sustained and intermittent hypoxia in the lung, and nuanced approaches to modeling human disease are likely needed in order to understand end-organ effects of hypoxic exposures.

In addition to these knowledge gaps, and given the often opposing cardiometabolic effects of intermittent and sustained hypoxemia, our group has explored superimposed sustained and intermittent hypoxic exposures in young C57BL/6J mice.[109] We found that this combined exposure causes elevated levels of hepatic malondialdehyde (a marker of redox burden), systemic and pulmonary hypertension, elevated serum low density lipoprotein/very low density lipoprotein (LDL/VLDL) cholesterol, and changes to glucose metabolism. Further studies are needed in this area to describe mechanisms of the observed findings, define tissue-specific effects of combined hypoxia, and understand which of the observed effects might be most durable or reversible and most responsible for poor outcomes in the clinical realm.

SUMMARY

Hypoxemia can have highly variable presentations and in several clinical instances can be represented as some combination of sustained and intermittent hypoxemia (**Fig. 1**). This combination can be described by several parameters from a nocturnal sleep study, but identifying the most clinically relevant markers of hypoxemia may depend on the specific clinical entity, other pathophysiological findings, and the specific outcomes of interest. Nonetheless, emerging data suggest that the severity of hypoxemia in these states may generally be associated with a variety of adverse effects. Clinical trials in states of combined hypoxemia are lacking, and additional research is needed to understand these relationships in a more mechanistic manner.

CLINICS CARE POINTS

- Hypoxemia can have a variety of presentations in conditions of respiratory disease or high altitude, with concurrent sleep-disordered breathing. Combined hypoxic states may be described by sustained and intermittent hypoxemia.

- Many single metrics of hypoxemia routinely obtained from polysomnography or home sleep apnea tests may not fully encapsulate states of combined hypoxemia. A relatively novel metric (hypoxic burden) correlates well with cardiovascular outcomes.

- In combined hypoxic states, outcomes are often poor and are related to the severity of hypoxemia.

- Optimal treatment is poorly defined, and randomized, controlled trials are lacking. Many patients with combined hypoxic diseases are treated for each condition separately. The effect of improving oxygenation alone is unclear.

- Combined sustained and intermittent hypoxia in a rodent model increases redox burden and worsens pulmonary hypertension and dyslipidemia. Additional study is needed to understand mechanisms underlying such changes.

FUNDING

Funding received from grants NIH K08HL143140 and UCSD RG104645 for support.

DISCLOSURE

The authors have no relevant disclosures.

REFERENCES

1. Rundo JV, Downey R. Chapter 25 - polysomnography [Internet]. Available at:. In: Levin KH, Chauvel P, editors. Handbook of clinical Neurology. Elsevier; 2019. p. 381–92 https://www.sciencedirect.com/science/article/pii/B9780444640321000254. [Accessed 11 December 2023].

2. El Shayeb M, Topfer L-A, Stafinski T, et al. Diagnostic accuracy of level 3 portable sleep tests versus level 1 polysomnography for sleep-disordered breathing: a systematic review and meta-analysis. CMAJ (Can Med Assoc J) 2014; 186(1):E25–51.

3. Boulos MI, Jairam T, Kendzerska T, et al. Normal polysomnography parameters in healthy adults: a systematic review and meta-analysis. Lancet Respir Med 2019;7(6):533–43.

4. Sánchez-de-la-Torre M, Sánchez-de-la-Torre A, Bertran S, et al. Effect of obstructive sleep apnoea and its treatment with continuous positive airway pressure on the prevalence of cardiovascular events in patients with acute coronary syndrome (ISAACC study): a randomised controlled trial. Lancet Respir Med 2020;8(4):359–67.

5. Peker Y, Glantz H, Eulenburg C, et al. Effect of positive airway pressure on cardiovascular outcomes in coronary Artery disease patients with Nonsleepy obstructive sleep apnea. The RICCADSA randomized controlled trial. Am J Respir Crit Care Med 2016;194(5):613–20.

6. McEvoy RD, Antic NA, Heeley E, et al. CPAP for Prevention of cardiovascular events in obstructive sleep apnea. N Engl J Med 2016;375(10):919–31.

7. Han B, Chen WZ, Li YC, et al. Sleep and hypertension. Sleep Breath 2020;24(1):351–6.

8. Wang L, Ou Q, Shan G, et al. Independent association between oxygen desaturation index and cardiovascular disease in non-Sleepy sleep-disordered breathing Subtype: a Chinese community-based study. Nat Sci Sleep 2022;14:1397–406.

9. Punjabi NM. COUNTERPOINT: is the apnea-hypopnea index the best way to quantify the severity of sleep-disordered breathing? No. Chest 2016;149(1):16–9.

10. Oldenburg O, Wellmann B, Buchholz A, et al. Nocturnal hypoxaemia is associated with increased mortality in stable heart failure patients. Eur Heart J 2016;37(21):1695–703.

11. Martinez-Garcia MA, Sánchez-de-la-Torre M, White DP, et al. Hypoxic burden in obstructive sleep apnea: present and future. Arch Bronconeumol 2023;59(1):36–43.

12. Cao W, Luo J, Xiao Y. A review of current tools used for evaluating the severity of obstructive sleep apnea. Nat Sci Sleep 2020;12:1023–31.

13. Azarbarzin A, Sands SA, Taranto-Montemurro L, et al. Hypoxic burden captures sleep apnoea-specific nocturnal hypoxaemia. Eur Heart J 2019; 40(35):2989–90.

14. Li C, Gao Y, Huang W, et al. The use of the sleep apnea-specific hypoxic burden to predict obstructive sleep apnea hypopnea syndrome: evidence from a large cross-sectional study. Sleep Med 2023;111:94–100.

15. Azarbarzin A, Sands SA, Stone KL, et al. The hypoxic burden of sleep apnoea predicts cardiovascular disease-related mortality: the Osteoporotic Fractures in Men Study and the Sleep Heart Health Study. Eur Heart J 2019;40(14):1149–57.

16. Azarbarzin A, Sands SA, Taranto-Montemurro L, et al. The sleep apnea-specific hypoxic burden predicts incident heart failure. Chest 2020;158(2): 739–50.

17. Trzepizur W, Blanchard M, Ganem T, et al. Sleep apnea-specific hypoxic burden, Symptom Subtypes, and risk of cardiovascular events and all-cause mortality. Am J Respir Crit Care Med 2022; 205(1):108–17.

18. Pinilla L, Esmaeili N, Labarca G, et al. Hypoxic burden to guide CPAP treatment allocation in patients with obstructive sleep apnoea: a post hoc study of the ISAACC trial. Eur Respir J 2023; 62(6):2300828.

19. Uataya M, Banhiran W, Chotinaiwattarakul W, et al. Association between hypoxic burden and common cardiometabolic diseases in patients with severe obstructive sleep apnea. Sleep Breath 2023;27(6):2423–8.

20. Esmaeili N, Labarca G, Hu W-H, et al. Hypoxic burden based on automatically Identified desaturations is associated with adverse health outcomes. Ann Am Thorac Soc 2023;20(11):1633–41.

21. Jun JC. Dying with OSA, or from it: a Cautionary note about novel hypoxia metrics. Am J Respir Crit Care Med 2022;206(12):1563–4.

22. Owens RL, Macrea MM, Teodorescu M. The overlaps of asthma or COPD with OSA: a focused review. Respirology 2017;22(6):1073–83.

23. Benjafield AV, Ayas NT, Eastwood PR, et al. Estimation of the global prevalence and burden of obstructive sleep apnoea: a literature-based analysis. Lancet Respir Med 2019;7(8):687–98.

24. Shawon MSR, Perret JL, Senaratna CV, et al. Current evidence on prevalence and clinical outcomes of co-morbid obstructive sleep apnea and chronic obstructive pulmonary disease: a systematic review. Sleep Med Rev 2017;32:58–68.

25. Soler X, Gaio E, Powell FL, et al. High prevalence of obstructive sleep apnea in patients with moderate to severe chronic obstructive pulmonary disease. Ann Am Thorac Soc 2015;12(8):1219–25.

26. McNicholas WT. Chronic obstructive pulmonary disease and obstructive sleep apnoea-the overlap syndrome. J Thorac Dis 2016;8(2):236–42.

27. McNicholas WT. COPD-OSA overlap syndrome: Evolving evidence regarding Epidemiology, clinical consequences, and management. Chest 2017; 152(6):1318–26.

28. Han MK, Agusti A, Calverley PM, et al. Chronic obstructive pulmonary disease phenotypes: the future of COPD. Am J Respir Crit Care Med 2010; 182(5):598–604.

29. Friedlander AL, Lynch D, Dyar LA, et al. Phenotypes of chronic obstructive pulmonary disease. COPD 2007;4(4):355–84.

30. Vestbo J. COPD: definition and phenotypes. Clin Chest Med 2014;35(1):1–6.

31. Dempsey JA, Veasey SC, Morgan BJ, et al. Pathophysiology of sleep apnea. Physiol Rev 2010;90(1): 47–112.

32. Eckert DJ, Malhotra A. Pathophysiology of adult obstructive sleep apnea. Proc Am Thorac Soc 2008;5(2):144–53.

33. Marin JM, Soriano JB, Carrizo SJ, et al. Outcomes in patients with chronic obstructive pulmonary disease and obstructive sleep apnea: the overlap syndrome. Am J Respir Crit Care Med 2010;182(3):325–31.

34. Kendzerska T, Leung RS, Aaron SD, et al. Cardiovascular outcomes and all-cause mortality in

patients with obstructive sleep apnea and chronic obstructive pulmonary disease (overlap syndrome). Ann Am Thorac Soc 2019;16(1):71–81.

35. Du W, Liu J, Zhou J, et al. Obstructive sleep apnea, COPD, the overlap syndrome, and mortality: results from the 2005-2008 National Health and Nutrition Examination Survey. Int J Chron Obstruct Pulmon Dis 2018;13:665–74.

36. Shah AJ, Quek E, Alqahtani JS, et al. Cardiovascular outcomes in patients with COPD-OSA overlap syndrome: a systematic review and meta-analysis. Sleep Med Rev 2022;63:101627.

37. Voulgaris A, Archontogeorgis K, Pataka A, et al. Burden of comorbidities in patients with OSAS and COPD-OSAS overlap syndrome. Medicina (Kaunas) 2021;57(11):1201.

38. Adler D, Bailly S, Benmerad M, et al. Clinical presentation and comorbidities of obstructive sleep apnea-COPD overlap syndrome. PLoS One 2020; 15(7):e0235331.

39. Starr P, Agarwal A, Singh G, et al. Obstructive sleep apnea with chronic obstructive pulmonary disease among Medicare Beneficiaries. Ann Am Thorac Soc 2019;16(1):153–6.

40. Papachatzakis I, Velentza L, Zarogoulidis P, et al. Comorbidities in coexisting chronic obstructive pulmonary disease and obstructive sleep apnea - overlap syndrome. Eur Rev Med Pharmacol Sci 2018;22(13):4325–31.

41. Hu W, Zhao Z, Wu B, et al. Obstructive sleep apnea increases the prevalence of hypertension in patients with chronic obstructive disease. COPD 2020;17(5):523–32.

42. Wang Y, Li B, Li P, et al. Severe obstructive sleep apnea in patients with chronic obstructive pulmonary disease is associated with an increased prevalence of mild cognitive impairment. Sleep Med 2020;75:522–30.

43. Wang J, Li X, Hou W-J, et al. Endothelial function and T-lymphocyte subsets in patients with overlap syndrome of chronic obstructive pulmonary disease and obstructive sleep apnea. Chin Med J (Engl) 2019;132(14):1654–9.

44. Sun W-L, Wang J-L, Jia G-H, et al. Impact of obstructive sleep apnea on pulmonary hypertension in patients with chronic obstructive pulmonary disease. Chin Med J (Engl) 2019;132(11):1272–82.

45. Akinnusi M, El-Masri AR, Lawson Y, et al. Association of overlap syndrome with incident atrial fibrillation. Intern Emerg Med 2021;16(3):633–42.

46. van Zeller M, Basoglu OK, Verbraecken J, et al. Sleep and cardiometabolic comorbidities in the obstructive sleep apnoea-COPD overlap syndrome: data from the European Sleep Apnoea Database. ERJ Open Res 2023;9(3):00676–2022.

47. Xie J, Li F, Wu X, et al. Prevalence of pulmonary embolism in patients with obstructive sleep apnea and chronic obstructive pulmonary disease: the overlap syndrome. Heart Lung 2019;48(3):261–5.

48. Stepan B, Cservid L, Raduna O, et al. Severity of oxygen desaturation in OSA–COPD overlap syndrome compared to OSA alone: an observational cohort study. Pneumologia 2022;71(1):22–7.

49. Zhang P, Chen B, Lou H, et al. Predictors and outcomes of obstructive sleep apnea in patients with chronic obstructive pulmonary disease in China. BMC Pulm Med 2022;22(1):16.

50. Steveling EH, Clarenbach CF, Miedinger D, et al. Predictors of the overlap syndrome and its association with comorbidities in patients with chronic obstructive pulmonary disease. Respiration 2014; 88(6):451–7.

51. Lacedonia D, Carpagnano GE, Patricelli G, et al. Prevalence of comorbidities in patients with obstructive sleep apnea syndrome, overlap syndrome and obesity hypoventilation syndrome. Clin Respir J 2018;12(5):1905–11.

52. Tondo P, Scioscia G, Sabato R, et al. Mortality in obstructive sleep apnea syndrome (OSAS) and overlap syndrome (OS): the role of nocturnal hypoxemia and CPAP compliance. Sleep Med 2023;112:96–103.

53. Stanchina ML, Welicky LM, Donat W, et al. Impact of CPAP use and age on mortality in patients with combined COPD and obstructive sleep apnea: the overlap syndrome. J Clin Sleep Med 2013; 9(8):767–72.

54. Sterling KL, Pépin J-L, Linde-Zwirble W, et al. Impact of positive airway pressure therapy Adherence on outcomes in patients with obstructive sleep apnea and chronic obstructive pulmonary disease. Am J Respir Crit Care Med 2022;206(2):197–205.

55. Machado M-CL, Vollmer WM, Togeiro SM, et al. CPAP and survival in moderate-to-severe obstructive sleep apnoea syndrome and hypoxaemic COPD. Eur Respir J 2010;35(1):132–7.

56. Srivali N, Thongprayoon C, Tangpanithandee S, et al. The use of continuous positive airway pressure in COPD-OSA overlap syndrome: a systematic review. Sleep Med 2023;108:55–60.

57. Khor YH, Gutman L, Abu Hussein N, et al. Incidence and prognostic significance of hypoxemia in Fibrotic interstitial lung disease: an International cohort study. Chest 2021;160(3):994–1005.

58. Pihtili A, Bingol Z, Kiyan E, et al. Obstructive sleep apnea is common in patients with interstitial lung disease. Sleep Breath 2013;17(4):1281–8.

59. Lee JH, Park CS, Song JW. Obstructive sleep apnea in patients with interstitial lung disease: prevalence and predictive factors. PLoS One 2020; 15(10):e0239963.

60. Cheng Y, Wang Y, Dai L. The prevalence of obstructive sleep apnea in interstitial lung disease: a systematic review and meta-analysis. Sleep Breath 2021;25(3):1219–28.

61. Fell CD. Idiopathic pulmonary fibrosis: phenotypes and comorbidities. Clin Chest Med 2012;33(1): 51–7.

62. Sauleda J, Núñez B, Sala E, et al. Idiopathic pulmonary fibrosis: Epidemiology, Natural history, phenotypes. Med Sci 2018;6(4):110.

63. Troy LK, Corte TJ. Sleep disordered breathing in interstitial lung disease: a review. World J Clin Cases 2014;2(12):828–34.

64. Corte TJ, Wort SJ, Talbot S, et al. Elevated nocturnal desaturation index predicts mortality in interstitial lung disease. Sarcoidosis Vasc Diffuse Lung Dis 2012;29(1):41–50.

65. Kolilekas L, Manali E, Vlami KA, et al. Sleep oxygen desaturation predicts survival in idiopathic pulmonary fibrosis. J Clin Sleep Med 2013;9(6):593–601.

66. Bosi M, Milioli G, Fanfulla F, et al. OSA and Prolonged oxygen desaturation during sleep are Strong predictors of poor outcome in IPF. Lung 2017;195(5):643–51.

67. Gille T, Didier M, Boubaya M, et al. Obstructive sleep apnoea and related comorbidities in incident idiopathic pulmonary fibrosis. Eur Respir J 2017; 49(6):1601934.

68. Bouloukaki I, Fanaridis M, Testelmans D, et al. Overlaps between obstructive sleep apnoea and other respiratory diseases, including COPD, asthma and interstitial lung disease. Breathe 2022;18(3):220073.

69. Kaw R, Wong J, Mokhlesi B. Obesity and obesity hypoventilation, sleep hypoventilation, and Postoperative respiratory failure. Anesth Analg 2021; 132(5):1265–73.

70. Balachandran JS, Masa JF, Mokhlesi B. Obesity hypoventilation syndrome Epidemiology and diagnosis. Sleep Med Clin 2014;9(3):341–7.

71. Masa JF, Pépin J-L, Borel J-C, et al. Obesity hypoventilation syndrome. Eur Respir Rev 2019; 28(151):180097.

72. Littleton SW, Tulaimat A. The effects of obesity on lung volumes and oxygenation. Respir Med 2017; 124:15–20.

73. Bülbül Y, Ayik S, Ozlu T, et al. Frequency and predictors of obesity hypoventilation in hospitalized patients at a tertiary health care institution. Ann Thorac Med 2014;9(2):87–91.

74. Kaw R, Hernandez AV, Walker E, et al. Determinants of hypercapnia in obese patients with obstructive sleep apnea: a systematic review and metaanalysis of cohort studies. Chest 2009; 136(3):787–96.

75. Mokhlesi B, Masa JF, Brozek JL, et al. Evaluation and Management of obesity hypoventilation syndrome. An Official American Thoracic Society clinical practice guideline. Am J Respir Crit Care Med 2019;200(3):e6–24.

76. Banerjee D, Yee BJ, Piper AJ, et al. Obesity hypoventilation syndrome: hypoxemia during continuous positive airway pressure. Chest 2007;131(6): 1678–84.

77. Nowbar S, Burkart KM, Gonzales R, et al. Obesity-associated hypoventilation in hospitalized patients: prevalence, effects, and outcome. Am J Med 2004; 116(1):1–7.

78. Castro-Añón O, Pérez de Llano LA, De la Fuente Sánchez S, et al. Obesity-hypoventilation syndrome: increased risk of death over sleep apnea syndrome. PLoS One 2015;10(2):e0117808.

79. Budweiser S, Riedl SG, Jörres RA, et al. Mortality and prognostic factors in patients with obesity-hypoventilation syndrome undergoing noninvasive ventilation. J Intern Med 2007;261(4):375–83.

80. Kakazu MT, Soghier I, Afshar M, et al. Weight loss Interventions as treatment of obesity hypoventilation syndrome. A systematic review. Ann Am Thorac Soc 2020;17(4):492–502.

81. Masa JF, Mokhlesi B, Benítez I, et al. Long-term clinical effectiveness of continuous positive airway pressure therapy versus non-invasive ventilation therapy in patients with obesity hypoventilation syndrome: a multicentre, open-label, randomised controlled trial. Lancet 2019;393(10182):1721–32.

82. Quiroga MÁS, Jiménez JFM, Mokhlesi B, et al. The Pickwick randomized clinical trial: long-term positive airway pressure therapy in obesity hypoventilation syndrome. European Respiratory Journal [Internet]. 2019. 54(suppl 63). Available at: https://erj.ersjournals.com/content/54/suppl_63/ PA2015. [Accessed 11 December 2023].

83. Tremblay JC, Ainslie PN. Global and country-level estimates of human population at high altitude. Proc Natl Acad Sci U S A 2021;118(18). e2102463118.

84. Rojas-Córdova S, Torres-Fraga MG, Rodríguez-Reyes YG, et al. Altitude and breathing during sleep in healthy Persons and sleep disordered patients: a systematic review. Sleep Sci 2023;16(1): 117–26.

85. Burgess KR, Ainslie PN. Central sleep apnea at high altitude. Adv Exp Med Biol 2016;903:275–83.

86. Pham LV, Meinzen C, Arias RS, et al. Cross-sectional Comparison of sleep-disordered breathing in Native Peruvian highlanders and Lowlanders. High Alt Med Biol 2017;18(1):11–9.

87. Bird JD, Kalker A, Rimke AN, et al. Severity of central sleep apnea does not affect sleeping oxygen saturation during ascent to high altitude. J Appl Physiol (1985) 2021;131(5):1432–43.

88. Heinzer R, Saugy JJ, Rupp T, et al. Comparison of sleep disorders between real and Simulated 3,450-m altitude. Sleep 2016;39(8):1517–23.

89. Ulrich S, Nussbaumer-Ochsner Y, Vasic I, et al. Cerebral oxygenation in patients with OSA: effects of

hypoxia at altitude and impact of acetazolamide. Chest 2014;146(2):299–308.

90. Lombardi C, Meriggi P, Agostoni P, et al. High-altitude hypoxia and periodic breathing during sleep: gender-related differences. J Sleep Res 2013; 22(3):322–30.

91. Frost S, E Orr J, Oeung B, et al. Improvements in sleep-disordered breathing during acclimatization to 3800 m and the impact on cognitive function. Physiol Rep 2021;9(9):e14827.

92. Latshang TD, Lo Cascio CM, Stöwhas A-C, et al. Are nocturnal breathing, sleep, and cognitive performance impaired at moderate altitude (1,630-2,590 m)? Sleep 2013;36(12):1969–76.

93. Pham LV, Miele CH, Schwartz NG, et al. Cardiometabolic correlates of sleep disordered breathing in Andean highlanders. Eur Respir J 2017;49(6): 1601705.

94. Miele CH, Schwartz AR, Gilman RH, et al. Increased cardiometabolic risk and worsening hypoxemia at high altitude. High Alt Med Biol 2016;17(2):93–100.

95. Fletcher EC, Lesske J, Qian W, et al. Repetitive, episodic hypoxia causes diurnal elevation of blood pressure in rats. Hypertension 1992;19(6 Pt 1): 555–61.

96. Fletcher EC. Invited review: physiological consequences of intermittent hypoxia: systemic blood pressure. J Appl Physiol (1985) 2001;90(4):1600–5.

97. Prabhakar NR, Kumar GK. Mechanisms of sympathetic activation and blood pressure elevation by intermittent hypoxia. Respir Physiol Neurobiol 2010;174(1–2):156–61.

98. Fagan KA. Selected Contribution: pulmonary hypertension in mice following intermittent hypoxia. J Appl Physiol (1985) 2001;90(6):2502–7.

99. Campen MJ, Shimoda LA, O'Donnell CP. Acute and chronic cardiovascular effects of intermittent hypoxia in C57BL/6J mice. J Appl Physiol 2005; 99(5):2028–35.

100. Nisbet RE, Graves AS, Kleinhenz DJ, et al. The role of NADPH oxidase in chronic intermittent hypoxia-induced pulmonary hypertension in mice. Am J Respir Cell Mol Biol 2009;40(5):601–9.

101. Savransky V, Nanayakkara A, Li J, et al. Chronic intermittent hypoxia induces atherosclerosis. Am J Respir Crit Care Med 2007;175(12):1290–7.

102. Jun J, Reinke C, Bedja D, et al. Effect of intermittent hypoxia on atherosclerosis in apolipoprotein E-deficient mice. Atherosclerosis 2010;209(2):381–6.

103. Arnaud C, Poulain L, Lévy P, et al. Inflammation contributes to the atherogenic role of intermittent hypoxia in apolipoprotein-E knock-out mice. Atherosclerosis 2011;219(2):425–31.

104. Gautier-Veyret E, Arnaud C, Bäck M, et al. Intermittent hypoxia-activated cyclooxygenase pathway: role in atherosclerosis. Eur Respir J 2013;42(2):404–13.

105. Fang G, Song D, Ye X, et al. Chronic intermittent hypoxia exposure induces atherosclerosis in ApoE knockout mice: role of NF-κB p50. Am J Pathol 2012;181(5):1530–9.

106. Polotsky VY, Li J, Punjabi NM, et al. Intermittent hypoxia increases insulin resistance in genetically obese mice. J Physiol 2003;552(Pt 1):253–64.

107. Drager LF, Li J, Reinke C, et al. Intermittent hypoxia exacerbates metabolic effects of diet-induced obesity. Obesity 2011;19(11):2167–74.

108. Iiyori N, Alonso LC, Li J, et al. Intermittent hypoxia causes insulin resistance in lean mice independent of autonomic activity. Am J Respir Crit Care Med 2007;175(8):851–7.

109. Zhen X, Moya EA, Gautane M, et al. Combined intermittent and sustained hypoxia is a novel and deleterious cardio-metabolic phenotype. Sleep 2022;45(6):zsab290.

110. Drager LF, Li J, Shin M-K, et al. Intermittent hypoxia inhibits clearance of triglyceride-rich lipoproteins and inactivates adipose lipoprotein lipase in a mouse model of sleep apnoea. Eur Heart J 2012; 33(6):783–90.

111. Jun JC, Shin M-K, Yao Q, et al. Acute hypoxia induces hypertriglyceridemia by decreasing plasma triglyceride clearance in mice. Am J Physiol Endocrinol Metab 2012;303(3):E377–88.

112. Yao Q, Shin M-K, Jun JC, et al. Effect of chronic intermittent hypoxia on triglyceride uptake in different tissues. J Lipid Res 2013;54(4):1058–65.

113. Hislop A, Reid L. New findings in pulmonary arteries of rats with hypoxia-induced pulmonary hypertension. Br J Exp Pathol 1976;57(5):542–54.

114. Stenmark KR, Meyrick B, Galie N, et al. Animal models of pulmonary arterial hypertension: the hope for etiological discovery and pharmacological cure. Am J Physiol Lung Cell Mol Physiol 2009;297(6):L1013–32.

115. Ioja S, Singamsetty S, Corey C, et al. Nocturnal hypoxia improves glucose Disposal, Decreases Mitochondrial Efficiency, and increases reactive oxygen species in the muscle and liver of C57BL/6J mice independent of weight change. Oxid Med Cell Longev 2018;2018:9649608.

116. Chen X-Q, Dong J, Niu C-Y, et al. Effects of hypoxia on glucose, insulin, glucagon, and modulation by corticotropin-releasing factor receptor type 1 in the rat. Endocrinology 2007;148(7):3271–8.

117. Hui AS, Striet JB, Gudelsky G, et al. Regulation of catecholamines by sustained and intermittent hypoxia in neuroendocrine cells and sympathetic neurons. Hypertension 2003;42(6):1130–6.

118. Lu H, Wu X, Fu C, et al. Lung injury and inflammation response by chronic intermittent hypoxia in rats. Sleep Science and Practice 2017;1(1):1.

119. Shi Z, Xu L, Xie H, et al. Attenuation of intermittent hypoxia-induced apoptosis and fibrosis in

pulmonary tissues via suppression of ER stress activation. BMC Pulm Med 2020;20(1):92.

120. Tuleta I, Pizarro C, Nickenig G, et al. Deleterious effects of intermittent hypoxia on lung tissue. Available at: European Respiratory Journal [Internet] 2016;48(suppl 60) https://erj.ersjournals.com/content/48/suppl_60/PA2070. [Accessed 24 December 2023].

121. Tuleta I, Stöckigt F, Juergens UR, et al. Intermittent hypoxia contributes to the lung damage by increased oxidative stress, inflammation, and Disbalance in Protease/Antiprotease system. Lung 2016;194(6):1015–20.

122. Gille T, Didier M, Rotenberg C, et al. Intermittent hypoxia increases the severity of bleomycin-induced lung injury in mice. Oxid Med Cell Longev 2018;2018:1240192.

123. Braun RK, Broytman O, Braun FM, et al. Chronic intermittent hypoxia worsens bleomycin-induced lung fibrosis in rats. Respir Physiol Neurobiol 2018;256:97–108.

124. Wu G, Lee YY, Gulla EM, et al. Short-term exposure to intermittent hypoxia leads to changes in gene expression seen in chronic pulmonary disease. Elife 2021;10:e63003.

125. Mirchandani AS, Jenkins SJ, Bain CC, et al. Hypoxia shapes the immune landscape in lung injury and promotes the persistence of inflammation. Nat Immunol 2022;23(6):927–39.

126. Chen T, Yang C, Li M, et al. Alveolar hypoxia-induced pulmonary inflammation: from Local initiation to Secondary Promotion by activated systemic inflammation. J Vasc Res 2016;53(5–6):317–29.

127. Pham K, Parikh K, Heinrich EC. Hypoxia and inflammation: Insights from high-altitude Physiology. Front Physiol 2021;12:676782.

128. Fröhlich S, Boylan J, McLoughlin P. Hypoxia-induced inflammation in the lung: a potential therapeutic target in acute lung injury? Am J Respir Cell Mol Biol 2013;48(3):271–9.

129. Araneda OF, Tuesta M. Lung oxidative damage by hypoxia. Oxid Med Cell Longev 2012;2012:856918.

130. Wu G, Xu G, Chen D-W, et al. Hypoxia exacerbates inflammatory acute lung injury via the toll-like receptor 4 signaling pathway. Available at: Front Immunol [Internet] 2018. 9. https://www.ncbi.nlm.nih.gov/pmc/articles/PMC6064949/. [Accessed 21 June 2020].

The Role of Obstructive Sleep Apnea in Hypercapnic Respiratory Failure Identified in Critical Care, Inpatient, and Outpatient Settings

Brian W. Locke, MD, MSCI*, Jeanette P. Brown, MD, PhD,
Krishna M. Sundar, MD

KEYWORDS

- Hypercapnia • Hypercapnic respiratory failure • Hypoventilation • Respiratory insufficiency
- Sleep apnea • Non-invasive ventilation • Positive airway pressure

KEY POINTS

- The diagnostic evaluation of patients with hypercapnic respiratory failure has typically focused on finding a single cause for the hypercapnia, but many patients have multiple contributing conditions.
- The prevalence of obstructive sleep apnea (OSA) in patients with hypercapnic respiratory failure is poorly recognized. Over two-thirds of patients with hypercapnia in acute settings have underlying OSA if tested, but only 10% to 25% are diagnosed in routine clinical care.
- While the importance of OSA in obesity hypoventilation syndrome is well-established, its role in contributing to hypercapnia in general is under-investigated. Addressing this knowledge gap is crucial because sleep apnea is treatable, and hypercapnic respiratory failure is common and associated with substantial morbidity and mortality.
- Epidemiologic research on hypercapnic respiratory failure faces several challenges, including inaccuracy of health record-based comorbidity assessment, substantial follow-up loss between inpatient and outpatient settings, and oversimplified attribution of the cause of respiratory failure.

CASE PRESENTATION

A 67-year-old female with no previously obtained spirometry or sleep testing presented with confusion. She was admitted to the intensive care unit (ICU) for non-invasive ventilation after a venous blood gas obtained in the emergency room showed a pH of 7.25 and a $Paco_2$ of 72 mm Hg. She is a current smoker and has a body mass index (BMI) of 36 kg/m^2. A chest computed tomography (CT) scan was negative for pulmonary embolism but showed mild centrilobular emphysema. An echocardiogram showed right ventricle enlargement, elevated left-ventricular diastolic filling pressures, and a normal ejection fraction. The patient improved with non-invasive ventilation, diuresis, steroids, and antibiotics. She was discharged on 1 L/min of supplemental oxygen. The sleep clinic is contacted to facilitate a sleep study. How important is it to diagnose co-morbid obstructive sleep apnea

Division of Respiratory, Critical Care, and Occupational Pulmonary Medicine, Department of Internal Medicine, University of Utah School of Medicine, Salt Lake City, UT, USA
* Corresponding author. Division of Respiratory, Critical Care, and Occupational Pulmonary Medicine, Department of Internal Medicine, University of Utah School of Medicine, 30 N Mario Capecchi Drive, North Salt Lake City, UT 84112.
E-mail address: brian.locke@hsc.utah.edu

Sleep Med Clin 19 (2024) 339–356
https://doi.org/10.1016/j.jsmc.2024.02.012
1556-407X/24/© 2024 Elsevier Inc. All rights reserved.

(OSA), and how urgently should a sleep study be performed?

INTRODUCTION

The health impact of hypercapnic respiratory failure (an increase in arterial blood carbon dioxide resulting from insufficient alveolar ventilation to match the metabolic production of carbon dioxide) is under-appreciated, irrespective of clinical circumstance. An emerging body of evidence suggests that hypercapnic respiratory failure is common[1] and associated with significant morbidity[2] and mortality risk.[3] One in four hospitalized patients who receive a diagnostic code for hypercapnic respiratory failure are readmitted within 30 days.[4] Even amongst inpatients whose arterial blood gas is consistent with compensated hypercapnia (normalization of blood pH), roughly 1 in 3 die within 1 year.[5]

Changes in the physiology of breathing during sleep usually lead to the appearance of hypercapnia first at night. An increasing body of research highlights the role of sleep-disordered breathing (SDB), particularly OSA, in developing hypercapnia. In this article, we review the pertinent physiologic principles governing the occurrence of hypercapnia. We then review the existing literature to answer the common clinical scenario outlined in the case presented earlier—when a patient is identified as having hypercapnic respiratory failure, what is the likely contribution of sleep apnea in the development of their condition? We also discuss challenges encountered in research assessing the impact of OSA on hypercapnic respiratory failure risk, which limit the strength of the current evidence on the role of OSA in hypercapnia seen in hospitalized settings.

BACKGROUND

Hypercapnic (synonymously, hypercarbic[6]) respiratory failure occurs when the amount of inhaled air participating in gas exchange (alveolar ventilation, V_A) is insufficient to match carbon dioxide production (VCO_2) from cellular metabolism. The resulting rise in the partial pressure of CO_2 in arterial blood ($Paco_2$) to above 45 mm Hg (at sea level) operationally defines hypercapnic respiratory failure. Numerous disease states can contribute to the development of hypercapnic respiratory failure through differing physiologic mechanisms (**Fig. 1**)[7].

1. Increasing the rate of CO_2 production that must be exhaled (increased VCO_2).
2. Reducing the efficiency of ventilation (by increasing dead space or reducing desired arterial CO_2 tension).

3. Increasing the work required for a given amount of ventilation due to either increased resistance to airflow (such as obstructive airway disease) or increased elastic or inertial loads (such as stiff lungs or excess chest wall mass, respectively).
4. Decreasing the capacity of the respiratory apparatus to do work (neuro-muscular disease or mechanical disadvantage).
5. Disrupting the usual feedback loops that lead to increased ventilation in response to rising blood CO_2.

Hypercapnic respiratory failure is difficult to diagnose. Except for the use of capnography in some procedural and intensive care settings, arterial CO_2 levels are not monitored or estimated as part of routine care. Clinicians must actively look for hypercapnia and order appropriate diagnostic testing. Signs and symptoms of hypercapnic respiratory failure, such as confusion, lethargy, tachycardia, and shortness of breath (or its absence), are non-specific. Furthermore, empiric supportive respiratory care often temporarily stabilizes patients without properly understanding the cause(s) of hypercapnia. Thus, hypercapnic respiratory failure is frequently missed in clinical practice.[8–10]

Hypercapnic respiratory failure and sleep are intertwined.[11] Several physiologic changes to the respiratory system promote the development of hypercapnia during sleep.[12,13] First, the respiratory control system becomes less responsive to increases in blood CO_2, particularly during rapid eye movement (REM) sleep.[14] Mechanical changes to the respiratory system also occur.[15] Supine positioning reduces lung volumes, particularly in patients with excess abdominal adiposity,[16] which predisposes the upper airway to narrowing or collapse and thereby causes obstructive hypopneas or apneas.[17] Skeletal muscles, except the diaphragm, are hypotonic during REM. In healthy individuals, this contributes to a 13% decrease in the tidal volume and minute ventilation.[18] The metabolic production of CO_2 drops during sleep, but the minute ventilation drops even more, resulting in a rise in blood CO_2 levels.[19] In healthy individuals, the arterial CO_2 tension can increase up to 4 to 6 mm Hg during sleep.[20] However, individuals who rely more on accessory muscles, such as those with muscular dystrophies, phrenic nerve injuries, or hyperinflation, experience a greater decrease in ventilation during REM sleep. Pathologic nocturnal hypoventilation is defined by an increase in CO_2 to 55 mm Hg (or above 50 mm Hg and more than 10 mm Hg above awake, supine CO_2) sustained for 10 or more minutes measured using end-tidal or transcutaneous CO_2 monitoring.[21]

High Ventilatory Need:
Increased CO2 Production

• Fever, Infection, or Inflammation
• Advanced malignancy
• Muscle activity
    • Seizures
    • Exercise
    • ↑↑ Work of breathing
• Toxic ingestion
• Obesity

High Ventilatory Need
Low Desired Arterial CO2
• Metabolic acidosis • Hypoxia

$$Arterial\ CO2 \propto \frac{Production\ of\ CO2}{(Ventilation - Deadspace)}$$

Decreased Ventilation		
Decreased Drive to Breathe:	Muscle weakness or inefficiency	Increased respiratory system loads

• Opiates and other sedatives
• Brainstem lesions
• Compensated hypercapnia
• Submissive Hypercapnia
• Sleep
• Metabolic alkalosis
	• Neuromuscular disease
	• Lung Hyperinflation
	• Respiratory muscle hypoxia
		• Elevated airway resistance
		    • COPD, Asthma
		    • Mucus
		    • Upper-airway obstruction
		• Stiff Lungs
		    • Parenchymal lung disease
		    • Pulmonary edema
		• Stiff Chest Wall
		    • Pleural disease
		    • Excess or stiff chest wall tissue

High Ventilatory Need:
Increased Deadspace "Wasted Ventilation"

• Anatomic
    • shallow breathing
• Physiologic
    • Pulmonary embolism
    • Pulmonary hypertension
    • Congestive heart failure
    • Parenchymal lung disease of any kind

Fig. 1. Determinants of the arterial blood CO_2 tension. The efficiency of ventilation refers to the portion of ventilation (air moved by the respiratory system) that participates in gas exchange. Deadspace (Vd) is synonymous with "wasted ventilation" that does not participate in gas exchange. Therefore, the unwasted ventilation is 1 minus the deadspace fraction (Vd/Vt, Vt refers to the overall tidal volume). The production of CO_2 (VCO2) depends on the overall metabolic rate, and the portion of that is aerobic versus anaerobic. Each condition can contribute to hypercapnia through multiple mechanisms (eg, COPD may result in elevated dead space, resistive respiratory system loads, and mechanical disadvantage from hyperinflation) and multiple diseases can contribute to each physiologic abnormality. (Berger KI, Rapoport DM, Ayappa I, Goldring RM. Pathophysiology of Hypoventilation During Sleep. Sleep Med Clin. 2014;9(3):289-300. https://doi.org/10.1016/j.jsmc.2014.05.014)

Nocturnal hypoventilation is often an initial manifestation of a disease state that will subsequently lead to daytime hypoventilation,[22,23] but SDB can also lead to hypercapnia on its own. Increases in blood CO_2 levels occur during obstructive apneas because ventilation halts while metabolic CO_2 production continues (**Fig. 2**). Ventilation must increase between apneic events to unload the accumulating CO_2. Otherwise, the blood CO_2 level will rise.[24] Hypercapnia develops when obstructive respiratory events are either frequent or prolonged enough or the inter-event increase in ventilation is limited.[12] Therefore, "pure" sleep hypoventilation and hypoventilation resulting from sleep apnea exist on a spectrum rather than as discrete categories, particularly in patients who do not appropriately increase their ventilation between apneas.[12] Obesity hypoventilation syndrome (OHS) epitomizes this spectrum. Patients with OHS and severe OSA resolve their hypercapnia following treatment of obstructive respiratory events by continuous positive airway pressure.[25] In contrast, patients with a more "pure hypoventilation" without significant OSA are recommended bilevel positive airway pressure.[26,27] A similar spectrum of resolution of hypercapnia in response to OSA treatment likely occurs in other "overlap syndromes," such as chronic obstructive pulmonary disease (COPD) and OSA,[28,29] though insufficient evidence exists for strong management recommendations.[30]

In summary, changes in the mechanics and regulation of breathing during sleep lead to the initial development of hypercapnia at night. Sleep apnea, mainly when severe or co-occurring with limited ability to increase inter-event alveolar ventilation, contributes to nocturnal CO_2 accumulation. In specific diseases, such as OHS with severe OSA, addressing sleep apnea prevents or resolves hypercapnic respiratory failure. Indirect evidence suggests that treating OSA might reduce or prevent respiratory decompensations in patients with other causes, multifactorial causes, or undifferentiated cases of hypercapnic respiratory failure.[31–33] However, the degree of benefit would depend on how large the contribution of OSA is amongst different etiologies of hypercapnic respiratory failure. The remainder of this article focuses on quantifying the role of untreated OSA in hypercapnic respiratory failure encountered in various clinical settings.

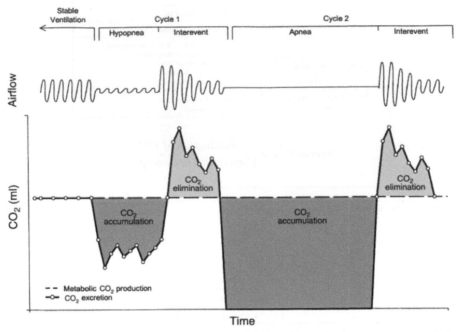

Fig. 2. CO_2 loading during apneas and hypopneas. Apneas and hypopneas can lead to an accumulation of CO_2 in the arterial blood, particularly if the inter-event ventilation is not able to increase because metabolic CO_2 production continues while alveolar ventilation drops. According to this model, more frequent events (a higher Apnea-Hypopnea Index), longer events, or a limited ability to increase the amount of ventilation between obstructions will lead to progressive nocturnal CO_2 accumulation. In combination with any underlying respiratory system abnormalities, bicarbonate retention by the kidneys to minimize the change to blood pH is then hypothesized to lessen the tendency to normalize the nocturnal loading, eventual leading to daytime hypercapnic respiratory failure. (*From* Berger and colleagues J Appl Physiol 88:257 to 264 (2000)[12,24]; with permission.)

EPIDEMIOLOGY

Research on hypercapnic respiratory failure has generally focused on what factors differ between patients with or without hypercapnia among patients who have specific diseases that can cause hypercapnic respiratory failure, such as COPD,[34] obesity with SDB (OHS[35–37]), restrictive chest wall disease,[38,39] or neuromuscular disease (NMD)[40,41]. However, clinicians often face an "inverse problem"[42,43] where hypercapnic respiratory failure has been identified, but the conditions that have led to hypercapnia must be determined (**Fig. 3**).

This question is important for clinicians because hypercapnic respiratory failure is often identified in acute care settings (ICU, emergency department, or inpatient ward), where definitive diagnostic studies such as spirometry, polysomnography, and electromyography have not been performed and cannot be obtained immediately. In the specific case of OSA, care must be transitioned to an outpatient sleep physician to diagnose and manage OSA, as the qualification criteria for respiratory assist devices (in the United States) limit empiric management.[44] The urgency of this referral depends on whether OSA is commonly an important cause of hypercapnia or not.

Both clinicians and researchers are interested in what portion of hypercapnic respiratory failure cases would be averted if OSA were prevented or treated because this guides the extent to which addressing SDB should be prioritized in this group. In each patient, OSA can be an important driver, a weak contributor, or unrelated to the development of hypercapnia. Frequent co-occurrence alone is, therefore, insufficient evidence that OSA is an important cause of hypercapnia. However, an important role is supported if OSA is more common in patients with hypercapnic respiratory failure than otherwise appropriately matched patients who do not have hypercapnia.[45,46] The current literature, with few exceptions,[47] does not contain matched control groups. Inferences about the excess risk caused by OSA therefore rely on implied comparisons, which limits the strength of evidence.

In the following section, the authors consider the evidence supporting OSA's role as a cause of hypercapnic respiratory failure in various settings. The patient mix and the methodologies of studies

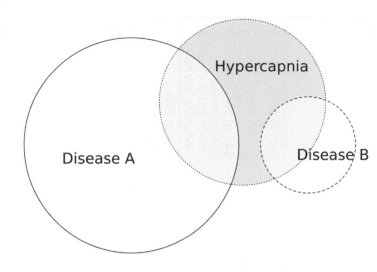

Fig. 3. Spatial representation of the "inverse problem" of conditional probability. The probability of having a disease among patients identified with hypercapnia (represented as: P [disease | hypercapnia] in statistical notation) may be much different from the probability that a patient with a disease develops hypercapnia (P[hypercapnia | disease]). This is an important difference because clinicians often recognize hypercapnia before knowing the cause, and thus, P (disease | hypercapnia) is the expected rate for finding that disease in subsequent investigations. In this case, only 1 in 5 cases of "Disease A" develop hypercapnia, while 1 in 2 cases of "Disease B" do. However, because disease A is much more common, the likelihood of hypercapnia being caused by disease A is double that of Disease B. It has been suggested that obesity hypoventilation syndrome is the most common current cause of hypercapnia (see **Table 3**), despite most patients with obesity and obstructive sleep apnea not developing hypercapnia.[37] (Adapted from Larsson J, Gustafsson P. A case study in fitting area-proportional euler diagrams with ellipses using eulerr. In: ; 2018:84-91.[94])

differ between the intensive care, inpatient, emergency, and outpatient settings. Thus, the authors have subdivided our discussion into those groups.

Intensive Care Unit

The diagnosis of hypercapnic respiratory failure is often made in the ICU, where patients with the most severe respiratory decompensation who require ventilatory support are encountered. A summary of studies evaluating comorbidities of patients with hypercapnic respiratory failure in the ICU is shown in **Table 1**.

All studies included patients using an arterial blood gas criterion (either a $Paco_2$ over 45 mm Hg or 6 kPa) and either a pH consistent with un-compensated respiratory acidosis (Contou and colleagues[48] and Ouanes-Besbes et al.[49]) or requirement that patients received non-invasive (NIV) or invasive mechanical ventilation (IMV) (Thille and colleagues[50] Adler and colleagues[51] Gursel and colleagues[52]). OSA/OHS was uncommon (12% of 230 patients) in the single study that relied on clinician attribution (Contou and colleagues[48]).

In contrast, moderate or severe OSA was very common in the 3 studies where patients underwent sleep testing ranging from 63% to 88% (75% of 37 patients in Adler and colleagues,[51] 88% of 16 patients in Thille and colleagues,[50] and 63% in Ouanes-Besbes et al.[49]). Notably, these 3 studies used either in-lab polysomnography 3 months after ICU discharge (Adler and colleagues[51] and Thille and colleagues[50]) or home

sleep apnea tests 3 weeks after discharge (Ouanes-Besbes et al.[49]). All had very low rates of follow-up among patients invited for testing (46%,[51] 47%,[50] and 76%,[49] respectively).

This low follow-up rate, even among the patients who consent to participate in research, suggests that many patients are lost when transitioning from inpatient to outpatient care and thus may not receive definitive evaluation in routine clinical care. These patients often encounter issues preventing timely access to follow-up, and recognition for the need for treatment may be lacking for both patients and providers. This is particularly problematic given the high likelihood of early readmissions for patients with hypercapnic respiratory failure.[4] Gursel and colleagues[52] reported that respiratory polygraphy during ICU admission identified OSA in 8 of 11 patients diagnosed with OHS and 12 of 21 patients with COPD and hypercapnia (overall rate of OSA of 64%). Alternatively, Adler and colleagues reported that the absence of hyperinflation (as assessed by plethysmography) might select survivors of hypercapnia with a particularly high likelihood of moderate-severe OSA.[53] However, plethysmography is also not easily performed in acute care settings.

Overall, OSA is identified in ICU patients with hypercapnic respiratory failure at a roughly 5-fold higher rate (63%–88%) when sleep testing is performed compared to when clinicians' assessment of the cause is used (12%). While OSA is likely common and unrecognized among all ICU patients (for example, Bucklin and colleagues[54] estimate that 40% of ICU patients have moderate or

Table 1
Prevalence of obstructive sleep apnea among intensive care unit survivors of hypercapnic respiratory failure

Author	Year, Location	Enrollment Criteria	Exclusion Criteria	Method of Assessment	Loss to Follow-up	Rate of Mod-Severe OSA
Prospective without Protocolized Comorbidity Assessment.						
Contou et al,[48] 2013	France, 2008–2011	pH < 7.35 and $Paco_2$ > 45 mm Hg	Invasive Mechanical Ventilation or DNI	Chart review	Not Applicable	30 of 242 (12%)
Prospective Studies with Protocolized Ascertainment						
Adler et al,[51] 2017	France 2012–2015	$Paco_2$ over 47.25 mm Hg. NIV or IMV treatment	neuromuscular disease, prognosis < 3 mo, iatrogenic hypercapnia, persistent confusion	PSG 3 mo after discharge	53%	28 of 37 (75%)
Thille et al,[50] 2018	Prior to 2018 (precise dates not reported)	pH < 7.35 and $Paco_2$ 45 mm Hg treated with NIV or IMV	none	PSG 3 mo after discharge	54%	14 of 16 (88%)
Ouanes-Besbes et al,[49] 2021	Tunisia, 2015–2018	pH < 7.35 and $Paco_2$ > 45 mm Hg	Previously diagnosed OSA.	HSAT 3 wk after discharge	24%	104+ of 164 (63%); 34 not tested (STOP-BANG < 3 points, indicating low risk)
Gursel et al,[52] 2015	Turkey, not reported.	Hypercapnia treated with NIV	None	Respiratory Polygraph during ICU	0%	20 of 31 (64%), hypopneas not assessed.

Abbreviations: DNI, do not intubate advanced directive; HSAT, home sleep apnea testing; IMV, invasive mechanical ventilation; Mod-Severe obstructive sleep apnea (OSA), apnea-hypopnea index over 15 events/hour; NIV, Non-Invasive Ventilation; $Paco_2$, arterial gas tension of CO_2; PSG, polysomnogram; STOP-BANG (Snoring, Tiredness, Observed Apneas, high blood Pressure, BMI over 35 kg/m2, Age over 50 years, Neck cirumfrence over 40cm, male Gender), risk stratification score for OSA.[112]

severe OSA), a more likely explanation is that OSA at least contributes to the development of hypercapnia in many more cases than are commonly recognized in practice or coded in documentation.

While it is common to document the "single cause" of hypercapnic respiratory failure, as encouraged by device-qualification practices (which often require the absence of other contributors in the United States, thus dissuading searching for and documenting their presence[44]), there is both physiologic and epidemiologic evidence that multiple conditions often contribute to the occurrence of hypercapnia. Physiologically, the model of CO_2 loading during apneas (see **Fig. 2**) predicts that limitations on the ability to increase interapnea ventilation will lead to the early development of hypercapnia.[24] This is corroborated empirically, as hypercapnia develops in patients with OSA-COPD overlap syndrome with milder obstruction than in the pure COPD case and milder obesity.[55] In the 3 prospective ICU cohorts, very high rates of multiple contributors were noted. Adler and colleagues found that 36% of their cohort had COPD and OSA, 61% had OSA and congestive heart failure (CHF), and 54% had CHF and COPD.[51]

In summary, the available evidence on ICU patients treated for hypercapnic respiratory failure suggests a very high rate of undiagnosed sleep apnea that is often not recorded as a contributor to hypercapnic respiratory failure. The prospective ascertainment of comorbidity status is a notable strength of these studies, though low follow-up rates for sleep studies limit the strength of conclusions.

Emergency Department and Inpatient Setting

Several studies have investigated hypercapnic respiratory failure in hospitalized and emergency room patients, mostly relying on retrospective health record data (**Table 2**).

Chung and colleagues leveraged data from a single hospital serving a defined population in Liverpool, Australia, to publish several informative studies.[1,47,56] They included patients with a measured arterial $Paco_2$ over 45 mm Hg within 24 hours of hospital presentation, after excluding iatrogenic causes, from 2013 to 2017. By standardizing the rate of hypercapnia to the region's demographics, they estimated the yearly period prevalence of hypercapnia in acute care settings to be 163 per 100,000 person-years, and the prevalence roughly doubling with each decade of age above 50[1].

Next, they investigated conditions that may have led to the development of hypercapnia. In the cohort, obstructive lung disease codes were the most common diagnostic code (n = 389, 44.6%), followed by CHF (n = 278, 31.8%).[56] In contrast to other studies, only 6.0% (n = 52) had a SDB diagnosis code, and only 13% had diagnostic codes for multiple contributing conditions.

They then selected a subset of patients with hypercapnia (cases) and a matched sample of patients in the community (controls) to determine which diseases occurred in excess among people with hypercapnic respiratory failure.[47] Among the subsample, 43% of patients with hypercapnia (vs 12% of controls) reported they had OSA. However, home sleep apnea tests found moderate-severe OSA at equivalent rates between cases and controls (28% cases, 34% controls). Response rates with follow-up testing were very low in both cases and controls (roughly 1 in 10), reinforcing the difficulty of establishing the diagnosis of OSA once patients are discharged from the hospital.

Comparatively little is known about the epidemiology of sleep-breathing disorders among hospitalized patients.[57,58] Several groups have attempted to estimate the prevalence of OSA among general inpatients, and compare it with the prevalence of OSA in those patients with hypercapnia. Using a screening program based on STOP-BANG (the presence of five or more of the following criteria: snoring, tiredness, observed apneas, high blood pressure, BMI over 35 kg/m2, age over 50 years, neck circumfrence over 40cm, and male gender; which is validated to predict a high risk of OSA) and high-resolution pulse oximetry, the estimated prevalence of sleep apnea among patients with obesity was 19.7% at a single center.[59] Higher rates (48%) are seen in patients with cardiovascular disease.[60] Among the subset of hospitalized patients referred for inpatient sleep testing, Johnson and colleagues[61] found that patients usually had either nocturnal or diurnal hypoventilation (65% of 326 patients) on inpatient polysomnogram with CO_2 monitoring. Patients also had high rates of sleep apnea (17% mild, 21% moderate, and 56% severe), OHS (59%, operationally defined as other factors not *entirely* explaining the hypoventilation), and other comorbidities (68% had CHF and 35% had COPD).

Several other studies show similar distributions of comorbidities as assessed by diagnostic codes. Rates of recognized OSA vary from 10% to 25%, with either COPD[2,3,62,63] or CHF[5] being the most common comorbidity. The frequency of obesity ranges from a mean BMI of 36.4 kg/m^2 (Meservey and colleagues[4]) to a median of 25.8 kg/m^2 (Cavalot and colleagues[2]) and age

Table 2
Prevalence of obstructive sleep apnea among patients presenting to the emergency room or admitted to the hospital with hypercapnic respiratory failure

Author	Year/Location	Enrollment Criteria	Exclusion Criteria	Method of Assessment	Loss to Follow-up	Prevalence of OSA
Prospective, arterial blood gas assessment in all patients, but no structured OSA assessment						
Nowbar et al,[8] 2004	USA, before 2004 (not stated)	Arterial blood gas $Paco_2 > 2$ SD above norm (elevation-adjusted).	Severe obstruction (FEV1/FVC < 0.5); lung resection	Inferred from lack of other identified causes	Not Applicable	31%
Retrospective, all patients received polysomnography						
Johnson et al,[61]	USA 2015–2018	Inpatient PSG ordered, $Paco_2 > 45$ mm Hg or $TcCO_2/EtCO_2 > 50$ mm Hg for 10+ minutes	No titration study performed	Inpatient PSG	None	65%[a]
Prospective with structured comorbidity ascertainment						
Chung et al,[47] 2023	Australia 2013–2017	$Paco_2$ over 45 mm Hg	Iatrogenic causes, trauma, post-arrest.	HSAT (case-control study)[b]	90%	28% in cases (vs 34% in controls)
Retrospective Studies						
Chung et al,[1] 2022; Chung et al,[56] 2022	Australia 2013–2017	$Paco_2$ over 45 mm Hg	Iatrogenic causes, trauma, post-arrest.	Diagnosis code	Not Applicable	6%
Cavalot et al,[2] 2021	Canada 2017	ABG: $CO_2 > 45$ mm Hg & pH < 7.35 or VBG: $CO_2 > 50$ mm Hg & pH < 7.34	Cystic fibrosis, neuromuscular disease, ILD, lung cancer, drug overdose, or tracheostomy.	Diagnosis code	Not Applicable	19.3%
Meservey et al,[4] 2020	USA 2016	Diagnostic Code for Hypercapnic Respiratory Failure	Advanced cancer, trauma, stroke, seizure, cardiac arrest, advanced neurologic disease, serious non-pulmonary illness.	Chart review	Not Applicable	24%

Study	Country / Years	Criteria	Exclusion	Ascertainment		OSA prevalence
Vonderbank et al,[3] 2020	Germany 2015–2016	Arterialized capillary blood gas $CO_2 > 45$ mm Hg	None	Health record review	Not Applicable	10.8%
Wilson et al,[5] 2021	USA 2018	$PaCO_2 > 50$ mm Hg and pH > 7.35	Admitted at psychiatric or inpatient rehabilitation hospitals.	EMR problem list	Not Applicable	22.4%
Domaradzki et al,[63] 2018	USA 2009–2015	Diagnostic code for chronic obstructive pulmonary disease (COPD) or respiratory failure & VBG	tracheostomy	Home CPAP (or BPAP)	Not Applicable	10% (and 5%)
Bülbül et al,[62]	Turkey 2009–2010	Initial and follow-up (stable) $PaCO_2 > 45$ mm Hg	Acute hypercapnia	Inferred from lack of other identified causes	Not Applicable	25%
Fox et al,[95] 2022	Israel 2012–2017	Referral for NIV on discharge	Death during admission	Chart Review	Not Applicable	5%
Calvo et al,[96] 2012	Spain 2008–2009	$PaCO_2$ over 45 mm Hg and pH < 7.35	None	Chart Review	Not Applicable	6%
Brandão et al,[97] 2016	Portugal 2012–2013	NIV use outside an ICU (90% Hypercapnic)	Elective admissions	Chart Review	Not Applicable	23%

Abbreviations: ABG, arterial blood gas; VBG, peripheral venous blood gas; ILD, interstitial lung disease; SD, standard deviation, FEV1/FVC: forced expiratory volume in 1s over forced vital capacity; EMR, electronic medical record; CPAP, constant positive airway pressure; BPAP, bilevel positive airway pressure.

a Only patients referred for inpatient sleep testing included.

b Cases come from the hospital, but controls are taken from the general population.

from the mean of 60.5 years in (Wilson and colleagues)[5] to median age of 70 years (Domardzki and colleagues[63]). All studies have shown high rates of death (1-year mortality of roughly 30% in Wilson and colleagues,[5] 25% in Vonderbank and colleagues[3]) and re-presentation to the hospital (23% were readmitted within 30 days, usually for recurrent hypercapnic respiratory failure[4]; 66% within 1 year[2]).

The unreliability of diagnostic codes is a significant challenge for this literature because many respiratory conditions are not diagnosed, and many are misdiagnosed, particularly in obese patients.[64-66] This makes it challenging to disentangle the influence of these conditions on each other, the rates of (mis) diagnosis, and the likelihood of hypercapnia.[67] In addition, the definition of OHS—hypercapnic respiratory failure occurring in the context of SDB and *in the absence of other contributing conditions*[26]—is particularly challenging to apply in health record-based epidemiologic research because OHS is under-recognized[8,66] and one cannot infer which contributing conditions have been considered and excluded, particularly in the presence of missing data.

Despite these limitations, several patterns emerge. First, hypercapnia is common in acute care settings, is associated with substantial morbidity, and often occurs in the context of multiple potentially contributing diagnoses, including OSA. Data on the excess rate of OSA among patients with hypercapnia are conflicting and vary substantially based on the method used for ascertaining OSA.

OUTPATIENTS

Determining the contribution of SDB to outpatient hypercapnic respiratory failure is particularly challenging because neither elevated arterial CO_2 levels nor sleep breathing abnormalities are reliably assessed in the outpatient population. One approach to investigating the community-dwelling population with hypercapnic respiratory failure is to evaluate the patients who receive home NIV. However, only a subset of patients receiving home NIV have hypercapnic respiratory failure, given that NIV is started before overt respiratory failure for conditions such as neuromuscular disease. Conversely, not all patients with hypercapnic respiratory failure qualify for, or obtain, home NIV.

Twenty-two identified studies evaluated the composition of patients enrolled in home mechanical ventilation programs and commented on OSA or the prevalence of related comorbidities

(**Table 3**). The estimated population prevalence of hypercapnia presenting to the hospital by Chung and colleagues (163 per 100,000)[1] is between 3 and 100 times higher than estimates of the prevalence of patients in domiciliary home ventilation programs (1–47 per 100,000[68]). It is reported that 25% to 50% of patients in home mechanical ventilation programs are enrolled after a hospitalization for acute (on chronic) respiratory failure.[69-72]

Mirroring the ICU and inpatient literature, studies with universal assessment of sleep breathing when home NIV is initiated generally show that most patients have OSA,[73,74] while studies relying on clinician documentation of the "primary cause" of hypercapnia result in much lower estimates. Several cohorts listed NMD, COPD, and OHS as the most common indications for non-invasive ventilation.

Longitudinal studies report an overall increase in the prevalence of patients receiving home mechanical ventilation over the past several decades and also an increase in the proportion of those patients who have OHS .[70,75,76] Demographic and comorbidity data suggest that OSA likely contributes to many more patients with hypercapnic respiratory failure than is documented. For example, the patients who are labeled as having "COPD" as their primary cause for home ventilation in these cohorts tend to have much higher BMI (generally, above 30 kg/m^2) and less severe airflow limitation on spirometry obstruction compared to the cohorts of patients with hypercapnia and COPD when OSA was excluded. For example, in the trials of home ventilation by Kohnlein and colleagues and in the subset of patients with hypercapnia in the National Emphysema Treatment (NETT) trial of lung volume reduction the mean BMI of included patients was 24 to 25 kg/m^2.[34,77,78] This pattern would be expected if many of these patients have an overlap syndrome, which results in hypercapnia at milder obstruction.[79]

Even among patients with neuromuscular disease, sleep apnea may contribute to the earlier occurrence of respiratory failure. Boentert and colleagues[41] showed that OSA was present in 45.6% of the patients with amyotrophic lateral sclerosis (ALS) before they developed an indication for NIV, and patients with OSA had 1.9 times higher odds of having nocturnal hypoventilation, which is known to predict the subsequent development of daytime hypoventilation.[23] Duchenne muscular dystrophy is another condition where OSA is highly prevalent early in the course of the disease but progresses to nocturnal hypoventilation and ultimately hypercapnic respiratory failure.[80,81] Lastly,

Table 3
Constitution of home non-invasive ventilation programs

Author	Location Year	Enrollment Criteria	Exclusion Criteria	Method of Assessment	Most Common Cause	Prevalence of OSA
Cohorts on Home NIV; Polysomnography Performed						
Poh Tan et al,[74] 2018	AUS, 2005–2010	Records review of a clinic, sole provider of services to their region.	Home mechanical or non-invasive prescribed	Routine PSG performed at NIV initiation.	neuromuscular disease (NMD)	15% 240 with obesity hypoventilation syndrome (OHS) as reason for Vent; but OSA present in most patients of all other classifications.
Patout et al,[73] 2020	UK and France, 2008–2014	Established via inpatient study at 2 centers (London and Rouen	CPAP, ASV, tracheostomy	Patients received inpatient titration studies at initiation	OHS	29.5% of 1746 with OHS. 12.7% with Overlap Syndrome. 10.5% with OSA (non-OHS) listed as a cause.
Cohorts on Home NIV; provider determination of cause or survey						
Cantero et al,[70] 2020	2016–2018, Switzerland	Receipt of Home NIV—which generally though not always requires hypercapnia. (all regional providers)	Adaptive servo ventilation, tracheostomy	Clinical determination of pulmonologist	COPD	26% OHS 11% COPD-Overlap 4% with OSA as part of 'other' SDB
Budweiser et al,[98] 2007	2002–2004 Germany	Home NIV for 3 or more months (single center)	None reported	Clinician diagnosis	COPD	30% of 231 with OHS or OVS
Neill et al,[76] 2022; Garner et al,[99] 2013	2018 New Zealand	Receipt of Home NIV (country-wide)	None reported	Clinician diagnosis	OHS	47.3% of 1188 with OHS additional 23% with Overlap Syndrome

(continued on next page)

Table 3
(continued)

Author	Location Year	Enrollment Criteria	Exclusion Criteria	Method of Assessment	Most Common Cause	Prevalence of OSA
Hannan et al,[100] 2016	2013, Australia	Provision of Home NIV	Non-English speaking, survey nonresponse (43.4%)	Patient self-report	NMD	31% with OHS
Hannan et al,[100] 2016	2013, Canada	Provision of Home NIV	Non-English speaking, survey nonresponse (43.4%)	Patient self-report	NMD	8.1% with OHS
Rose et al,[101] 2015	Canada, 2012–2013	Ventilation provision (Service providers identified prescribers, then surveyed)	None	Provider determination	NMD	14% with OHS
Maquillon et al,[102] 2021	Chile, 2008–2017	Admission for inpatient initiation of NIV (Nationwide)	Smoking, drug use, lack of power or resources at home.	Provider determination	COPD	23.9% with OHS
Schwarz et al,[103] 2005	UK, 2008–2018	Death while enrolled in a large weaning and HMV service; $Paco_2 > 45$ mm Hg	Still alive (roughly half of enrolled patients)	Provider determination	NMD	17% with OHS 4% with Overlap Syndrome
Lloyd-Owen et al,[68]	16 European countries, 2002	Survey estimates of NIV or IMV for 3+ months delivered at home.	Negative pressure vent, phrenic stim, positional therapies.	Provider determination.	COPD	<31% OHS (lumped with "chest wall restriction")
Laub and Midgren[71] 2007	Sweden, 1995–2005	National register of patient receiving Home Ventilation	None	Diagnosis provided to register	OHS	28% of 422 OHS

Study	Location, years	Setting	Exclusions	Method	Condition	Result
Nasilowsky et al,[104] 2015	Poland, 2000–2010	Treated at an Experienced HMV program	None	Provider determination; survey	NMD	11% with hypoventilation syndromes[a]
Valko et al,[105] 2018	Hungary, 2018	Survey to centers providing HMV	None	Provider determination; survey	OHS	60% with hypoventilation syndromes[a]
Windisch et al[106] 2003	Germany, prior to 2003	4 hospitals, established in HMV clinic	First visit with HMV clinic, acute decompensation, tracheostomy	Provider determination	COPD	5.3% OHS of 226
Biggelaar et al,[107] 2022	Netherlands 1991–2020	4 centers that provision home NIV	None	Diagnosis provided to register	NMD	~15% 'Sleep Disorders' indication.
Cohorts on Home NIV; Documentation of Comorbidity present						
Jimenez, Akrivo, et al,[108] 2023	Mich. USA, 2012–2021	$Paco_2/PtCO_2$ 45+mm Hg and pH over 7.35;	Tracheostomy, not on NIV at first visit.	Diagnostic Codes	NMD	14% of 48 OHS
Povitz et al,[72] 2017	Canada 2000–2012.	Request for NIV or IMV equipment from provincial administrative data	Private acquisition of supplies; long-term care facility residents	Diagnostic codes;	NMD	15.9% 'Obesity' (OSA and OHS not directly assessed)
Borel et al,[69] 2013	France 2003–2008	Initiation of NIV at one of five facilities; obesity is the main explanation of NIV.	Neuromuscular disorder, severe pulmonary fibrosis, $FEV_1/VC < 30\%$	Chart review	OHS	67% of 107 OHS
Tissot et al[109] 2015	France 2009–2014	Referral for NIV (3 hospitals)	Death or loss to follow-up within 6 mo	Patient survey	OHS	42% of 264 OHS
Poh Tan et al,(b)[110] 2019	Singapore, 2009–2015	Single center HMV service	None	Chart Review	NMD (ALS)	2% of 112 with OSA listed as contributor
Rentala et al,[111] 2021	Finland, 2012–2015	Referral for home NIV	None	Chart Review	OHS	47.3% OHS 57.1% OSA as contributor

$PtCO_2$, transcutaneous partial pressure of CO_2; ASV, Adaptive Servo-Ventilation; HMV, home mechanical ventilation; SDB, sleep-disordered breathing.

[a] Includes obesity hypoventilation, congenital central hypoventilation syndrome, and central apneas.

extremely high rates of SDB (above 60%[82]) and nocturnal hypoventilation (30%[83,84]) are seen in patients with spinal cord injuries, where PAP treatment has been shown to improve respiratory events and autonomic symptoms.[85] While the complex respiratory control abnormalities[86] and simultaneous onset SDB and muscle weakness hamper the ability to isolate the contribution of OSA, both the epidemiologic and physiologic evidence support the role of OSA in accelerating the development of hypercapnia in patients with spinal cord injury. However, under recognition of SDB likely results from challenges accessing traditional sleep lab testing due to complex care needs of patients with neuromuscular disease.[87] Innovative management pathways may facilitate early recognition of patients with nocturnal hypoventilation,[88] who are difficult to identify with clinical criteria[83] and have been shown to benefit from NIV in randomized trials.[89]

In summary, though significant limitations exist with applying the data from home-mechanical ventilation to the question of OSA's contribution to hypercapnia in outpatients, the available data suggest that OSA is frequently present in patients who providers have not labeled as having OHS as their primary indication. Furthermore, both the prevalence of domiciliary ventilation and the diagnosis of OHS are increasing, likely as a result of the increasing prevalence of obesity.[90]

SUMMARY

A burgeoning literature describing the epidemiology of hypercapnic respiratory failure has developed over the last 2 decades. Sleep apnea is prevalent among patients recognized to have hypercapnia in a variety of settings but is often not diagnosed. Both physiologic understanding and epidemiologic evidence support that OSA is a contributing cause in many cases, though better ascertainment of potentially contributing conditions would improve the strength of evidence. Additionally, hypercapnic respiratory failure is common (167 per 100,000 persons in Chung and colleagues,[1] which, for frame of reference, is roughly as common as decompensated cirrhosis[91]), occurs in patients with multiple morbidities,[92] and is associated with high health care expenditure,[93] morbidity, and mortality. As sleep apnea is treatable and likely contributes to the occurrence of hypercapnic respiratory failure with consequent increases in health care burden, determining the exact contribution of OSA and the effectiveness of improved identification or management of OSA in this population should be a public health priority.

CLINICS CARE POINTS

- Hypercapnic respiratory failure is common, becoming more prevalent, and sleep apnea contributes to its development.
- Sleep apnea is found in most patients with hypercapnic respiratory failure if sleep testing is sought, though far fewer are recognized to have OSA during routine clinical care.
- Patients who have OSA and other causes of hypercapnia tend to develop hypercapnia at a milder stage of the disease, suggesting OSA contributes to its occurrence.
- While the current documentation requirements and the existing evidence base encourage categorizing patients as having a single cause, recognizing that many patients with hypercapnic respiratory failure have multiple contributing comorbidities may allow more patients to receive beneficial treatments.
- Significant loss to follow-up is seen in all studies when patients identified in acute settings are recommended to return for sleep testing after discharge, suggesting that approaches to encourage higher follow-up rates or more immediate testing are needed for clinical care and research.

DISCLOSURE

B.W. Locke. receives research funding from the American Thoracic Society ASPIRE Fellowship and the National Institutes of Health under the Ruth L. Kirschstein National Research Service Award 5T32HL105321 J.P. Brown. no conflicts of interest. K.M. Sundar is co-founder of Hypnoscure LLC—a software application for population management of sleep apnea through the University of Utah Technology Commercialization Office.

REFERENCES

1. Chung Y, Garden FL, Marks GB, et al. Population prevalence of hypercapnic respiratory failure from any cause. Am J Respir Crit Care Med 2022; 205(8):966–7.
2. Cavalot G, Dounaevskaia V, Vieira F, et al. One-year readmission following undifferentiated acute hypercapnic respiratory failure. COPD J Chronic Obstr Pulm Dis 2021;18(6):602–11.
3. Vonderbank S, Gibis N, Schulz A, et al. Hypercapnia at hospital admission as a predictor of

mortality. Open Access Emerg Med OAEM 2020; 12:173–80.

4. Meservey AJ, Burton MC, Priest J, et al. Risk of re-admission and mortality following hospitalization with hypercapnic respiratory failure. Lung 2020; 198(1):121–34.

5. Wilson MW, Labaki WW, Choi PJ. Mortality and health-care utilization of patients with compensated hyper-capnia. Ann Am Thorac Soc 2021;18(12):2027–32.

6. Lewis GM. "Hypercapnia" versus "Hypercarbia.". Anesthesiology 1961;22(2):324. https://doi.org/10.1097/00000542-196103000-00030.

7. Kapitan KS. Ventilatory failure. Can you sustain what you need? Ann Am Thorac Soc 2013;10(4): 396–9.

8. Nowbar S, Burkart KM, Gonzales R, et al. Obesity-associated hypoventilation in hospitalized patients: prevalence, effects, and outcome. Am J Med 2004; 116(1):1–7.

9. Randerath W, Ahmed S, BaHammam AS. Over-looking obesity hypoventilation syndrome: the need for obesity hypoventilation syndrome staging and risk stratification. Ann Am Thorac Soc 2020; 17(10):1211–2.

10. Krishnan V. Holding our breath: exploring the causes of hypercapnic respiratory failure resulting in mortality. Respirology 2023;28(2):97–8.

11. Kryger MH. Sleep apnea: from the needles of dio-nysius to continuous positive airway pressure. JAMA Intern Med 1983;143(12):2301–3.

12. Berger KI, Rapoport DM, Ayappa I, et al. Patho-physiology of hypoventilation during sleep. Sleep Med Clin 2014;9(3):289–300.

13. Piper AJ, Yee BJ. Hypoventilation syndromes. Compr Physiol 2014;4(4):1639–76.

14. Guyenet PG, Bayliss DA. Neural control of breathing and CO2 homeostasis. Neuron 2015;87(5):946–61.

15. McCartney A, Phillips D, James M, et al. Ventilatory neural drive in chronically hypercapnic patients with COPD: effects of sleep and nocturnal noninvasive ventilation. Eur Respir Rev 2022;31(165):220069. https://doi.org/10.1183/16000617.0069-2022.

16. Hegewald MJ. Impact of obesity on pulmonary function: current understanding and knowledge gaps. Curr Opin Pulm Med 2020;27(2):132–40.

17. Owens RL, Malhotra A, Eckert DJ, et al. The influ-ence of end-expiratory lung volume on measure-ments of pharyngeal collapsibility. J Appl Physiol 2010;108(2):445–51.

18. Stradling J, Chadwick GA, Chadwick GA, et al. Changes in ventilation and its components in normal subjects during sleep. Thorax 1985;40(5):364–70.

19. Lin CK, Lin CC, Lin CC. Work of breathing and res-piratory drive in obesity. Respirology 2012;17(3): 402–11.

20. Robin ED, Whaley RD, Crump CH, et al. Alveolar gas tensions, pulmonary ventilation, and blood

pH during physiologic sleep in normal subjects. Surv Anesthesiol 1959;3(2). https://doi.org/10.1097/00132586-195904000-00006.

21. Troester M, Quan S, Berry R, et al. The AASM manual for the scoring of sleep and associated events: rules, terminology and technical specifica-tions. Version 3. Darien, IL: American Academy of Sleep Medicine; 2023.

22. Hillman DR, Singh B, McArdle N, et al. Relation-ships between ventilatory impairment, sleep hypo-ventilation and type 2 respiratory failure. Respirol Carlton Vic 2014;19(8):1106–16.

23. Orlikowski D, Prigent H, Quera Salva MA, et al. Prognostic value of nocturnal hypoventilation in neuromuscular patients. Neuromuscul Disord 2017;27(4):326–30.

24. Berger KI, Ayappa I, Sorkin IB, et al. CO(2) homeo-stasis during periodic breathing in obstructive sleep apnea. J Appl Physiol Bethesda Md 1985 2000;88(1):257–64.

25. Masa JF, Mokhlesi B, Benítez Iván, et al. Long-term clinical effectiveness of continuous positive airway pressure therapy versus non-invasive ventilation therapy in patients with obesity hypoventilation syndrome: a multicentre, open-label, randomised controlled trial. Lancet 2019;393(10182):1721–32.

26. Mokhlesi B, Masa JF, Brozek JL, et al. Evaluation and management of obesity hypoventilation syn-drome. An official American thoracic society clin-ical practice guideline. Am J Respir Crit Care Med 2019;200(3):e6–24.

27. Masa JF, Corral J, Caballero C, et al. Non-invasive ventilation in obesity hypoventilation syndrome without severe obstructive sleep apnoea. Thorax 2016;71(10):899.

28. Zheng Y, Yee BJ, Wong K, et al. A pilot randomized trial comparing CPAP versus bilevel PAP sponta-neous mode in the treatment of hypoventilation dis-order in patients with obesity and obstructive airway disease. J Clin Sleep Med 2021;18(1):99–107.

29. Borel JC, Pepin JL, Pison C, et al. Long-term adher-ence with non-invasive ventilation improves prog-nosis in obese COPD patients. Respirology 2014; 19(6):857–65.

30. Nowalk NC, Neborak JM, Mokhlesi B. Is bilevel PAP more effective than CPAP in treating hyper-capnic obese patients with COPD and severe OSA? J Clin Sleep Med 2022;18(1):5–7.

31. Pépin JL, Timsit JF, Tamisier R, et al. Prevention and care of respiratory failure in obese patients. Lancet Respir Med 2016;4(5):407–18.

32. Kaw R, Bhateja P, y Mar HP, et al. Postoperative complications in patients with unrecognized obesity hypoventilation syndrome undergoing elective noncardiac surgery. Chest 2016;149(1):84–91.

33. Channick JE, Jackson NJ, Zeidler MR, et al. Effects of obstructive sleep apnea and obesity on 30-day

readmissions in patients with chronic obstructive pulmonary disease: a cross-sectional mediation analysis. Ann Am Thorac Soc 2022;19(3):462–8.

34. Mathews AM, Wysham Nicholas G, Wysham NG, et al. Hypercapnia in advanced chronic obstructive pulmonary disease: a secondary analysis of the national emphysema treatment trial. Chronic Obstr Pulm Dis J COPD Found 2020;7(4):336–45.

35. Mokhlesi B, Tulaimat A, Faibussowitsch I, et al. Obesity hypoventilation syndrome: prevalence and predictors in patients with obstructive sleep apnea. Sleep Breath 2007;11(2):117–24.

36. Tran K, Wang L, Gharaibeh S, et al. Elucidating predictors of obesity hypoventilation syndrome in a large bariatric surgery cohort. Ann Am Thorac Soc 2020;17(10):1279–88.

37. Kaw R, Hernandez AV, Walker E, et al. Determinants of hypercapnia in obese patients with obstructive sleep apnea: a systematic review and metaanalysis of cohort studies. Chest 2009; 136(3):787–96.

38. Branthwaite MA. Cardiorespiratory consequences of unfused idiopathic scoliosis. Br J Dis Chest 1986;80:360–9.

39. Sawicka EH, Branthwaite MA. Respiration during sleep in kyphoscoliosis. Thorax 1987;42(10):801.

40. Tilanus TBM, Groothuis JT, TenBroek-Pastoor JMC, et al. The predictive value of respiratory function tests for non-invasive ventilation in amyotrophic lateral sclerosis. Respir Res 2017;18(1):144.

41. Boentert M, Glatz C, Helmle C, et al. Prevalence of sleep apnoea and capnographic detection of nocturnal hypoventilation in amyotrophic lateral sclerosis. J Neurol Neurosurg Psychiatry 2018; 89(4):418–24.

42. Llewelyn H, Ang HA, Lewis K, et al. Making the diagnostic process evidence-based. In: Llewelyn H, Ang HA, Lewis K, Al-Abdullah A, editors. *Oxford handbook of clinical diagnosis*. Oxford University Press; 2014. https://academic.oup.com/book/31795.

43. Fienberg SE. When did Bayesian inference become"Bayesian" ? Bayesian Anal 2006;1(1):1–40.

44. Gay PC, Owens RL, Wolfe LF, et al. Executive summary: optimal NIV medicare access promotion: a technical expert panel report from the American college of chest physicians, the American association for respiratory care, the American academy of sleep medicine, and the American thoracic society. Chest 2021;160(5):1808–21.

45. Suzuki E, Yamamoto E, Tsuda T. On the relations between excess fraction, attributable fraction, and etiologic fraction. Am J Epidemiol 2012;175(6): 567–75.

46. Pearl J. Probabilities of Causation: Three Counterfactual Interpretations and Their Identification. Synthese 1999;121:93–149.

47. Chung Y, Garden FL, Marks GB, et al. Causes of hypercapnic respiratory failure: a population-based case-control study. BMC Pulm Med 2023. https://doi.org/10.1186/s12890-023-02639-6.

48. Contou D, Fragnoli C, Córdoba-Izquierdo A, et al. Noninvasive ventilation for acute hypercapnic respiratory failure: intubation rate in an experienced unit. Respir Care 2013;58(12):2045–52.

49. Ouanes-Besbes L, Hammouda Z, Besbes S, et al. Diagnosis of sleep apnea syndrome in the intensive care unit: a case series of survivors of hypercapnic respiratory failure. Ann Am Thorac Soc 2021;18(4):727–9.

50. Thille AW, Córdoba-Izquierdo A, Maitre B, et al. High prevalence of sleep apnea syndrome in patients admitted to ICU for acute hypercapnic respiratory failure: a preliminary study. Intensive Care Med 2018;44(2):267–9.

51. Adler D, Pépin JL, Dupuis-Lozeron E, et al. Comorbidities and subgroups of patients surviving severe acute hypercapnic respiratory failure in the intensive care unit. Am J Respir Crit Care Med 2017; 196(2):200–7.

52. Gursel G, Zerman A, Aydogdu M, et al. Diagnosis of obstructive sleep apnea with respiratory polygraph in hypercapnic ICU patients. Crit Care 2015;19:1–201.

53. Adler D, Dupuis-Lozeron E, Janssens JP, et al. Obstructive sleep apnea in patients surviving acute hypercapnic respiratory failure is best predicted by static hyperinflation. PLoS One 2018;13(10):e0205669.

54. Bucklin AA, Ganglberger W, Quadri SA, et al. High prevalence of sleep-disordered breathing in the intensive care unit — a cross-sectional study. Sleep Breath 2022. https://doi.org/10.1007/s11325-022-02698-9.

55. Resta O, Barbaro MPF, Brindicci C, et al. Hypercapnia in overlap syndrome: possible determinant factors. Sleep Breath Schlaf Atm 2002;6(1):11–7.

56. Chung Y, Garden FL, Marks GB, et al. Causes of hypercapnic respiratory failure and associated in-hospital mortality. Respirology 2022. https://doi.org/10.1111/resp.14388.

57. Sharma SK, Stansbury R. How we do it: sleep disordered breathing in hospitalized patients - a game changer? Chest 2021. https://doi.org/10.1016/j.chest.2021.10.016.

58. Sharma SK. Hospital sleep medicine: the elephant in the room? J Clin Sleep Med 2014;10(10):1067–8.

59. Sharma S, Mukhtar U, Kelly C, et al. Recognition and treatment of sleep-disordered breathing in obese hospitalized patients may improve survival. The HoSMed database. Am J Med 2017;130(10): 1184–91.

60. Suen C, Wong J, Ryan CM, et al. Prevalence of undiagnosed obstructive sleep apnea among patients hospitalized for cardiovascular disease and

associated in-hospital outcomes: a scoping review. J Clin Med 2020;9(4):989.

61. Johnson KG, Rastegar V, Scuderi N, et al. PAP therapy and readmission rates after in-hospital laboratory titration polysomnography in patients with hypoventilation. J Clin Sleep Med 2022;18(7): 1739–48. https://doi.org/10.5664/jcsm.9962.

62. Bülbül Y, Ayik S, Ozlu T, et al. Frequency and predictors of obesity hypoventilation in hospitalized patients at a tertiary health care institution. Ann Thorac Med 2014;9(2):87–91.

63. Domaradzki L, Gosala S, Iskandarani K, et al. Is venous blood gas performed in the Emergency Department predictive of outcome during acute on chronic hypercarbic respiratory failure? Clin Respir J 2018;12(5):1849–57.

64. Collins BF, Collins BF, Ramenofsky DH, et al. The association of weight with the detection of airflow obstruction and inhaled treatment among patients with a clinical diagnosis of COPD. Chest 2014; 146(6):1513–20.

65. Scott S, Currie J, Albert P, et al. Risk of misdiagnosis, health-related quality of life, and BMI in patients who are overweight with doctor-diagnosed asthma. Chest 2012;141(3):616–24.

66. Marik PE, Chen C. The clinical characteristics and hospital and post-hospital survival of patients with the obesity hypoventilation syndrome: analysis of a large cohort. Obes Sci Pract 2016;2(1):40–7.

67. Manuel DG, Rosella LC, Stukel TA. Importance of accurately identifying disease in studies using electronic health records. BMJ 2010;341:c4226.

68. Lloyd-Owen SJ, Donaldson GC, Ambrosino N, et al. Patterns of home mechanical ventilation use in Europe: results from the Eurovent survey. Eur Respir J 2005;25(6):1025–31.

69. Borel JC, Burel B, Tamisier R, et al. Comorbidities and mortality in hypercapnic obese under domiciliary noninvasive ventilation. PLoS One 2013;8(1):e52006. https://doi.org/10.1371/journal.pone.0052006.

70. Cantero C, Adler D, Pasquina P, et al. Long-Term noninvasive ventilation in the Geneva lake area: indications, prevalence, and modalities. Chest 2020; 158(1):279–91.

71. Laub M, Midgren B. Survival of patients on home mechanical ventilation: a nationwide prospective study. Respir Med 2007;101(6):1074–8.

72. Povitz M, Rose L, Shariff SZ, et al. Home mechanical ventilation: a 12-year population-based retrospective cohort study. Respir Care 2017;63(4):380–7.

73. Patout M, Lhuillier E, Kaltsakas G, et al. Long-term survival following initiation of home non-invasive ventilation: a European study. Thorax 2020;75(11): 965–73.

74. Tan GP, Tan GP, McArdle N, et al. Patterns of use, survival and prognostic factors in patients receiving home mechanical ventilation in Western Australia: a single centre historical cohort study. Chron Respir Dis 2018;15(4):356–64.

75. Escarrabill J, Tebé C, Espallargues Mireia, et al. Variabilidad en la prescripción de la ventilación mecánica a domicilio. Arch Bronconeumol 2015; 51(10):490–5.

76. Neill AM, Tristram RI, Perry Meredith, et al. Noninvasive ventilation in New Zealand: a national prevalence survey. Intern Med J 2022;3. https://doi.org/ 10.1111/imj.15960.

77. Wijkstra PJ, Duiverman ML. Home mechanical ventilation: a fast-growing treatment option in chronic respiratory failure. Chest 2020;158(1): 26–7.

78. Köhnlein T, Windisch W, Windisch W, et al. Noninvasive positive pressure ventilation for the treatment of severe stable chronic obstructive pulmonary disease: a prospective, multicentre, randomised, controlled clinical trial. Lancet Respir Med 2014;2(9):698–705.

79. Verbraecken J, McNicholas WT. Respiratory mechanics and ventilatory control in overlap syndrome and obesity hypoventilation. Respir Res 2013;14(1):132.

80. Hoque R. Sleep-disordered breathing in Duchenne muscular dystrophy: an assessment of the literature. J Clin Sleep Med 2016;12(6):905–11.

81. Li L, Umbach DM, Li Y, et al. Sleep apnoea and hypoventilation in patients with five major types of muscular dystrophy. BMJ Open Respir Res 2023; 10(1):e001506.

82. Chiodo A, Sitrin RG, Bauman Kristy A, et al. Sleep disordered breathing in spinal cord injury: a systematic review. J Spinal Cord Med 2016;39(4): 374–82.

83. Graco M, Ruehland W, Schembri R, et al. Prevalence of central sleep apnoea in people with tetraplegic spinal cord injury: a retrospective analysis of research and clinical data. Sleep 2023. https://doi. org/10.1093/sleep/zsad235.

84. Bauman Kristy A, Bauman KA, Kurili A, et al. Simplified approach to diagnosing sleep-disordered breathing and nocturnal hypercapnia in individuals with spinal cord injury. Arch Phys Med Rehabil 2016;97(3):363–71.

85. Brown JP, Bauman Kristy A, Bauman KA, et al. Positive airway pressure therapy for sleep-disordered breathing confers short-term benefits to patients with spinal cord injury despite widely ranging patterns of use. Spinal Cord 2018;56(8):777–89.

86. Sankari A, Vaughan S, Bascom AT, et al. Sleep-disordered breathing and spinal cord injury: a state-of-the-art review. Chest 2019;155(2):438–45.

87. Wolfe LF, Benditt JO, Aboussouan L, et al. Optimal NIV Medicare access promotion: patients with thoracic restrictive disorders: a technical expert panel report from the American College of chest

physicians, the American association for respiratory care, the American Academy of sleep medicine, and the American thoracic Society. Chest 2021;160(5):e399–408.

88. Graco M, Gobets David F, O'Connell C, et al. Management of sleep-disordered breathing in three spinal cord injury rehabilitation centres around the world: a mixed-methods study. Spinal Cord 2022; 60(5):414–21.

89. Ward S, Chatwin M, Heather S, et al. Randomised controlled trial of non-invasive ventilation (NIV) for nocturnal hypoventilation in neuromuscular and chest wall disease patients with daytime normocapnia. Thorax 2005;60(12):1019.

90. Finkelstein EA, Khavjou O, Thompson HF, et al. Obesity and severe obesity forecasts through 2030. Am J Prev Med 2012;42(6):563–70.

91. Sepanlou SG, Sepanlou SG, Safiri S, et al. The global, regional, and national burden of cirrhosis by cause in 195 countries and territories, 1990-2017 : a systematic analysis for the Global Burden of Disease Study 2017. Lancet Gastroenterol Hepatol 2020;5(3):245–66.

92. Adler D, Cavalot G, Brochard L. Comorbidities and readmissions in survivors of acute hypercapnic respiratory failure. Semin Respir Crit Care Med 2020;41(06):806–16.

93. Toussaint M, Wijkstra PJ, McKim D, et al. Building a home ventilation programme: population, equipment, delivery and cost. Thorax 2022;77(11):1140–8.

94. Larsson J, Gustafsson P. A Case Study in Fitting Area-Proportional Euler Diagrams with Ellipses Using Eulerr." In Proceedings of International Workshop on Set Visualization and Reasoning, 2116:84-91. Edinburgh, UK: CEUR Workshop Proceedings.

95. Fox BD, Bondarenco M, Shpirer I, et al. Transitioning from hospital to home with non-invasive ventilation: who benefits? Results of a cohort study. BMJ Open Respir Res 2022;9(1):e001267. https://doi.org/10.1136/bmjresp-2022-001267.

96. Segrelles Calvo G, Zamora García E, Girón Moreno R, et al. Non-invasive ventilation in an elderly population admitted to a respiratory monitoring unit: causes, complications and one-year evolution. Arch Bronconeumol 2012;48(10):349–54.

97. Brandão ME, Conde B, Silva JC, et al. Non-invasive ventilation in the treatment of acute and chronic exacerbated respiratory failure: what to expect outside the critical care units? Rev Port Pneumol Engl Ed 2016;22(1):54–6.

98. Budweiser S, Hitzl AP, Jörres RA, et al. Health-related quality of life and long-term prognosis in chronic hypercapnic respiratory failure: a prospective survival analysis. Respir Res 2007;8(1):92.

99. Garner DJ, Berlowitz DJ, Douglas J, et al. Home mechanical ventilation in Australia and New Zealand. Eur Respir J 2013;41(1):39–45.

100. Hannan LM, Sahi H, Road J, et al. Care practices and health-related quality of life for individuals receiving assisted ventilation. A cross-national study. Ann Am Thorac Soc 2016;13(6):894–903.

101. Rose L, McKim DA, Katz SL, et al. Home mechanical ventilation in Canada: a national survey. Respir Care 2015;60(5):695–704.

102. Maquilon C, Antolini M, Valdés N, et al. Results of the home mechanical ventilation national program among adults in Chile between 2008 and 2017. BMC Pulm Med 2021;21(1):394.

103. Schwarz EI, Mackie Mike, Mackie M, et al. Time-to-death in chronic respiratory failure on home mechanical ventilation: a cohort study. Respir Med 2020;162:105877. https://doi.org/10.1016/j.rmed.2020.105877.

104. Nasiłowski J, Wachulski M, Trznadel W, et al. The evolution of home mechanical ventilation in Poland between 2000 and 2010. Respir Care 2015;60(4):577–85.

105. Valkó L, Baglyas S, Gál J, et al. National survey: current prevalence and characteristics of home mechanical ventilation in Hungary. BMC Pulm Med 2018;18(1):190.

106. Windisch W, Freidel K, Schucher B, et al. The Severe Respiratory Insufficiency (SRI) Questionnaire: a specific measure of health-related quality of life in patients receiving home mechanical ventilation. J Clin Epidemiol 2003;56(8):752–9.

107. van den Biggelaar RJM, Hazenberg A, Cobben NAM, et al. Home mechanical ventilation: the Dutch approach. Pulmonology 2022;28(2):99–104.

108. Jimenez JV, Ackrivo J, Hsu JY, et al. Lowering PCO2 with non-invasive ventilation is associated with improved survival in chronic hypercapnic respiratory failure. Respir Care 2023;respcare:10813. https://doi.org/10.4187/respcare.10813.

109. Tissot A, Jaffre S, Jaffre Sandrine, et al. Home non-invasive ventilation fails to improve quality of life in the elderly: results from a multicenter cohort study. PLoS One 2015;10(10):e0141156. https://doi.org/10.1371/journal.pone.0141156.

110. Tan GP, Soon LHY, Ni B, et al. The pattern of use and survival outcomes of a dedicated adult Home Ventilation and Respiratory Support Service in Singapore: a 7-year retrospective observational cohort study. J Thorac Dis Vol 2019;11(3). https://jtd.amegroups.org/article/view/27412. [Accessed 2 January 2019].

111. Rantala HA, Leivo-Korpela S, Kettunen S, et al. Survival and end-of-life aspects among subjects on long-term noninvasive ventilation. Eur Clin Respir J 2021;8(1):1840494. https://doi.org/10.1080/20018525.2020.1840494.

112. Chung F, Subramanyam R, Liao P, et al. High STOP-Bang score indicates a high probability of obstructive sleep apnoea. Br J Anaesth 2012; 108(5):768–75.

Targeting Hypercapnia in Chronic Lung Disease and Obesity Hypoventilation
Benefits and Challenges

Lee K. Brown, MD*

KEYWORDS

- Hypercapnia • Respiratory insufficiency • Pulmonary Disease, Chronic Obstructive
- Noninvasive ventilation • Continuous positive airway pressure • Obesity hypoventilation syndrome
- Sleep apnea

KEY POINTS

- Arterial puncture with blood gas analysis remains the most reliable tool for detecting hypercapnia and acid–base status. The use of venous samples for this purpose is discouraged.
- End-tidal CO_2 ($PetCO_2$) and transcutaneous CO_2 ($PtcCO_2$) measurements can take the place of an arterial puncture but both have limitations that must be understood. Both are important tools for monitoring arterial partial pressure of carbon dioxide ($Paco_2$) during sleep.
- Chronic obstructive pulmonary disease with hypoventilation will usually respond to noninvasive ventilation (NIV), but the long-term utility of use of NIV at home is still unclear. Domiciliary use of high-flow nasal oxygen is still under investigation.
- Treatment of obesity hypoventilation syndrome virtually always requires positive airway pressure therapy whether obstructive sleep apnea (OSA) is either present or not present. In many patients, particularly those with moderate-to-severe OSA, continuous positive airway pressure rather than ventilatory support modalities will suffice.

INTRODUCTION

Hypoventilation, as evidenced by arterial hypercapnia, is a ubiquitous finding in medical practice. Hypoventilation has a myriad of causes, can be acute, chronic, or acute on chronic, and occurs in both the inpatient and outpatient arenas. Moreover, hypercapnia can be an expected response to metabolic alkalosis, although the effect is often masked by complicating medical conditions that induce hyperventilation.[1] Nevertheless, Chung and colleagues, in 2 publications, attempted to discern overall prevalence and to identify specific medical conditions that were likely to be causative.[2,3] Their most comprehensive investigation was a cross-sectional study of 873 patients admitted to the Liverpool, Australia hospital, with hypercapnic respiratory failure between 2013 and 2017.[3] The cause(s) of hypercapnia were identified based on recorded diagnoses from the medical record: chronic obstructive pulmonary disease (COPD) was the presumed cause in 45% of cases and chronic congestive heart failure in 32%. Lower on the list were opioids and benzodiazepines (6.5% and 3%, respectively), sleep-disordered breathing in 6%, and neuromuscular disease in less than 2%. Thirty percent of the patients with COPD had comorbid congestive heart failure, while 42% of

Division of Pulmonary, Critical Care, and Sleep Medicine, Department of Internal Medicine, University of New Mexico School of Medicine, Albuquerque, NM, USA
* Corresponding author. UNM Sleep Disorders Center, 1101 Medical Arts Avenue NE, Building 2, Albuquerque, NM 87102.
E-mail address: lkbrown@salud.unm.edu

Sleep Med Clin 19 (2024) 357–369
https://doi.org/10.1016/j.jsmc.2024.02.014
1556-407X/24/© 2024 Elsevier Inc. All rights reserved.

the subjects with congestive heart failure had comorbid COPD.

DETECTING AND MONITORING HYPERCAPNIA

The targeted treatment of hypoventilation requires (1) defining a value of arterial partial pressure of carbon dioxide ($Paco_2$) above which constitutes hypoventilation; (2) measuring $Paco_2$ using reliable methodology so as to identify the patient who presents with or develops hypoventilation; and (3) continuous or intermittent measurement of $Paco_2$, again using reliable methodology, to assess the effect of the management strategies being employed. Hypoventilation is virtually always defined as a $Paco_2$ greater than 45 mm Hg and using this value as the upper limit of normal is based upon published mean values for awake $Paco_2$ of about 38 mm Hg, associated with an upper 95% confidence limit of approximately 45 mm Hg at sea level.[4,5]

Identifying the presence of hypoventilation during wakefulness in an adult is best determined from an arterial puncture or withdrawing a sample from an arterial line. The sample is then assayed for pH, Pco_2, and Po_2, along with a number of other derived values such as base excess. There is an increasing tendency to obtain a venous blood gas (VBG), possibly because it takes far less skill and time to perform a venipuncture than an arterial puncture, and/or due to an element of increased risk of bleeding or other complications when performing an arterial puncture. However, the validity of VBG results may reasonably be questioned due to the metabolic activity of the tissues distal to the point of venipuncture, whether the blood sample is withdrawn with the tourniquet in place, or even whether sufficient time has passed after tourniquet removal for the restoration of normal blood flow.[6] A meta-analysis of 18 studies reporting on a total of 1768 subjects examined venous Pco_2 ($PvCO_2$) obtained from a peripheral vein and found that the 95% prediction interval of bias for $PvCO_2$ was unacceptably wide (−10.7 mm Hg to +2.4 mm Hg) and could not be used for clinical decision-making.[6] Bloom and colleagues performed a meta-analysis examining the same issue in the emergency department setting and concluded that agreement between $PvCO_2$ from a peripheral vein and $Paco_2$ was not reliable, but that a normal peripheral $PvCO_2$ generally indicated a normal $Paco_2$ in terms of negative predictive value, and consequently $PvCO_2$ could be used to exclude ventilatory failure.[7] Kelly studied the same issue, again in the emergency department, and reported that the 95% limits of agreement were as high as ±20 mm Hg and that peripheral $PvCO_2$ values

were not clinically useful.[8] Finally, Lim and colleagues performed a meta-analysis examining the issue as to whether a peripheral $PvCO_2$ could be used in patients with COPD presenting with acute exacerbations in the emergency department in order to decide upon proper management. However, the 95% limits of agreement were −17 to 26 mm Hg, and therefore of little clinical utility.[9]

A direct measurement from an arterial puncture or catheter during sleep is impractical given the disruption in sleep from the procedure as well as the fact that it is a rare sleep laboratory that has access to arterial blood gas equipment. Designating a particular value as abnormal during sleep is subject to the indirect manner in which $Paco_2$ must be measured. Consequently, $Paco_2$ is measured either by monitoring end-tidal Pco_2 ($PetCO_2$) or by using transcutaneous Pco_2 ($PtcCO_2$) technology. Both techniques result in approximations for $Paco_2$ rather than exact values, and both are associated with drawbacks that limit either their utility or their accuracy. $PetCO_2$ generally cannot be used concurrent with oxygen administration or positive airway pressure treatment that involves a continuous flow of air, due to dilution of the quantity of exhaled CO_2 by the flow of oxygen or room air. However, there has become available a full face-mask interface designed to circumvent this limitation, but it has not been widely adopted.[10] While $PetCO_2$ can be reasonably accurate in patients with normal lungs (underestimating $Paco_2$ by 2–5 mm Hg), accuracy deteriorates with low ventilation/perfusion (V/Q) values, as well as in respiratory disorders such as acute respiratory distress syndrome.[11] Also, if exhalation time is too short to reach the alveolar plateau (phase III of the $PetCO_2$ vs time capnograph waveform) due to incomplete emptying of lung units distal to obstructed airways, $PetCO_2$ will underestimate $Paco_2$. This commonly occurs in COPD and asthma; usage in these patients mandates that the capnograph signal be included in the montage displayed when interpreting a polysomnogram. Alternatively, if significant obstructive ventilatory impairment is suspected or known, $PtcCO_2$ rather than $PetCO_2$ monitoring should be employed.

$PtcCO_2$ has developed a reputation as being the more reliable surrogate for the measurement of $Paco_2$, but it also has technical issues that must be addressed and the literature comparing $PtcCO_2$ to simultaneous $Paco_2$ has not always confirmed its reliability. One technical issue relates to the tendency to potentially overestimate $Paco_2$ due to CO_2 produced by the metabolic activity of the heated skin underneath the sensor.[12] To some extent, this has been mitigated by using somewhat lower sensor temperatures and by applying an empirically derived correction factor. $PtcCO_2$ values may drift upward during prolonged periods of monitoring, and correction of the reported value may be required when this is known to occur; alternatively, it is not uncommon that the sensor must be removed and reapplied approximately midway through the night when used during polysomnography or during other extended periods. Unlike $PetCO_2$, $PtcCO_2$ values do not immediately reflect changes in $Paco_2$ but rather require an equilibration period that can vary between 2 minutes to as long as 15 minutes.[13]

With respect to accuracy, Aarrestad and colleagues have reported their own results as well as compiling a table of 36 studies listing the level of agreement (LoA) reported in studies comparing $Paco_2$ and $PtcCO_2$ published between 2005 and 2015.[13] They employed the manufacturer's recommended best practices and found LoAs of -2.4 ± 5.9 mm Hg; no paired values exceeded a difference of 7.5 mm Hg. For the subgroup of subjects with $Paco_2$ greater than 45 mm Hg, LoAs were -2.8 ± 6.3 mm Hg. Examination of 36 previous studies demonstrated a maximum bias of -6.0 mm Hg and LoAs of -19.5 to -11.2 mm Hg; however, many studies reported positive values of bias and/or acceptable LoAs. One may conclude from the report of Aarrestad and colleagues that $PtcCO_2$ tends to underestimate $Paco_2$, but other investigations reported that $PtcCO_2$ may underestimate as well as overestimate $Paco_2$, and this tendency is unpredictable.[14] It is best for the clinician to interpret single values obtained by these methods with due regard to the patient's overall clinical picture; during treatment, the trend in these values may be of greater utility.

NATURE OF THE PROBLEM

When targeting hypercapnia in chronic lung disease or obesity hypoventilation syndrome (OHS), one must be cognizant of the why, and not just the how, of the need to address an abnormally elevated $Paco_2$. When $Paco_2$ levels reach extreme degrees and are associated with decreased levels of consciousness or even coma, the age-old adage of CO_2 narcosis is often invoked. Whether this entity truly exists or is the result of comorbidities can be questioned.[15–17] In contrast, hypercapnia in and of itself has been shown to be responsible for adverse effects on the normal function of a variety of organ systems. These effects were well summarized recently by Almanza-Hurtado and colleagues.[18] Hypercapnia increases cerebral blood flow, which can ultimately result in cerebral edema[19] and is associated with adverse outcomes in stroke, traumatic brain injury, or following cardiopulmonary arrest.[20]

Cardiovascular effects include reducing systemic vascular resistance and cardiac contractility; with increasing severity, the result may be arrhythmias or hemodynamic instability.[21] Patients presenting for inpatient care due to hypercapnia experience higher likelihoods of readmission and mortality that vary depending on underlying etiology.[22]

TARGETING HYPERCAPNIA IN CHRONIC OBSTRUCTIVE LUNG DISEASE

COPD is a generic term that has evolved to an increasingly complex range of phenotypes that consider a vast array of features[23]; various combinations of these features are thought to define specific phenotypes that may or may not be useful in the management of an individual patient, and for that reason, the concept of "treatable traits" has entered the lexicon of phenotyping and are meant to guide therapy; hence the exercise of phenotyping has practical value.[24] One treatable trait that has emerged as deserving of particular attention is hypercapnia, and therefore, the discussion herein has significant relevance.

All phenotypes incorporate various degrees of airways obstruction and as forced expiratory volume in 1 second (FEV_1) falls, the capacity to sustain adequate alveolar ventilation declines resulting in hypercapnia that can progress to sleep-associated, and then diurnal, hypercapnia. Initially, hypercapnia may exhibit a distinct pattern of occurrence every 60 to 120 minutes, corresponding to the loss of accessory muscle contributions to inspiratory effort during rapid eye movement sleep, but as the disease progresses, hypercapnia will manifest on a more continuous basis.[25] Patients with COPD may also suffer from obstructive sleep apnea (OSA), a combination that has been termed by Flenley as the "overlap syndrome."[25] While it was originally hypothesized that some manner of causal relationship between COPD and OSA existed, it now seems clear that both of these disorders co-occur because they share certain demographic characteristics.[26,27] The estimated prevalence of overlap syndrome in patients with COPD varies widely depending on the characteristics of the population being studied. A recent systematic review reported a prevalence ranging between 30% and 50% if defined as apnea–hypopnea index (AHI) of 15/h or greater.[28] Compared with patients diagnosed with OSA alone, those with overlap syndrome exhibit greater degrees of hypoxia and higher prevalence of hypertension, ischemic heart disease, and heart failure.[29] Overlap syndrome patients exhibit diurnal hypercapnia more frequently,[30] and concomitant COPD is likely to be an important cause of acute-on-chronic ventilatory failure in patients with severe

OSA, a so-called critical care syndrome.[31] Gothi and colleagues reported that patients hospitalized for acute exacerbations of COPD (AECOPD) without comorbid OSA more commonly experienced mild or moderate exacerbations, while those with overlap syndrome were more likely to endure severe, very severe, or life-threatening exacerbations.[32] Marin and colleagues prospectively studied patients with COPD alone or with overlap syndrome for a median duration of 9.4 years (range, 3.3–12.7 years).[33] Participants with overlap syndrome exhibited significantly higher mortality and time to a first severe AECOPD (defined as requiring hospital admission) compared to those with COPD alone. In addition, a third group of patients with overlap syndrome had similar outcomes to those with COPD alone when treated with continuous positive airway pressure (CPAP).[33]

In addition to optimizing medical management, long-term oxygen treatment (LTOT) for at least 15 h/d, including during all sleep periods, has been the standard of care for hypoxemia in stable patients with COPD, based on 2 studies performed approximately 40 years ago.[34,35] Both studies appeared to include some patients with hypercapnia as well as hypoxemia, but the specific outcomes of LTOT in patients with hypercapnia are difficult to extract. One trial, comparing 12 hour nocturnal oxygen administration to continuous oxygen therapy, reported mean $Paco_2$ values of 43.9 and 43.4 mm Hg, respectively, but did provide a graphic demonstrating that subjects with $Paco_2$ greater than 43 mm Hg had strikingly higher mortality when receiving nocturnal oxygen administration alone compared to continuous oxygen treatment.[35] Over the ensuing years, the validity of these early trials has been questioned, although the standard of care had consistently incorporated the use of LTOT greater than 15 h/d for patients demonstrating nocturnal hypoxemia with or without diurnal hypoxemia. Oswald-Mammosser and colleagues studied 84 patients with COPD and hypoxemia treated with LTOT who had undergone right heart catheterizations and found that pulmonary hypertension affected survival but hypercapnia did not.[36] Aida and colleagues prospectively recorded the mortality of 4552 patients with COPD and hypoxemia (at rest, during exercise, or while asleep), who received LTOT from 1985 to 1993.[37] All subjects were considered to have been stable during at least 4 weeks prior to enrollment and were receiving the standard medical therapy available during that time period. They reported no significant difference in survival using Cox regression analysis when comparing patients with hypercapnia ($Paco_2 \geq 45$ mm Hg) versus those who were eucapnic. Age, sex, forced vital capacity percent predicted (%FVC), and Pao_2 were independent predictors of mortality.

Subsequently, most research involving patients with hypercapnia and COPD reported on outcomes involving noninvasive ventilation (NIV) or high flow nasal oxygen (HFNO), since either modality could augment CO_2 clearance as well as provide oxygenation. Initially used in acute care venues to delay or prevent mechanical ventilation, it was not long before these new noninvasive technologies were trialed in patients with stable COPD and hypercapnia in the domiciliary setting and interest in examining LTOT alone waned.

As studies of nocturnal NIV in patients with COPD and hypercapnia accumulated, it became possible to perform meta-analyses; 5 such studies have been published. Wickstra and colleagues incorporated the 4 publications that met inclusion criteria at the time of the meta-analysis in 2003.[38] Three months of NIV in patients with stable COPD did not improve lung function, gas exchange, or sleep efficiency. Liao and colleagues performed a meta-analysis of 7 studies involving a total of 810 subjects.[39] Overall mortality, oxygenation, frequency of acute exacerbations, lung and respiratory muscle function, and exercise capacity showed no improvement attributable to the use of NIV. In a sub-analysis of patients who experienced a significant reduction in $Paco_2$, NIV was found to improve mortality when it was targeted at substantial reductions in $Paco_2$. Struik and colleagues published a meta-analysis of 7 trials of moderate-to-high quality treated with NIV for 3 to 12 months and found no overall improvement in $Paco_2$ and Pao_2, 6 minute walking distance, health-related quality of life (HRQL), FEV_1 and FVC, maximal inspiratory pressure, or sleep efficiency.[40] Wu and colleagues and Raveling and colleagues published the most recent meta-analyses, thus incorporating the most recent and largest number of trials.[41,42] Raveling and colleagues published a Cochrane review in 2021 and were able to analyze 21 randomized controlled trials (RCTs).[41] Four RCTs included in the analysis involved patients receiving domiciliary NIV after an admission for an acute exacerbation. In the stable COPD group, $Paco_2$ was lower in the NIV patients at both 3 and 12 months, with evidence judged as of high certainty. There was little effect on Pao_2 at 12 months. Mortality was reduced in the NIV group with evidence of moderate certainty. Patients treated with NIV after discharge for an acute exacerbation also demonstrated a reduction in $Paco_2$ at 3 and 12 months, and frequency of hospital admissions for acute exacerbations declined although mortality did not. Wu and colleagues were able to analyze 19 trials involving 1482 patients, representing an approximately equal number of patients and controls.[42] Notably, mortality rates were lower in the patients treated with domiciliary NIV (relative risk, 0.76, 95% CI 0.61–0.95) and other important outcomes also improved: frequency of hospital admissions, $Paco_2$, Pao_2, dyspnea, exercise capacity, and HRQL. Interestingly, those participants with a higher baseline $Paco_2$ ($\geq$55 mm Hg) demonstrated improved mortality compared to subjects with lower degrees of baseline hypercapnia. It should be noted that the American Thoracic Society (ATS) published clinical practice guidelines in 2020 specifically addressing NIV in chronic stable COPD.[43] Based on a conditional recommendation with moderate certainty, NIV plus usual care was suggested as the standard of care for patients with chronic stable COPD complicated by hypercapnia.

With the development of HFNO via nasal cannula,[44] NIV may no longer remain the only option for domiciliary care of patients with chronic stable COPD with hypercapnia. HFNO is an open circuit modality and does not directly enhance tidal volume. However, evidence suggests that HFNO alters ventilatory physiology in a manner that enhances CO_2 clearance, primarily by reducing anatomic dead space, thus reducing the dead space to tidal volume (Vd/Vt) ratio for each tidal breath. Patients treated with HFNO assume a lower respiratory rate but alveolar ventilation, as assessed by $Paco_2$, remains stable in normal subjects. In patients with hypercapnia, $Paco_2$ can decrease after optimal settings are achieved. Despite the use of an open circuit, high flow from the nasal cannula resists the ability to exhale and thereby increases airway pressure, effectively applying a degree of positive end expiratory pressure. HFNO is now in regular use in adult critical care, most frequently to prevent the need for intubation and mechanical ventilation in critically ill patients with hypercapnia. Three meta-analyses have provided data suggesting that HFNO may be used at home in patients with COPD and hypercapnia. Bonnevie and colleagues sought to answer the specific question as to whether HFNO could substitute for NIV in patients with COPD at home.[45] They identified 6 studies involving 339 subjects and reported a significant reduction of $Paco_2$ in 2 long-term studies and 2 short-term studies. There was a significant improvement in HRQL in 2 studies and a reduced rate of acute exacerbations at 1 year in one study. A more recent meta-analysis failed to demonstrate an advantage when HFNO was compared to NIV with respect to preventing intubation but was superior to conventional oxygen therapy in patients with COPD exacerbations, consistent with its use in intensive care.[46] When assessed for domiciliary use in stable hypercapnic COPD, HFNO was associated with improved HRQL only. The third meta-analysis, also recent, compared HFNO to conventional oxygen administration in treating COPD exacerbations as well as for use in stable patients with COPD at home.[47] HFNO was found to reduce $Paco_2$ and prevent intubation in acute respiratory failure, and decreased hospital admissions when used at home. While HFNO certainly shows promise for domiciliary use in hypercapnic COPD, many clinicians may be unfamiliar with this therapeutic modality unless they have had extensive experience practicing critical care, and there appears to be an element of increased complexity in arriving at the proper settings for any given patient compared to prescribing NIV and oxygen.

Finally, lung reduction surgery (LVRS), in those individuals deemed suitable candidates, has also been shown to ameliorate hypercapnia, with patients having the highest preoperative levels of $Paco_2$ seeming to benefit the most at 3 to 6 months of follow-up.[48,49] The seminal National Emphysema Treatment Trial (NETT) excluded patients with the most severe degrees of hypoventilation, despite original entrance criteria that accepted $Paco_2$ up to 60 mm Hg; $Paco_2$ averaged only 43 mm Hg in the NETT.[50] A Cochrane Database Systematic Review published in 2016 (13 years after the NETT) confirmed higher short-term mortality for LVRS than for control, apparently related to persistent air leaks, pneumonia, or cardiovascular issues.[51] However, long-term mortality favored LVRS in 2 studies with moderate-quality evidence.

TARGETING HYPERCAPNIA IN OBESITY HYPOVENTILATION SYNDROME

The widely accepted definition of OHS consists of diurnal hypercapnia in an individual who is considered obese. The World Health Organization has been the arbiter of what constitutes obesity and has classified degrees of obesity based on body mass index (BMI), with values of 30 kg/m^2 or greater transitioning an individual from "overweight" to obese.[52] An awake $Paco_2$ greater than 45 mm Hg and BMI of 30 kg/m^2 or greater (in adults) establishes the suspicion for OHS; history, physical examination, and appropriate laboratory testing must exclude other reasons for hypercapnia such as obstructive airways disease, restrictive ventilatory impairment, opioid use (especially with concomitant use of gabapentinoids or benzodiazepines), or adult onset congenital central hypoventilation syndrome.[53] The "Pickwickian syndrome," a term coined by Burwell and colleagues in a 1956 case report, is often used as a synonym for

OHS.[54] Burwell and colleagues coined this appellation from Dickens' description of "Joe the Fat Boy" in "The Posthumous Papers of the Pickwick Club,"[55] but there do exist competing diagnoses that might possibly apply to poor Joe, including OSA without OHS, OHS without OSA, narcolepsy, Prader–Willi syndrome, or Klein–Levin syndrome. There are also earlier reports that may well have described individuals with OHS that predate Burwell's description. In 1781, Fothergill reported 2 obese individuals complaining of somnolence whose symptoms remitted following substantial weight loss.[56]

The co-occurrence of obesity, alveolar hypoventilation, and hypersomnia as what is now categorized as OHS was recognized in 1972 in an article by Douglas Carroll,[57] but current thinking divides OHS into categories that are particularly important in driving proper evaluation and management. These include OHS with OSA that responds to treatment of OSA alone; OHS with OSA that does not respond to effective and compliant treatment of OSA; and OHS that is not accompanied by significant OSA.[58] The symptoms and signs of each of these OHS entities are not particularly different from those described by Fothergill and Burwell: excessive sleepiness and obesity, frequently accompanied by plethora (polycythemia) and *cor pulmonale* (Dickens in one passage described Joe as "young dropsy," dropsy being an archaic term for edema).[55]

EPIDEMIOLOGY

The prevalence of obesity in the United States remains disturbingly high based on 2017 to 2018 National Center for Health Statistics data, and the trend predicts that stage 1 obesity will become more ubiquitous over time.[59] The current estimate is 42.4% of the US population, and even more disturbing is the estimate of class 3 obesity, at 9.2%. Not surprisingly, the difficulty in measuring arterial $Paco_2$ in population surveys has precluded direct estimates of OHS prevalence. A variety of approaches have been used to arrive at estimates that are not population-based, usually after referral for pulmonology or sleep medicine consultation or hospital admission for acute on chronic ventilatory failure. Data on the population prevalence of OHS have not been definitively reported. Mokhlesi estimated a prevalence of OHS in the adult population with BMI of 40 kg/m^2 or greater of 0.15% to 0.3% using a complex calculation from individual prevalence values of the population prevalence of BMI 40 kg/m^2 or greater, the prevalence of OSA in this cohort, and the prevalence of OHS in patients with OSA with BMI of 40 kg/m^2 or greater.[60] The same group later published a revised value of 0.6%, using a higher prevalence of BMI of 40 kg/m^2 or greater in their calculations.[61]

PATHOGENESIS: "CANNOT BREATHE" VERSUS "WILL NOT BREATHE"
Respiratory System Mechanics and Gas Exchange: "Cannot Breathe"

Obesity, particularly morbid obesity, profoundly affects the mechanical properties of the ventilatory pump. Consequently, OHS pathogenesis was initially considered to result from impairments and adaptations to these mechanical restrictions such that the elevated work of breathing and a certain degree of hypercapnia could coexist. The mechanical impairments include reduced respiratory system compliance and increased tissue resistance from obesity. More recently, obesity has also been associated with airways obstruction, including in one comprehensive meta-analysis.[62,63] Whether there is an intrinsic abnormality in diaphragmatic contractility due to obesity that leads to OHS has been of considerable interest. However, even in patients with overt OHS, the ability to voluntarily increase minute ventilation (and achieve eucapnia) is preserved as long as significant airways obstruction is not present.[64]

Gas Exchange

Obesity is known to affect several aspects of gas exchange that may further stress ventilatory capacity. Obesity impairs distribution of ventilation, especially with respect to reduced ventilation to dependent lung zones, an effect partly attributed to atelectatic lung compressed by abdominal adipose tissue; the reduction in functional residual capacity (FRC) attendant to obesity, which may decline to below closing capacity (CC; the lung volume at which small airways collapse), also plays a role. Under these conditions, each tidal breath will descend to below CC, small airways will close, and the equivalent of a shunt will develop.[65–67] This manifests as hypoxemia and an increased alveolar-arterial Po_2 gradient.[68,69]

Control of Breathing: "Cannot Breathe"

Physiologists and clinicians dating back to the 1950s have attempted to relate these changes in respiratory system mechanics and gas exchange to the development of OHS, without success. Consequently, abnormalities in ventilatory control ("will not breathe") has emerged as the underlying basis for OHS in the majority of cases. Initially, there was a suspicion that patients with OHS had an inherited defect in ventilatory control. The existence of inherited defects in ventilatory control by testing close relatives of patients with OHS has not supported the existence of an inherited control of breathing defect.[70,71]

The vast majority of patients with OHS are found to also have OSA, with only a distinct minority exhibiting AHI of less than 5; these patients have in the past been named "Pickwickian syndrome, Auchincloss' type."[72] It is estimated that approximately 70% of cases have severe OSA, while 90% of patients with OHS have at least mild OSA.[73] For the 70% of patients with OHS with at least moderate-to-severe OSA, treatment of OSA results in resolution of OHS in most individuals.[74] Almost 40 years later, research by Berger, Ayappa, Sorkin, Norman, Rapoport, and Goldring have built a case for the cumulative effect of impaired nocturnal CO_2 clearance as the mechanism for OHS pathogenesis in patients with OSA.[75–80] They have demonstrated that inadequate compensatory ventilation between obstructive apneas and hypopneas leads to the gradual accumulation of high levels of nocturnal $Paco_2$. In response, renal reabsorption and generation of bicarbonate occurs during the night leading to metabolic alkalosis. Reversal of this process is too slow to be completed on the following day, and metabolic alkalosis persists and worsens over time. These investigators have also identified a temporal mismatch between the timing of CO_2 presentation at the alveolar–capillary interface and the time course of alveolar ventilation, creating a further defect in CO_2 elimination.[75] The metabolic alkalosis induced by persistently high levels of serum bicarbonate acts to blunt respiratory drive, particularly in response to hypercapnia, and maintains awake hypoventilation.[81–83] For the remaining 10% of patients with OHS, Rapoport and colleagues have suggested that these individuals be designated as the "true Pickwickians," which as noted above, has also been called "Pickwickian syndrome, Auchincloss' type."[72] The pathogenesis for this variety of OHS remains obscure, although as late as 1975 Carroll still attributed it to increased work of breathing.[84]

The adipokine leptin has been implicated as possibly involved in the pathogenesis of OHS. Leptin is synthesized in adipose tissue and consequently plasma levels reflect the degree of obesity in any given individual. Leptin has been found to have respiratory stimulant properties,[85] and patients with OHS have leptin levels even higher than in weight-matched obese subjects with eucapnia.[86] Consequently, some have concluded that leptin resistance in breathing control centers may also be involved in OHS pathogenesis.[87,88] In addition, there is speculation that other neurohumeral agents related to obesity may play a role, as reviewed by Pillar and Shehadeh.[88]

Diagnosis

At its simplest, the diagnosis of OHS only requires calculation of a BMI greater than 30 kg/m^2 plus an arterial blood gas determination yielding a $Paco_2$ greater than 45 mm Hg. Other causes for hypercapnia must be excluded, which usually entails pulmonary function testing and chest radiography. If pulmonary function testing reveals obstructive ventilatory impairment (eg, from COPD), the degree of obstruction must be sufficiently minor to exclude the possibility that it contributes significantly to hypercapnia. Unfortunately, this is a difficult judgment to make, although an FEV_1 less than 1 L has been suggested as an independent risk factor for hypercapnia in COPD.[89] Urine toxicology should be considered to exclude the use of ventilatory depressant drugs, specifically opioids and any concomitant use of gabapentinoids or benzodiazepines. In addition, due to the importance of OSA in the pathogenesis of most OHS, nocturnal polysomnography or at least home sleep apnea testing (HSAT) is essential; if OSA is present, CPAP or bilevel positive airway pressure (bilevel PAP) is indicated (see later discussion).

In lieu of measuring $Paco_2$, the noninvasive measurement of $Paco_2$ by means of $PetCO_2$ or $PtcCO_2$ can be useful, since such equipment is usually present in any well-equipped sleep laboratory. Another approach consists of using serum bicarbonate values. Since the positive predictive value of serum bicarbonate at 27 mmol/L or greater approximates only 50%, this metric should be combined with other clinical data in order to decide the likelihood of OHS; note that the negative predictive value of serum bicarbonate less than 27 mmol/L approaches 100%.[89]

TREATMENT
Positive Airway Pressure

The use of CPAP for the treatment of OSA and OHS emerged from a report by Sullivan and colleagues and the work of Rapoport and coworkers in the 1980s.[74,90] Noninvasive application of positive airway pressure has since become the treatment of choice for patients with OHS with or without moderate-to-severe OSA, although the latter group, probably not having OSA as a causative factor, is best treated with bilevel PAP or another ventilatory support mode. This latter point was the conclusion reached in a study by Ojeda Castillejo and colleagues, which compared outcomes for patients with OHS with or without OSA (AHI >5/h) managed with bilevel PAP-S/T at home.[91] Efficacy was demonstrated in terms of reduced 1 year and 5 year mortalities and improved spirometric variables, $Paco_2$, and Pao_2, with similar results for those without, as well as with, OSA. It follows that patients with only a modest degree of OSA may not develop the metabolic alkalosis implicated as the etiology of OHS and consequently may not respond to CPAP alone. Much has been written in the recent past concerning the optimum choice of PAP modality for the treatment of OHS. The various modalities that have been studied include CPAP, bilevel PAP in spontaneous mode (bilevel PAP-S), bilevel PAP in spontaneous/timed mode (bilevel PAP-S/T) with and without high backup rates, adaptive servo-ventilation (ASV) with fixed expiratory positive airway pressure (EPAP), ASVauto (both pressure support and EPAP are automatically titrated in this mode), and average volume-assured pressure support (AVAPS). Several technologies are not recommended for the treatment of OHS: ASV in either fixed pressure support or auto EPAP mode titrates to achieve an average minute ventilation or average peak inspiratory flow as measured over a period of minutes prior to making an adjustment; consequently, both devices will target what may already be an inadequate degree of minute ventilation. The objective in treating OHS in patients who are not critically ill is to eliminate OSA as the causative factor. These patients will respond to either CPAP or bilevel PAP-S; although the immediate response from most clinicians is to order a ventilatory support mode, this is frequently not necessary. Howard and colleagues published a multicenter, parallel, double-blind trial comparing CPAP and bilevel PAP as the initial treatment of OHS with OSA and found no significant difference in effect on ventilatory failure, HRQL, or adherence.[92] Masa and colleagues compared lifestyle modifications to CPAP or AVAPS and found no difference in the degree of improvement of daytime $Paco_2$ between these positive pressure modalities.[93] Fortunately, there is little need to continue describing the multitude of comparative studies that have been published over the ensuing years, since there are 2 meta-analyses and one network meta-analysis now available. The most recent meta-analysis concluded that NIV/bilevel PAP-S/T improved hypercapnia to a small extent compared to no PAP treatment (average, 2.4 mm Hg).[94] The second meta-analysis, published 1 year earlier, concluded that NIV/bilevel PAP-S/T may result in a greater improvement in hypercapnia than CPAP alone; remarkably, the improvement also averaged 2.4 mm Hg.[95] The third meta-analysis is particularly useful; as a network meta-analysis, the authors were able to generate comparisons between different PAP modalities as to the primary outcome variables, which were changes in $Paco_2$ and Epworth Sleepiness Scale (ESS) score, without the benefit of head-to-head studies.[96] The results indicated that $Paco_2$ improvement was superior for AVAPS and bilevel PAP-S/T compared to control, and only CPAP was inferior compared to the other modalities. AVAPS improved ESS more than control, but ESS was no better or worse when the PAP modalities were compared with each other. Consequently, it is difficult to argue against implementing a bilevel PAP mode in patients with more severe degrees of hypercapnia or who are beginning treatment after an admission for an acute exacerbation of chronic ventilatory failure from OHS. Given the low quality of evidence and the failure to conclusively identify the best PAP modality in any given situation, an in-laboratory titration polysomnogram would seem to be the best strategy when treating any individual patient.

Weight Loss

Substantial weight loss has been the most obvious treatment of OHS, dating back to the earliest descriptions of the entity.[56] Unfortunately, it is well known that weight loss is not only difficult to achieve by diet and exercise but also difficult to sustain. More recently, bariatric surgery also provides a perhaps more effective option since patients with OHS can be considered as suffering from a life-threatening condition. However, bariatric procedures in patients with OHS may experience higher complication rates than those without OHS.[97] Bariatric surgical technique currently encompasses a wide variety of procedures, both open and laparoscopic, with a strong tendency at present to choose a laparoscopic approach. Several meta-analyses have been published comparing different techniques with respect to their efficacy and early and late complication rates. It can be concluded that, overall, Roux-en-Y gastric bypass results in greater degrees of weight loss; sleeve gastrectomy was safer than Roux-en-Y gastric bypass in the elderly; and both Roux-en-Y gastric bypass and sleeve gastrectomy were safe and effective options in adolescents. The European Association for Endoscopic Surgery Bariatric Guidelines Group has recently published guidelines concerning preferred choices for technique in severe obesity with metabolic diseases, and concluded that sleeve gastrectomy or laparoscopic Roux-en-Y gastric bypass were better choices than adjustable gastric banding, biliopancreatic diversion with duodenal switch or gastric plication.[98] The American Academy of

Sleep Medicine commissioned a meta-analysis that included bariatric surgery as a treatment of OSA, and based on moderate quality of evidence, the task force concluded that bariatric surgery offered benefits in terms of a reduction in obstructive respiratory events, improved blood pressure, reduced oxyhemoglobin desaturation index, lesser degrees of excessive sleepiness, lower BMI, reduced snoring, lower effective CPAP levels, and an increase in lowest oxyhemoglobin saturation.[99] The ATS also published a systematic review in part addressing the role of bariatric surgery in patients with OHS.[100] The task force confirmed that weight loss of 15% to 64.6% as well as improvement in OSA severity in terms of AHI (18%–44%), and improved $Paco_2$ (17%–20%) were achievable and that resolution of OHS was ultimately possible. Adverse effects occurred in approximately 20% of patients, but serious adverse effects were rare. Common sense would dictate that OHS should be adequately treated with a positive airway pressure modality prior to contemplating bariatric surgery; thus, polysomnography or HSAT is routinely part of the preoperative evaluation in these patients.

Respiratory Stimulants

Medroxyprogesterone and the carbonic anhydrase inhibitor acetazolamide have both been suggested as possible treatments for OHS in view of their properties as stimulants of central ventilatory drive. There are few data to support long-term use of medroxyprogesterone.[101,102] Since the advent of positive pressure modalities, there has been little impetus to use this drug in OHS particularly in view of potential side effects such as thromboembolic disease. Acetazolamide has the potential to counter the elevated bicarbonate levels that represent an important mechanism leading to OHS in patients with OSA. One randomized study is available trialing acetazolamide early in the course of mechanical ventilation in patients for either OHS or COPD and found no advantage in length of ventilatory support in these individuals.[103] Another trial of acetazolamide in 8 patients with OHS found a significant decrease in their plasma bicarbonate (31.6 $\pm$ 2.9 mmol/L at baseline), falling by 8.4 $\pm$ 3.0 mmol/L as well as a shift to the left of their ventilatory response to CO_2 curve; however, there was no change in the absolute value of ventilatory response to CO_2.[82] Further research with respect to using this drug in OHS does not appear to be a popular subject at this time.

Outcomes

Untreated, OHS increases morbidity and mortality when compared to individuals with only OSA. In one study, mortality in OHS was about 2 times that of individuals with OSA alone, predominantly due to cardiovascular causes.[104] A study examining the Danish National Patient Registry found that diabetes, hypertension, atrial fibrillation, congestive heart failure, COPD, and asthma were highly prevalent in the 3 years prior to a diagnosis of OHS.[105] OHS is commonly associated with type 3 pulmonary hypertension, which may persist after positive airway pressure treatment due to vascular remodeling.[106] Although after effective treatment, patients with OHS still carry the elevated risk of morbidity and mortality associated with remaining obese, there does exist a significant improvement in many outcomes. Of great relevance is a study of mortality in patients with OHS with and without OSA treated with NIV, which assessed mortality rates during a follow-up period of 12 years.[91] Overall mortality, despite NIV treatment, was 21.7%; no difference was found between participants with or without OSA. Mean survival time was 8.47 years. The only factor predicting survival was forced vital capacity (FVC), with higher FVC translating into longer survival.

SUMMARY

The unifying message conveyed in this article is that of hypoventilation complicating 2 prevalent disorders: COPD and OHS. The nuances of detecting hypoventilation are discussed, particularly with respect to alternatives to arterial puncture and blood gas analysis. COPD is a common cause of hypoventilation, as is OHS by definition. Both can respond to NIV, but both require additional treatment measures, particularly when they present to the inpatient service with acute on chronic hypoventilation. COPD is a distressingly common disease in our population, and obesity has become epidemic. Therefore, treating hypoventilation in both disorders will remain a common challenge for pulmonary and sleep medicine physicians. Home NIV may prove to be of advantage in patients with COPD as opposed to oxygen alone, but the evidence proving that NIV should routinely be prescribed is not yet mature. Achieving compliance with NIV therapy can be challenging. With respect to OHS, a high index of suspicion should be maintained when candidates for this disorder present themselves, and serum bicarbonate has proved to be helpful in this regard. Moreover, a high degree of clinical acumen is required to exclude other causes of hypoventilation and, when employing positive pressure therapy, to foster compliance with treatment. Major advances have been made in elucidating the pathogenesis of OHS when it is accompanied by moderate-to-severe OSA, but when OSA is not present or is quite mild, the mechanisms leading to ventilatory failure remain obscure. Both disorders can be difficult to manage for clinicians not familiar with the various modes of NIV or settings of HFNO. OHS continues to be a fascinating subject for research in control of breathing, respiratory physiology, and the practice of respiratory care.

CLINICS CARE POINTS

- Arterial puncture with blood gas analysis remains the most reliable tool for detecting hypercapnia and acid–base status. The use of $PvCO_2$ in the place of $Paco_2$ is discouraged.

- $PetCO_2$ and $PtcCO_2$ to estimate $Paco_2$ have limitations that must be understood. However, both are important tools for monitoring $Paco_2$ during sleep.

- Domiciliary LTOT remains the standard of care for patients with COPD and hypoxemia. COPD with hypoventilation will usually respond to NIV, but the question of adding NIV in patients with hypoxemia and hypercapnia remains unsettled.

- Treatment of OHS virtually always requires positive airway pressure therapy whether OSA is either present or not present. In many patients, CPAP rather than ventilatory support modalities will suffice.

DISCLOSURE

Dr L.K. Brown coedits the Sleep and Respiratory Neurobiology section of Current Opinion in Pulmonary Medicine and is a coauthor of an article on positive airway pressure treatment for OSA in UpToDate. Dr L.K. Brown is a member of the Council of the New Mexico Medical Society and serves on the Board of Trustees of the Greater Albuquerque Medical Association. He chairs the Polysomnography Practice Advisory Committee of the New Mexico Medical Board and chairs the New Mexico Advisory Board for Respiratory Care. Dr L.K. Brown chairs the Board of Directors of GAMA-PAC, the political action committee of the Greater Albuquerque Medical Association.

REFERENCES

1. Javaheri S, Shore NS, Rose B, et al. Compensatory hypoventilation in metabolic alkalosis. Chest 1982; 81:296–301.
2. Chung Y, Garden FL, Marks GB, et al. Causes of hypercapnic respiratory failure: a population-based case-control study. BMC Pulm Med 2023;23:347.
3. Chung Y, Garden FL, Marks GB, et al. Causes of hypercapnic respiratory failure and associated in-hospital mortality. Respirology 2023;28:176–82.
4. Diem K, Lentner C. Respiration. In: Scientific tables. Basel: CIBA-GEIGY limited; 1970. p. 545–570.
5. Grebstad JA, Svendsen L. Gulsvik. Precision of arterial blood gases and cutaneous oxygen saturation in healthy non-smokers. Scand J Clin Lab Invest 1989;49:265–8.
6. Byrne AL, Bennett M, Chatterji R, et al. Peripheral venous and arterial blood gas analysis in adults: are they comparable? A systematic review and meta-analysis. Respirology 2014;19:168–75.
7. Bloom BM, Grundlingh J, Bestwick JP, et al. The role of venous blood gas in the emergency department: a systematic review and meta-analysis. Eur J Emerg Med 2014;21:81–8.
8. Kelly A-M. Review article: Can venous blood gas analysis replace arterial in emergency medical care. Emerg Med Australas. 2010;22:493–8.
9. Lim BL, Kelly AM. A meta-analysis on the utility of peripheral venous blood gas analyses in exacerbations of chronic obstructive pulmonary disease in the emergency department. Eur J Emerg Med 2010;17:246–8.
10. Baba Y, Takatori F, Inoue M, et al. A novel mainstream capnometer system for non-invasive positive pressure ventilation. Annu Int Conf IEEE Eng Med Biol Soc. 2020;2020:4446–9.
11. Wahba RWM, Tessler MJ. Misleading end-tidal CO_2 tensions. Can J Anaesth 1996;43:862–6.
12. Eberhard P. The design, use, and results of transcutaneous carbon dioxide analysis: current and future directions. Anesth Analg 2007;105(6 Suppl):S48–52.
13. Aarrestad S, Tollefsen E, Kleiven AL, et al. Validity of transcutaneous PCO2 in monitoring chronic hypoventilation treated with non-invasive ventilation. Respir Med 2016;112:112–8.
14. Palmisano BW, Severinghaus JW. Transcutaneous PCO2 and PO2: a multicenter study of accuracy. J Clin Monit 1990;6:189–95.
15. Drechsler M, Morris J. Carbon dioxide narcosis. [Updated 2023 jan 9]. In: StatPearls [Internet]. Treasure Island (FL): StatPearls publishing. 2023. Available at: https://www.ncbi.nlm.nih.gov/books/NBK551620/. [Accessed 25 December 2023].
16. Aberegg SK, Carr J. Carbon dioxide Narcosis or sleep Deprivation? Ann Am Thorac Soc. 2019;16: 777.
17. Sieker HO. HickamJB. Carbon dioxide intoxication: the clinical syndrome, its etiology and management with particular reference to the use of mechanical respirators. Medicine (Baltimore). 1956; 35:389–423.
18. Almanza-Hurtado A, Polanco Guerra C, Martínez-Ávila MC, et al. Hypercapnia from Physiology to practice. Int J Clin Pract 2022;2022:2635616.

19. Pollock JM, Deibler AR, Whitlow CT, et al. Hypercapnia-induced cerebral hyperperfusion: an underrecognized clinical entity. AJNR Am J Neuroradiol 2009;30:378–85.

20. Tiruvoipati R, Pilcher D, Botha J, et al. Association of hypercapnia and hypercapnic acidosis with clinical outcomes in mechanically ventilated patients with cerebral injury. JAMA Neurol 2018;75:818–26.

21. Crystal GJ. Carbon Dioxide and the heart: Physiology and clinical Implications. Anesth Analg 2015;121:610–23.

22. Meservey AJ, Burton MC, Priest J, et al. Risk of readmission and mortality following hospitalization with hypercapnic respiratory failure. Lung 2020; 198:121–34.

23. Christenson SA. COPD phenotyping. Respir Care 2023;68:871–80.

24. McDonald VM, Holland AE. Treatable traits models of care. Respirology 2024;29:24–35.

25. Flenley DC. Sleep in chronic obstructive lung disease. Clin Chest Med 1985;6:651–61.

26. Adler D, Bailly S, Benmerad M, et al. Clinical presentation and comorbidities of obstructive sleep apnea-COPD overlap syndrome. PLoS One 2020; 15. e0235331.

27. Bednarek M, Plywaczewski R, Jonczak L, et al. There is no relationship between chronic obstructive pulmonary disease and obstructive sleep apnea syndrome: a population study. Respiration 2005;72:142–9.

28. Czerwaty K, Dżaman K, Sobczyk KM, et al. The overlap Syndrome of obstructive sleep Apnea and chronic obstructive pulmonary disease: a systematic review. Biomedicines 2022;11(1):16.

29. van Zeller M, Basoglu OK, Verbraecken J, et al. European Sleep Apnoea Database study group. Sleep and cardiometabolic comorbidities in the obstructive sleep apnoea-COPD overlap syndrome: data from the European Sleep Apnoea Database. ERJ Open Res. 2023;9(3):00676–2022.

30. Bradley TD, Rutherford R, Lue F, et al. Role of diffuse airway obstruction in the hypercapnia of obstructive sleep apnea. Am Rev Respir Dis 1986;134:920–4.

31. Fletcher EC, Shah A, Qian W, et al. "Near miss" death in obstructive sleep apnea: a critical care syndrome. Crit Care Med 1991;19:1158–64.

32. Gothi D, Gupta SS, Kumar N, et al. Impact of overlap syndrome on severity of acute exacerbation of chronic obstructive pulmonary disease. Lung India 2015;32:578–83.

33. Marin JM, Soriano JB, Carrizo SJ, et al. Outcomes in patients with chronic obstructive pulmonary disease and obstructive sleep apnea: the overlap syndrome. Am J Respir Crit Care Med 2010;182: 325–31.

34. Report of the Medical Research Council Working Party. Long term domiciliary oxygen therapy in chronic hypoxic cor pulmonale complicating chronic bronchitis and emphysema. Lancet 1981;1:681–6.

35. Nocturnal Oxygen Therapy Trial Group. Continuous or nocturnal oxygen therapy in hypoxemic chronic obstructive lung disease: a clinical trial. Ann Intern Med 1980;93:391–8.

36. Oswald-Mammosser M, Weitzenblum E, Quoix E, et al. Prognostic factors in COPD patients receiving long-term oxygen therapy. Importance of pulmonary artery pressure. Chest 1995;107:1193–8.

37. Aida A, Miyamoto K, Nishimura M, et al. Prognostic value of hypercapnia in patients with chronic respiratory failure during long-term oxygen therapy. Am J Respir Crit Care Med 1998;158:188–93.

38. Wijkstra PJ, Lacasse Y, Guyatt GH. A meta-analysis of nocturnal noninvasive positive pressure ventilation in patients with stable COPD. Chest 2003; 124:337–43.

39. Liao H, Pei W, Li H, et al. Efficacy of long-term noninvasive positive pressure ventilation in stable hypercapnic COPD patients with respiratory failure: a meta-analysis of randomized controlled trials. Int J Chron Obstruct Pulmon Dis 2017;12: 2977–85.

40. Struik FM, Lacasse Y, Goldstein RS, et al. Nocturnal noninvasive positive pressure ventilation in stable COPD: a systematic review and individual patient data meta-analysis. Respir Med 2014;108:329–37.

41. Raveling T, Vonk J, Struik FM, et al. Chronic noninvasive ventilation for chronic obstructive pulmonary disease. Cochrane Database Syst Rev 2021; 8:CD002878.

42. Wu Z, Luo Z, Luo Z, et al. Baseline level and reduction in PaCO2 are associated with the treatment effect of long-term home noninvasive positive pressure ventilation in stable hypercapnic patients with COPD: a systematic review and meta-analysis of randomized controlled trials. Int J Chronic Obstr Pulm Dis 2022;17:719–33.

43. Macrea M, Oczkowski S, Rochwerg B, et al. Long-term noninvasive Ventilation in chronic stable hypercapnic chronic obstructive pulmonary disease. An Official American Thoracic Society clinical practice guideline. Am J Respir Crit Care Med 2020; 202(4):e74–87.

44. Dysart K, Miller TL, Wolfson MR, et al. Research in high flow therapy: mechanisms of action. Respir Med 2009;103:1400–5.

45. Bonnevie T, Elkins M, Paumier C, et al. Nasal high Flow for stable Patients with chronic obstructive pulmonary disease: a systematic Review and meta-analysis. COPD 2019;16:368–77.

46. Yang H, Huang D, Luo J, et al. The use of high-flow nasal cannula in patients with chronic obstructive pulmonary disease under exacerbation and stable phases: a systematic review and meta-analysis. Heart Lung 2023;60:116–26.

47. Zhang L, Wang Y, Ye Y, et al. Comparison of high-flow nasal Cannula with conventional oxygen Therapy in Patients with hypercapnic chronic obstructive pulmonary disease: a systematic Review and meta-analysis. Int J Chron Obstruct Pulmon Dis. 2023;18: 895–906.

48. Mitsui K, Kurokawa Y, Kaiwa Y, et al. Thoracoscopic lung volume reduction surgery for pulmonary emphysema patients with severe hypercapnia. Jpn J Thorac Cardiovasc Surg 2001;49:481–8.

49. Shade D Jr, Cordova F, Lando Y, et al. Relationship between resting hypercapnia and physiologic parameters before and after lung volume reduction surgery in severe chronic obstructive pulmonary disease. Am J Respir Crit Care Med 1999;159:1405–11.

50. National Emphysema Treatment Trial Research Group. A randomized trial comparing lung-volume-reduction surgery with medical therapy for severe emphysema. N Engl J Med 2003;348:2059–73.

51. Tiong LU, Davies R, Gibson PG, et al. Lung volume reduction surgery for diffuse emphysema. Cochrane Database Syst Rev 2006;(4):CD001001.

52. World Health Organization. Obesity: preventing and managing the global epidemic. Report of a WHO consultation. World Health Organ Tech Rep Ser 2000;894:1–253.

53. American Academy of Sleep Medicine. International classification of sleep disorders, 3rd ed-TR. Darien, IL: American Academy of Sleep Medicine; 2023.

54. Burwell CS, Robin ED, Whaley RD, et al. Extreme obesity associated with alveolar hypoventilation - a Pickwickian syndrome. Am J Med 1956;21:811–8.

55. Dickens C. The posthumous papers of the Pickwick Club. London: Chapman & Hall, 1837.

56. Fothergill J. Case of an angina pectoris. In: Elliot J, ed. Complete Collection of the Medical and Philosophical works. London: John Walker; 1781:525.

57. Carroll D. Nosology of "Pickwickian syndrome." Bull Physiopathol Respir 1972;8:1241–7.

58. Rapoport DM. Obesity hypoventilation syndrome: More than just severe sleep apnea. Sleep Med Rev 2011;15:77–8.

59. Hales CM, Carroll MD, Fryar CD, et al. Prevalence of obesity and severe obesity among adults: United States, 2017–2018. NCHS Data Brief, no 360. Hyattsville, MD: National Center for Health Statistics; 2020.

60. Mokhlesi B. Obesity hypoventilation syndrome: a state of the art review. Respir Care 2010;55:1347–62.

61. Balachandran JS, Masa JF, Mokhlesi B. Obesity hypoventilation syndrome epidemiology and diagnosis. Sleep Med Clin 2014;9:341–7.

62. Chan R, Lipworth B. Clinical impact of obesity on oscillometry lung mechanics in adults with asthma. Ann Allergy Asthma Immunol 2023;131:338–42.

63. Parasuaraman G, Ayyasamy L, Aune D, et al. The association between body mass index, abdominal fatness, and weight change and the risk of adult asthma: a systematic review and meta-analysis of cohort studies. Sci Rep 2023;13:7745.

64. Leech J, Onal E, Aronson R, et al. Voluntary hyperventilation in obesity hypoventilation. Chest 1991; 100:1334–8.

65. Holley HS, Milic-Emili J, Becklake MR, et al. Regional distribution of pulmonary ventilation and perfusion in obesity. J Clin Invest 1967;46:475–81, 49.

66. Barrera F, Reidenberg MM, Winters WL, et al. Ventilation-perfusion relationships in the obese patient. J Appl Physiol 1969;26:420–6.

67. Rivas E, Arismendi E, Agustí A, et al. Ventilation/ Perfusion distribution abnormalities in morbidly obese subjects before and after bariatric surgery. Chest 2015;147:1127–34.

68. Farebrother MJ, McHardy GJ, Munro JF. Relation between pulmonary gas exchange and closing volume before and after substantial weight loss in obese subjects. Br Med J 1974;3:391–3.

69. Hedenstierna G, Santesson J, Norlander O. Airway closure and distribution of inspired gas in the extremely obese, breathing spontaneously and during anaesthesia with intermittent positive pressure ventilation. Acta Anaesthesiol Scand 1976;20:334–42.

70. Jokic R, Zintel T, Sridhar G, et al. Ventilatory responses to hypercapnia and hypoxia in relatives of patients with the obesity hypoventilation syndrome. Thorax 2000;55:940–5.

71. Javaheri S, Colangelo G, Corser B, et al. Familial respiratory chemosensitivity does not predict hypercapnia of patients with sleep apnea-hypopnea syndrome. Am Rev Respir Dis 1992;145:837–40.

72. Auchincloss JH Jr, Cook E, Renzetti AD. Clinical and physiological aspects of a case of obesity, polycythemia and alveolar hypoventilation. J Clin Invest 1955;34:1537–45.

73. Masa JF, Pépin JL, Borel JC, et al. Sánchez-Quiroga MÁ. Obesity hypoventilation syndrome. Eur Respir Rev 2019;28(151):180097.

74. Rapoport DM, Garay SM, Epstein H, et al. Hypercapnia in the obstructive sleep apnea syndrome. A reevaluation of the "Pickwickian syndrome". Chest 1986;89:627–35.

75. Rapoport DM, Norman RG, Goldring RM. CO2 homeostasis during periodic breathing: predictions from a computer model. J Appl Physiol 1993;75: 2302–9.

76. Berger KI, Ayappa I, Sorkin IB, et al. CO2 homeostasis during periodic breathing in obstructive sleep apnea. J Appl Physiol 2000;88:257–64.

77. Berger KI, Ayappa I, Sorkin IB, et al. Postevent ventilation as a function of CO(2) load during respiratory events in obstructive sleep apnea. J Appl Physiol 2002;93:917–24.

78. Ayappa I, Berger KI, Norman RG, et al. Hypercapnia and ventilatory periodicity in obstructive sleep

apnea syndrome. Am J Respir Crit Care Med 2002; 166:1112–5.

79. Berger KI, Ayappa I, Chatr-Amontri B, et al. Obesity hypoventilation syndrome as a spectrum of respiratory disturbances during sleep. Chest 2001;120:1231–8.

80. Norman RG, Goldring RM, Clain JM, et al. Transition from acute to chronic hypercapnia in patients with periodic breathing: predictions from a computer model. J Appl Physiol 2006;100:1733–41.

81. Javaheri S, Simbarti LA. Respiratory determinants of diurnal hypercapnia in obesity hypoventilation syndrome what does weight have to do with it? Ann Am Thorac Soc. 2014;11:945–50.

82. Raurich JM, Rialp G, Ibáñez J, et al. Hypercapnic respiratory failure in obesity-hypoventilation syndrome: CO_2 response and acetazolamide treatment effects. Respir Care 2010;55:1442–8.

83. Oren A, Whipp BJ, Wasserman K. Effects of chronic acid-base changes on the rebreathing hypercapnic ventilatory response in man. Respiration 1991;58:181–5.

84. Carroll D. Pickwickian syndrome, 20 years later. Trans Am Clin Climatol Assoc 1975;86:112–27.

85. Tankersley CG, O'Donnell C, Daood MJ. Leptin attenuates respiratory complications associated with the obese phenotype. J Appl Physiol 1998;85: 2261–9.

86. Ryan S, Crinion SJ, McNicholas WT. Obesity and sleep-disordered breathing-when two 'bad guys' meet. Q J Med 2014;107:949–54.

87. Campo A, Frühbeck G, Zulueta JJ, et al. Hyperleptinaemia, respiratory drive and hypercapnic response in obese patients. Eur Respir J 2007;30:223–31.

88. Pillar G, Shehadeh N. Abdominal fat and sleep apnea: the chicken or the egg? Diabetes Care 2008; 2(7):S303–9, 31 Suppl.

89. Mokhlesi B, Tulaimat A, Faibussowitsch I, et al. Obesity hypoventilation syndrome: prevalence and predictors in patients with obstructive sleep apnea. Sleep Breath 2007;11:117–24.

90. Sullivan CE, Berthon-Jones M, Issa FG. Remission of severe obesity-hypoventilation syndrome after short-term treatment during sleep with nasal continuous positive airway pressure. Am Rev Respir Dis 1983;128:177–81.

91. Ojeda Castillejo E, de Lucas Ramos P, Martin SL. Noninvasive mechanical ventilation in patients with obesity hypoventilation syndrome. Long-term outcome and prognostic factors. Arch Bronconeumol 2015;51:61–8.

92. Howard ME, Piper AJ, Stevens B, et al. A randomised controlled trial of CPAP versus noninvasive ventilation for initial treatment of obesity hypoventilation syndrome. Thorax 2017;72:437–44.

93. Masa JF, Corral J, Alonso ML. Efficacy and different treatment alternatives for obesity hypoventilation syndrome: Pickwick study. Am J Respir Crit Care Med 2015;192:86–95.

94. Afshar M, Brozek JL, Soghier I, et al. The Role of positive airway pressure Therapy in Adults with obesity hypoventilation syndrome. A systematic Review and meta-analysis. Ann Am Thorac Soc. 2020;17:344–60.

95. Soghier I, Brozek JL, Afshar M, et al. Noninvasive Ventilation versus CPAP as Initial Treatment of Obesity Hypoventilation Syndrome. An Am Throac Soc 2019;16:1295–303.

96. Iftikhar IH, Greer M, Wigger GW, et al. A network meta-analysis of different positive airway pressure interventions in obesity hypoventilation syndrome. J Sleep Res 2021;30:e13158.

97. Martí-Valeri C, Sabaté A, Masdevall C, et al. Improvement of associated respiratory problems in morbidly obese patients after open Roux-en-Y gastric bypass. Obes Surg 2007;17:1102–10.

98. Carrano FM, Iossa A, Di Lorenzo N, et al. EAES Bariatric Surgery Guidelines Group. EAES rapid guideline: systematic review, network meta-analysis, CINeMA and GRADE assessment, and European consensus on bariatric surgery-extension 2022. Surg Endosc 2022;36:1709–25.

99. Kent D, Stanley J, Aurora RN, et al. Referral of adults with obstructive sleep apnea for surgical consultation: an American Academy of Sleep Medicine systematic review, meta-analysis, and GRADE assessment. J Clin Sleep Med 2021;17:2507–31.

100. Kakazu MT, Soghier I, Afshar M, et al. Weight loss Interventions as Treatment of obesity hypoventilation syndrome. A systematic review. Ann Am Thorac Soc. 2020;17:492–502.

101. McKenzie R, Wadhwa RK. Progesterone for the Pickwickian syndrome: respiratory implications: a case report Anesth Analg 1977;56:133–5.

102. Sutton FD Jr, Zwillich CW, Creagh CE, et al. Progesterone for outpatient treatment of Pickwickian syndrome. Ann Intern Med 1975;83:476–9.

103. Rialp Cervera G, Raurich Puigdevall JM, Chorro JM, et al. Effects of early administration of acetazolamide on the duration of mechanical ventilation in patients with chronic obstructive pulmonary disease or obesity-hypoventilation syndrome with metabolic alkalosis. A randomized trial. Pulm Pharmacol Ther 2017;44:30–7.

104. Castro-Anon O, Perez de Llano LA, De la Fuente Sanchez S, et al. Obesity-hypoventilation syndrome: Increased risk of death over sleep apnea syndrome. PLoS One 2015;10(2). e0117808.

105. Jennum P, Ibsen R, Kjellberg J. Morbidity prior to a diagnosis of sleep-disordered breathing: a controlled national study. J Clin Sleep Med 2013;9:103–8.

106. Kauppert CA, Dvorak I, Kollert F, et al. Pulmonary hypertension in obesity-hypoventilation syndrome. Respir Med 2013;107:2061–70.

Dyspnea and Quality of Life Improvements with Management of Comorbid Obstructive Sleep Apnea in Chronic Lung Disease

Kori Ascher, DO, Shirin Shafazand, MD, MS, ATSF*

KEYWORDS

- Overlap syndrome • OSA • Asthma • COPD • Interstitial lung disease • Health-related quality of life
- Positive airway pressure therapy • Patient-reported health outcomes

KEY POINTS

- The co-existence of obstructive sleep apnea (OSA) and chronic lung disease, "overlap syndromes," (COPD, asthma, and interstitial lung disease) has been associated with worse patient-reported outcomes (sleep quality, quality of life measures, mental health) than each condition occurring independently.
- Observational studies suggest that patients with overlap syndrome who are adherent to positive airway pressure therapy report improved quality of life and daytime symptoms.
- Randomized controlled trials are needed to solidify the growing observational evidence that supports the early diagnosis and management of OSA in patients with chronic lung disease.

INTRODUCTION

Obstructive sleep apnea (OSA) has emerged as a significant and prevalent comorbidity associated with chronic respiratory diseases, including chronic obstructive pulmonary disease (COPD), asthma, and interstitial lung diseases (ILDs). The term "overlap syndrome" encompasses the concurrent presence of chronic respiratory disease and OSA within the same individual. While these overlap syndromes have historically been understudied, emerging data underscore their association with increased morbidity and mortality compared to either condition in isolation.

Health-related quality of life (HRQOL) is a multidimensional self-report of an individual's perception of their functioning and well-being in physical, mental, and social domains of life.[1] It is considered one of the most important patient-centered outcomes and included in clinical trials as a valuable clinical endpoint. Individually, chronic lung disease[2–4] and OSA[5,6] have each been associated with impairments in HRQOL. In this article, we will discuss the best evidence, to date, for treatment of co-morbid OSA in the setting of chronic lung disease and the potential impact on HRQOL and dyspnea.

CHRONIC OBSTRUCTIVE PULMONARY DISEASE AND OBSTRUCTIVE SLEEP APNEA
Prevalence

The term "overlap syndrome (OS)," referring to the co-existence of COPD and OSA in an individual patient was initially described by Flenley[7] and now has extended to include overlap with other chronic lung diseases. The prevalence of COPD and OSA overlap varies according to the population studied and diagnostic criteria used but is

Division of Pulmonary, Critical Care, and Sleep Medicine, University of Miami, Miller School of Medicine
* Corresponding author. Division of Pulmonary, Critical Care, and Sleep Medicine (D-60), University of Miami, Miller School of Medicine, (D-60), PO Box 016960, Miami, FL 33101.
E-mail address: sshafazand@med.miami.edu

Sleep Med Clin 19 (2024) 371–378
https://doi.org/10.1016/j.jsmc.2024.02.013
1556-407X/24/© 2024 Published by Elsevier Inc.

estimated to range from 1.0% to 3.6% in the general population, according to a systematic review.[8] Notably, several studies have demonstrated a significantly higher prevalence of OSA in patients diagnosed with COPD and vice versa, compared to the general population. Specifically, the prevalence of OSA in COPD patients is estimated to range from 2.9% to 65.9%,[9] while the prevalence of COPD in patients with OSA ranges from 7.6% to 55.7%.[10]

Health-Related Quality of Life in Obstructive Sleep Apnea and Chronic Obstructive Pulmonary Disease

Given that both OSA and COPD have independently been associated with impairments in HRQOL[6,11,12] and increased global economic burden.[13,14] It is likely then that the co-existence of the 2 diagnoses will lead to greater impairments in physical domains of HRQOL, and worse daytime functioning.[15] Indeed existing evidence from observational studies confirm that in COPD patients with moderate resting or exertional desaturation and with intermediate-to-high risk of OSA, there is an increased risk of hospitalization and higher mortality.[16,17] COPD exacerbations are increased in OSA patients compared with COPD alone and patients report worsened quality of life in both COPD- specific and generic measures of HRQOL.[18]This suggests a potential role for the early diagnosis and management of OSA in COPD patients with the aim of reducing symptoms of OSA, decreasing the frequency of COPD exacerbations, and improving overall HRQOL.

Obstructive Sleep Apnea Therapy and Its Impact on Patient-Reported Outcomes

Positive airway pressure (PAP) remains the mainstay of therapy for moderate and severe OSA. However, while observational studies have shed some light on the potential benefits of PAP in patients with overlap syndrome, there is a paucity of high-quality randomized controlled trials (RCTs) supporting the role of PAP therapy in improving objective and subjective outcomes in overlap syndrome, including HRQOL and dyspnea.

In a small study of 24 hospitalized patients with COPD exacerbation, early recognition and treatment of OSA was associated with reduced 6-month hospital readmission rates and emergency room visits for those patients who were adherent to PAP therapy.[19] Observational studies additionally suggest that patients with COPD who are adherent to PAP have reduced COPD exacerbation rates,[20,21] improved arterial blood gases,[9] 6-minute walk results,[21,22] values of forced expiratory volume in 1 second (FEV1),[21,23] respiratory muscle strength, exercise capacity, and mean pulmonary artery pressures.[24] These physiologic improvements will likely translate to better HRQOL and less dyspnea, although patient-reported outcomes were not specifically measured in most studies.

ASTHMA AND OBSTRUCTIVE SLEEP APNEA
Prevalence

Asthma and OSA have a bi-directional relationship with the prevalence of OSA in asthmatic patients estimated at 50% in a meta-analysis of 26 studies and the odds of having OSA 2.6 times higher in asthmatic patients than non-asthmatic patients.[25] Teodorescu and colleagues reported an increased incidence of OSA among subjects with asthma in the Wisconsin Sleep Cohort Study during 4-year follow-up, while asthma duration increased the OSA risk in a dose-dependent manner.[26] Furthermore, as the severity of asthma increases, so does the likelihood of coexisting sleep apnea. In a small observational study, the prevalence of OSA was 88% in patients with severe asthma and 58% in those with moderate asthma.[27]

Ostructive Sleep Apnea and Its Impact on Asthma Symptoms, Lung Function, and Health-Related Quality of Life

Untreated sleep apnea can contribute to poor asthma control, making sleep health a pivotal factor to consider routinely in the management of asthma. In a study, patients with asthma who were identified as high-risk for sleep apnea or had been diagnosed with OSA were significantly more likely to report daytime asthma symptoms.[28]

An analysis of National Health Nutrition Examination Survey (NHANES) data found that patients with asthma are significantly more likely to sleep less than 6 hours compared to those without asthma.[29] Using NHANES data, Luyster and colleagues[30] reported that asthmatics with short sleep duration and poor sleep quality are 1.5 times more likely to experience asthma attacks, daytime or nighttime symptoms, and have worse HRQOL scores compared to those with normal sleep duration. Independent of its association with asthma, OSA has been associated with fragmented sleep and poor sleep quality making it a likely risk factor for worsened quality of life in asthmatic patients. Indeed, several cross-sectional studies have shown a correlation between OSA diagnosis and reduced quality of life, increased exacerbation rates, and poor asthma control.[31]

There may be a physiologic basis to the worsening daytime symptoms noted in asthmatic patients with untreated sleep apnea as they often experience an accelerated annual decline in FEV1, an important measure of lung function and daytime asthma symptoms.[32]

Obstructive Sleep Apnea Therapy and Its Impact on Patient-Reported Outcomes

The use of PAP has been associated with improved daytime and nighttime asthma symptoms, decrease in the use of rescue bronchodilators, decreased frequency of exacerbations, and improvements in quality of life.[33] In addition, there appears to be a dose-dependent improvement in asthma control and asthma-related quality of life with the biggest impact in patients with moderate-severe persistent asthma or severe OSA (respiratory disturbance index > 30)[33,34]

While PAP therapy's primary purpose is to treat sleep apnea, there is a multifaceted impact on asthmatic patient-reported outcomes. Effective sleep apnea treatment reduces intermittent nocturnal hypoxia, dramatic swings in intrathoracic pressure, and arousal index. The aforementioned factors improved by PAP are individually known triggers of asthma attacks and symptoms.[30,35,36] The reduction of these events through PAP therapy may lead to a decrease in the frequency and severity of asthma attacks. It is likely then that implementation of treatment for sleep apnea, a treatment that improves sleep quality and lung mechanics, will improve asthma exacerbations and HRQOL scores.

There have been no RCTs supporting the observational and physiologic data reviewed herein. **Table 1** summarizes the key studies that provide the evidence base in support of OSA screening and treatment for asthma patients to date. Kauppi and colleagues demonstrated a significant decrease in the use of rescue inhalers in asthmatics after initiating PAP therapy[37] suggesting that PAP therapy has a positive impact on the overall management of asthma that extends beyond nighttime asthma symptoms. Similarly, Teodorescu, and colleagues found that patient self-reported daytime asthma symptoms significantly improved with PAP compared to baseline.[28] In a prospective cohort study following ninety-nine uncontrolled asthmatic patients who received 6-month PAP therapy, the prevalence of uncontrolled asthmatics significantly decreased from 41% to 17%. This finding may in part be related to the significant improvement that was also noted in secondary outcomes including gastroesophageal reflux and rhinitis symptoms in patients using PAP therapy.[33]

Nocturnal symptoms pose unique challenges to asthmatic patients. In a small study of 9 asthmatic patients, Chan and colleagues[38] demonstrated an association between OSA and nocturnal asthma symptoms and noted that PAP therapy was effective in reducing nocturnal asthma attacks, a valuable insight into improving asthma-related clinical outcomes. Other observational studies have shown similar improvements in nocturnal symptoms post PAP therapy.[39] Frequency of reported nocturnal asthma symptoms leading to poor sleep quality is correlated with patient reports of worsening quality of life.[40] Reduction in nocturnal asthma attacks achieved with PAP therapy likely plays a role in overall improvement of HRQOL.

Impact of Positive Airway Pressure Therapy on Lung Function in Asthmatics with Obstructive Sleep Apnea

In a retrospective study of 77 patients with asthma who had 5 years of follow-up data, asthmatic patients with severe OSA, adherent to PAP therapy, showed a significant reduction in the rate of decline of FEV1; the annual FEV1 decline rate reduced from 69 mL per year to 41 mL per year.[32] Other studies with shorter follow-up time (weeks to months) have not demonstrated improvement in lung function when compared to baseline.[34,39] Results, while promising, should be interpreted with caution and require additional prospective studies and randomized trials. It is possible that the impact of PAP on the rate of FEV1 decline cannot be detected in a short time interval and several years of consistent PAP use are needed to detect a significant difference.

Positive Airway Pressure Therapy and Health-Related Quality of Life in Asthma Patients with Comorbid Sleep Apnea

Several studies have explored the relationship between asthma control, OSA, and overall quality of life (see **Table 1**). Studies vary by the questionnaires used, sample size, and duration of PAP therapy and are observational in nature. The asthma control test (ACT) has been used as a surrogate for evaluating quality of life in asthma patients. In a study involving approximately 5,600 asthmatic individuals, a higher score on the ACT was associated with improved physical and mental health-related quality of life.[41] This correlation translated to reduced emergency room visits and health care costs for well-controlled asthmatics. Studies with small sample sizes have shown an improvement in ACT in patients with asthma and co-morbid OSA.[37] In a systematic review of 12 quasi-experimental and observational

Table 1
Key studies evaluating patient-reported outcomes in treatment of asthma-obstructive sleep apnea overlap

Study	Design and Outcomes Studied	Patients	Key Findings	Limitations
Ng, et al,[43] 2018	RCT; CPAP vs conservative therapy; single center; 3-mo follow-up; primary outcome: ACT; secondary outcomes: ESS, AQLQ, Short Form (SF-36)	37 patients with uncontrolled nocturnal asthma symptoms and AHI ≥10/h on PSG; 17 received CPAP and 10 in control group	No significant change in ACT score; significant improvement in secondary outcomes: ESS, AQLQ score, and vitality domain of SF-36 after 3 mo of CPAP	Single center; small sample size
Davies et al,[42] 2018	Systematic review of 12 quasi-experimental and observational studies with a mean 19.5 wk of CPAP use; outcomes evaluated: AQLQ, ACT, forced expiratory volume in 1 second (FEV1), nocturnal and daytime symptoms	*Asthma-specific quality of life studies* n=119 from 2 studies combined, including mild to severe persistent asthma with moderate to severe obstructive sleep apnea (OSA) treated with CPAP. *Asthma symptoms and control* (n=515 from 9 studies). Studies measured different outcomes and varied in sample size, asthma and OSA severity, duration of CPAP use *Lung Function* n = 242 from 5 studies	Significant improvement in AQLQ Most studies showed a significant improvement in ACT, nocturnal symptoms, and asthma exacerbation rates No significant changes noted in FEV1 pre and post variable duration of CPAP use in a meta-analysis	Observational studies; varying duration of treatment and CPAP adherence; heterogeneous asthma population; a high risk of bias due to confounding was present in at least 4/12 studies with unclear evidence in 3/12
Teodorescu et al,[28] 2012	Cross-sectional: historical diagnosis of OSA, some with PSG, physician-diagnosed asthma; daytime asthma symptoms reported	n = 132 with OSA, 75 on CPAP	Improvement in daytime symptom reports for those on CPAP	Cross-sectional: CPAP adherence not reported

Abbreviations: ACT, asthma control test, a survey instrument to assess asthma control; AHI, apnea hypopnea index; AQLQ, asthma quality of life questionnaire; CPAP, continuous positive airway pressure; ESS, epworth sleepiness score; PSG, polysomnography; RCT, randomized controlled trial.

studies with a mean 19.5 weeks of PAP use, Davies and colleagues[42] report an overall improvement in quality-of-life measures in asthma patients using PAP for sleep apnea treatment. In the only RCT published to date, using intention-to-treat analysis among 37 patients with apnea hypopnea index (AHI) $\geq$10/h (17 patients in continuous positive airway pressure [CPAP] group vs 20 patients in control group), there was no significant difference in ACT score but those who received CPAP reported a significant improvement in daytime sleepiness, asthma quality of life questionnaire scores, and the vitality domain in the SF-36 questionnaire after 3 months of follow-up. Patients randomized into CPAP group used CPAP for an average of 5 hours at 3 months, with 70.5% of the participants using CPAP for more than 4 hours/day.[43]

OSA is prevalent in patients with asthma, especially in those with severe asthma. Untreated OSA has been associated with asthma exacerbations, poorly controlled nighttime symptoms, and worse quality of life. The treatment of sleep apnea using PAP therapy has a dual purpose in asthmatic patients: improving sleep quality and enhancing asthma-specific measures thereby improving overall HRQOL. Effective management of obstructive sleep apnea in asthmatics with PAP therapy should emphasize the interconnected nature of these 2 conditions and the positive impact that such management can have on patients' well-being and overall health. More research is needed in understanding the magnitude of improvement in asthma control, quality of life and possibly even lung function, whether other OSA treatment modalities are just as effective, and the duration of therapy needed to bring about improvements.

INTERSTITIAL LUNG DISEASE AND OBSTRUCTIVE SLEEP APNEA
Prevalence

ILDs are a large and heterogeneous group of restrictive lung disorders with significant impact on patient health outcomes and quality of life. Studies have suggested that one of the most common comorbidities associated with ILD is OSA.[44,45] Prevalence estimates range from 28% to 88% with the best estimate from a meta-analysis of 11 studies closer to 61%.[44] Lee and colleagues[46] observed a higher prevalence of OSA at 64.9% in a subgroup of idiopathic pulmonary fibrosis (IPF) patients compared to the 53.5% prevalence in the overall ILD study cohort. Similarly, the study by Pereira and colleagues[47] focused on patients with ILD and BMI less than

30 with an 83.3% prevalence of OSA in the IPF subgroup, surpassing the 68% prevalence in the broader ILD group.

Sarcoidosis, characterized by unique pathophysiological features, poses an increased risk of OSA, particularly in patients with granulomatous involvement of the upper airway, known as sarcoidosis of the upper airway (SURT). Baughman and colleagues[48] indicated that SURT may elevate the risk of OSA, and sarcoidosis patients with pulmonary involvement are significantly more likely to have coexisting OSA, with a reported prevalence of 88.2% in cases with lung involvement.[49]

Health-Related Quality of Life in Obstructive Sleep Apnea and Interstitial Lung Disease

Most studies evaluating HRQOL have predominantly focused on IPF or sarcoidosis with comorbid OSA. Mavroudi, and colleagues[50] studied 19 patients with IPF, and 21 patients with sarcoidosis stage II/III. They were compared with 15 healthy subjects. More than 70% of the chronic lung disease population was diagnosed with OSA. The participants with IPF or sarcoidosis reported worsened HRQOL (measured by SF-36) especially in the physical domain compared to healthy controls. Worse HRQOL scores were positively correlated with OSA severity measures. In a study of 34 patients with IPF who were not using supplemental oxygen, 50% of the patients with co-morbid OSA reported a reduced quality of life (measured by St. George Respiratory Questionnaire [SGRQ]) with the impairment significantly worse in patients with co-morbid OSA and nocturnal hypoxemia. In the stepwise multiple regression analysis, 75% of SGRQ score variability was significantly predicted by values of forced vital capacity % and diffusion capacity, sleep quality, and daytime sleepiness.[51] These findings underscore the important role that sleep quality and sleep apnea in particular play in the quality of life of IPF patients.

Positive Airway Pressure Therapy and Health-Related Quality of Life in Interstitial Lung Disease Patients with Comorbid Sleep Apnea

PAP therapy has been associated with improvements in HRQOL in IPF patients with OSA. In a study of 60 patients with IPF and OSA who were offered PAP therapy and followed for 1 year, the group with good PAP adherence (37 patients) showed statistically significant improvement in all quality-of-life measures, fatigue, daytime sleepiness, and sleep quality. The non-adherent group, however, did not show any consistent improvement in quality of life.[52] In another study of 45 participants, the 38 patients with IPF OSA overlap reported more severe functional impairments in the General Health component of the Short Form (SF)-36 life questionnaire. At 7-year follow-up, patients with more than 6 hours of PAP use had better survival compared with patients who were less adherent; significant improvement was observed in measures of sleepiness, fatigue, depression scores, and sleep quality. However, there was no statistically significant difference noted in quality-of-life measures (SF-36 questionnaire) regardless of PAP adherence.[53]

Other therapies, such as positional therapy, supplemental oxygen, and oral appliances, have not yet been studied in ILD and IPF patients with OSA. The bulk of the evidence to date, albeit more concentrated on IPF, highlights the prevalence of OSA as a co-morbidity and provides valuable insights into the impact of OSA treatment on the overall well-being of ILD patients. The studies, despite variations in methodologies and small sample size, demonstrate mostly positive patient-reported outcomes associated with OSA treatment with PAP. Further research, including well-designed RCTs that recruit subtypes of ILD and larger sample sizes are needed to better understand the role of OSA treatment on patient morbidity and mortality.

CLINICS CARE POINTS

- OSA is a prevalent condition in patients with chronic lung disease but is underdiagnosed.

- The co-existence of OSA and chronic lung disease, "overlap syndromes," is associated with worse patient-reported outcomes (sleep quality, quality of life measures, mental health) than each condition independently.

- Observational studies suggest that patients with overlap syndrome who are adherent to PAP therapy report improved quality of life, sleep quality, depression, and daytime symptoms.

- There may be an improvement in lung function in asthmatic and COPD patients with co-morbid OSA who are adherent to PAP therapy.

- There may be a reduction in COPD and asthma exacerbations and hospitalizations in those adherent to PAP therapy.

- Much of what is known to date about the impact of OSA treatment on patient-reported outcomes in chronic lung disease is from single center, observational studies with a small number of participants.

- There is a paucity of studies on the benefits of other OSA treatment modalities in patients who are unable to tolerate PAP therapy.

- RCTs are needed to solidify the growing observational evidence base that supports the early diagnosis and management of OSA in patients with chronic lung disease.

REFERENCES

1. Kaplan RM, Hays RD. Health-related quality of life measurement in public health. Annu Rev Publ Health 2022;43:355–73.
2. Collaborators GBDCRD. Global burden of chronic respiratory diseases and risk factors, 1990-2019: an update from the Global Burden of Disease Study 2019. EClinicalMedicine 2023;59:101936.
3. Kushwaha S, Singh SK, Manar M, et al. Health-related quality of life of chronic obstructive pulmonary disease patients: a hospital-based study. J Fam Med Prim Care 2020;9:4074–8.
4. Swigris JJ, Andrae DA, Churney T, et al. Development and initial validation analyses of the living with idiopathic pulmonary fibrosis questionnaire. Am J Respir Crit Care Med 2020;202:1689–97.
5. Krishnan S, Chai-Coetzer CL, Grivell N, et al. Comorbidities and quality of life in Australian men and women with diagnosed and undiagnosed high-risk obstructive sleep apnea. J Clin Sleep Med 2022; 18:1757–67.
6. Pierobon A, Vigore M, Taurino E, et al. Subjective HRQoL in patients with sleep apnea syndrome who underwent PAP therapy in a rehabilitation setting: a longitudinal study. J Clin Med 2023;12.
7. Flenley DC. Sleep in chronic obstructive lung disease. Clin Chest Med 1985;6:651–61.
8. Shawon MS, Perret JL, Senaratna CV, et al. Current evidence on prevalence and clinical outcomes of co-morbid obstructive sleep apnea and chronic obstructive pulmonary disease: a systematic review. Sleep Med Rev 2017;32:58–68.
9. Schreiber A, Cemmi F, Ambrosino N, et al. Prevalence and predictors of obstructive sleep apnea in patients with chronic obstructive pulmonary disease undergoing inpatient pulmonary rehabilitation. COPD 2018;15:265–70.
10. Lacedonia D, Carpagnano GE, Patricelli G, et al. Prevalence of comorbidities in patients with obstructive sleep apnea syndrome, overlap syndrome and obesity hypoventilation syndrome. Clin Res J 2018; 12:1905–11.
11. Moyer CA, Sonnad SS, Garetz SL, et al. Quality of life in obstructive sleep apnea: a systematic review of the literature. Sleep Med 2001;2:477–91.
12. Kharbanda S, Anand R. Health-related quality of life in patients with chronic obstructive pulmonary

disease: a hospital-based study. Indian J Med Res 2021;153:459–64.

13. Tarasiuk A, Reuveni H. The economic impact of obstructive sleep apnea. Curr Opin Pulm Med 2013;19:639–44.

14. May SM, Li JT. Burden of chronic obstructive pulmonary disease: healthcare costs and beyond. Allergy Asthma Proc 2015;36:4–10.

15. Mermigkis C, Kopanakis A, Foldvary-Schaefer N, et al. Health-related quality of life in patients with obstructive sleep apnoea and chronic obstructive pulmonary disease (overlap syndrome). Int J Clin Pract 2007;61:207–11.

16. Donovan LM, Feemster LC, Udris EM, et al. Poor outcomes among patients with chronic obstructive pulmonary disease with higher risk for undiagnosed obstructive sleep apnea in the LOTT cohort. J Clin Sleep Med 2019;15:71–7.

17. Omachi TA, Blanc PD, Claman DM, et al. Disturbed sleep among COPD patients is longitudinally associated with mortality and adverse COPD outcomes. Sleep Med 2012;13:476–83.

18. Marin JM, Soriano JB, Carrizo SJ, et al. Outcomes in patients with chronic obstructive pulmonary disease and obstructive sleep apnea: the overlap syndrome. Am J Respir Crit Care Med 2010;182:325–31.

19. Konikkara J, Tavella R, Willes L, et al. Early recognition of obstructive sleep apnea in patients hospitalized with COPD exacerbation is associated with reduced readmission. Hosp Pract (1995) 2016;44: 41–7.

20. Jaoude P, El-Solh AA. Predictive factors for COPD exacerbations and mortality in patients with overlap syndrome. Clin Res J 2019;13:643–51.

21. Voulgaris A, Archontogeorgis K, Anevlavis S, et al. Effect of compliance to continuous positive airway pressure on exacerbations, lung function and symptoms in patients with chronic obstructive pulmonary disease and obstructive sleep apnea (overlap syndrome). Clin Res J 2023;17:165–75.

22. Wang TY, Lo YL, Lee KY, et al. Nocturnal CPAP improves walking capacity in COPD patients with obstructive sleep apnoea. Respir Res 2013;14:66.

23. de Miguel J, Cabello J, Sanchez-Alarcos JM, et al. Long-term effects of treatment with nasal continuous positive airway pressure on lung function in patients with overlap syndrome. Sleep Breath 2002;6:3–10.

24. Suri TM, Suri JC. A review of therapies for the overlap syndrome of obstructive sleep apnea and chronic obstructive pulmonary disease. FASEB Bioadv 2021;3:683–93.

25. Kong DL, Qin Z, Shen H, et al. Association of obstructive sleep apnea with asthma: a meta-analysis. Sci Rep 2017;7:4088.

26. Teodorescu M, Barnet JH, Hagen EW, et al. Association between asthma and risk of developing obstructive sleep apnea. JAMA 2015;313:156–64.

27. Julien JY, Martin JG, Ernst P, et al. Prevalence of obstructive sleep apnea-hypopnea in severe versus moderate asthma. J Allergy Clin Immunol 2009;124: 371–6.

28. Teodorescu M, Polomis DA, Teodorescu MC, et al. Association of obstructive sleep apnea risk or diagnosis with daytime asthma in adults. J Asthma 2012; 49:620–8.

29. Yang G, Han YY, Sun T, et al. Sleep duration, current asthma, and lung function in a nationwide study of U.S. Adults. Am J Respir Crit Care Med 2019;200: 926–9.

30. Luyster FS, Shi X, Baniak LM, et al. Associations of sleep duration with patient-reported outcomes and health care use in US adults with asthma. Ann Allergy Asthma Immunol 2020;125:319–24.

31. Prasad B, Nyenhuis SM, Imayama I, et al. Asthma and obstructive sleep apnea overlap: what has the evidence taught us? Am J Respir Crit Care Med 2020;201:1345–57.

32. Wang TY, Lo YL, Lin SM, et al. Obstructive sleep apnoea accelerates FEV(1) decline in asthmatic patients. BMC Pulm Med 2017;17:55.

33. Serrano-Pariente J, Plaza V, Soriano JB, et al. Asthma outcomes improve with continuous positive airway pressure for obstructive sleep apnea. Allergy 2017;72:802–12.

34. Lafond C, Series F, Lemiere C. Impact of CPAP on asthmatic patients with obstructive sleep apnoea. Eur Respir J 2007;29:307–11.

35. Ahmad T, Kumar M, Mabalirajan U, et al. Hypoxia response in asthma: differential modulation on inflammation and epithelial injury. Am J Respir Cell Mol Biol 2012;47:1–10.

36. Alkhalil M, Schulman E, Getsy J. Obstructive sleep apnea syndrome and asthma: what are the links? J Clin Sleep Med 2009;5:71–8.

37. Kauppi P, Bachour P, Maasilta P, et al. Long-term CPAP treatment improves asthma control in patients with asthma and obstructive sleep apnoea. Sleep Breath 2016;20:1217–24.

38. Chan CS, Woolcock AJ, Sullivan CE. Nocturnal asthma: role of snoring and obstructive sleep apnea. Am Rev Respir Dis 1988;137:1502–4.

39. Ciftci TU, Ciftci B, Guven SF, et al. Effect of nasal continuous positive airway pressure in uncontrolled nocturnal asthmatic patients with obstructive sleep apnea syndrome. Respir Med 2005;99:529–34.

40. Luyster FS, Teodorescu M, Bleecker E, et al. Sleep quality and asthma control and quality of life in non-severe and severe asthma. Sleep Breath 2012;16:1129–37.

41. Williams SA, Wagner S, Kannan H, et al. The association between asthma control and health care utilization, work productivity loss and health-related quality of life. J Occup Environ Med 2009;51: 780–5.

42. Davies SE, Bishopp A, Wharton S, et al. Does Continuous Positive Airway Pressure (CPAP) treatment of obstructive sleep apnoea (OSA) improve asthma-related clinical outcomes in patients with co-existing conditions?- A systematic review. Respir Med 2018;143:18–30.

43. Ng SSS, Chan TO, To KW, et al. Continuous positive airway pressure for obstructive sleep apnoea does not improve asthma control. Respirology 2018;23: 1055–62.

44. Cheng Y, Wang Y, Dai L. The prevalence of obstructive sleep apnea in interstitial lung disease: a systematic review and meta-analysis. Sleep Breath 2021;25:1219–28.

45. Pihtili A, Bingol Z, Kiyan E, et al. Obstructive sleep apnea is common in patients with interstitial lung disease. Sleep Breath 2013;17:1281–8.

46. Lee JH, Park CS, Song JW. Obstructive sleep apnea in patients with interstitial lung disease: prevalence and predictive factors. PLoS One 2020;15: e0239963.

47. Pereira N, Cardoso AV, Mota PC, et al. Predictive factors of obstructive sleep apnoea in patients with fibrotic lung diseases. Sleep Med 2019;56:123–7.

48. Baughman RP, Lower EE, Tami T. Upper airway. 4: sarcoidosis of the upper respiratory tract (SURT). Thorax 2010;65:181–6.

49. Mari PV, Pasciuto G, Siciliano M, et al. Obstructive sleep apnea in sarcoidosis and impact of cpap treatment on fatigue. Sarcoidosis Vasc Diffuse Lung Dis 2020;37:169–78.

50. Mavroudi M, Papakosta D, Kontakiotis T, et al. Sleep disorders and health-related quality of life in patients with interstitial lung disease. Sleep Breath 2018;22: 393–400.

51. Bosi M, Milioli G, Parrino L, et al. Quality of life in idiopathic pulmonary fibrosis: the impact of sleep disordered breathing. Respir Med 2019;147:51–7.

52. Mermigkis C, Bouloukaki I, Antoniou K, et al. Obstructive sleep apnea should be treated in patients with idiopathic pulmonary fibrosis. Sleep Breath 2015;19:385–91.

53. Papadogiannis G, Bouloukaki I, Mermigkis C, et al. Patients with idiopathic pulmonary fibrosis with and without obstructive sleep apnea: differences in clinical characteristics, clinical outcomes, and the effect of PAP treatment. J Clin Sleep Med 2021;17:533–44.

Moving?

Make sure your subscription moves with you!

To notify us of your new address, find your **Clinics Account Number** (located on your mailing label above your name), and contact customer service at:

Email: journalscustomerservice-usa@elsevier.com

800-654-2452 (subscribers in the U.S. & Canada)
314-447-8871 (subscribers outside of the U.S. & Canada)

Fax number: 314-447-8029

Elsevier Health Sciences Division
Subscription Customer Service
3251 Riverport Lane
Maryland Heights, MO 63043

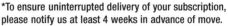

*To ensure uninterrupted delivery of your subscription, please notify us at least 4 weeks in advance of move.

Moving?

Make sure your subscription moves with you!

To notify us of your new address, find your Clinics Account Number (located on your mailing label above your name), and contact customer service at:

Email: journalscustomerservice-usa@elsevier.com

800-654-2452 (subscribers in the U.S. & Canada)
314-447-8871 (subscribers outside of the U.S. & Canada)

Fax number: 314-447-8029

Elsevier Health Sciences Division
Subscription Customer Service
3251 Riverport Lane
Maryland Heights, MO 63043

Printed and bound by CPI Group (UK) Ltd, Croydon, CR0 4YY
03/10/2024
01040363-0018